Anti-personnel Weapons

sipri

Stockholm International Peace Research Institute

SIPRI is an independent institute for research into problems of peace and conflict, with particular attention to the problems of disarmament and arms regulation. It was established in 1966 to commemorate Sweden's 150 years of unbroken peace.

The Institute is financed by the Swedish Parliament. The staff, the Governing Board and the Scientific Council are international. As a consultative body, the Scientific Council is not responsible for the views expressed in the publications of the Institute.

Governing Board

Governor Rolf Edberg, Chairman (Sweden)
Professor Robert Neild, Vice-Chairman
  (United Kingdom)
Mr Tim Greve (Norway)
Academician Ivan Málek (Czechoslovakia)
Professor Leo Mates (Yugoslavia)
Professor Gunnar Myrdal (Sweden)
Professor Bert Röling (Netherlands)
The Director

Director

Dr Frank Barnaby (United Kingdom)

sipri

Stockholm International Peace Research Institute

Sveavägen 166, S-113 46 Stockholm, Sweden
Cable: Peaceresearch, Stockholm
Telephone: 08–15 09 40

Anti-personnel Weapons

sipri

Stockholm International Peace Research Institute

Taylor & Francis Ltd
London
1978

First published 1978 by Taylor & Francis Ltd
10–14 Macklin St, London WC2B 5NF

Copyright © 1978 by SIPRI
Sveavägen 166, S-113 46 Stockholm

Distributed in the United States of America by
Crane, Russak & Company, Inc.
347 Madison Avenue, New York, N.Y. 10017
and in Scandinavia by
Almqvist & Wiksell International,
26 Gamla Brogatan,
S-101 20 Stockholm, Sweden

ISBN 0 85066 128 5

Text set in 11/12 pt Photon Times,
printed by photolithography, and bound in Great Britain
at The Pitman Press, Bath

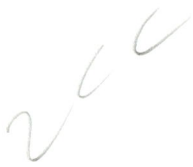

Preface

This book describes the development, uses and effects of conventional anti-personnel weapons such as rifles and machine-guns, grenades, bombs, shells and mines. It is intended as a contribution to the ongoing efforts to prohibit or restrict the use of some of the more inhumane and indiscriminate of these weapons.

The most urgent requirement for the modernization of international humanitarian law is a rule prohibiting the use of nuclear weapons and other means of mass destruction, including chemical weapons. There is also a need to prohibit or restrict the use of certain so-called 'conventional' weapons. The most immediate requirements are as follows:

(*a*) a rule prohibiting the use of napalm and other incendiary weapons (including white phosphorus) against personnel, the human habitat and natural resources;

(*b*) a rule prohibiting high-velocity small arms projectiles designed to yaw significantly, break up or deform within 150 mm of soft tissue or tissue simulant;

(*c*) a rule prohibiting the use of cluster bombs and shells and other area fragmentation munitions within a specified range of inhabited areas; and

(*d*) a rule requiring that all remotely delivered delayed-action weapons, including mines, should be fitted with a reliable neutralizing device, and prohibiting their use in inhabited areas.

In addition the implications of the development of fuel–air explosives, uranium projectiles, laser weapons and other wave-propagation devices must be carefully considered.

This book was written by Dr Malvern Lumsden, a SIPRI Research Fellow.

Acknowledgements

Eric Prokosch, a visiting researcher at SIPRI in 1975, has made many invaluable contributions, notably in chapter 5. The editorial assistance of Rajesh Kumar is gratefully acknowledged.

March 1978   *Frank Barnaby*
                                                                    Director

Abbreviations, Acronyms and Conventions

Abbreviations and acronyms

AC	Aircraft Cannon
AR	Assault Rifle
CDDH	Diplomatic Conference on the Reaffirmation and Development of International Humanitarian Law Applicable in Armed Conflicts
CEP	Circular Error Probable
ECM	Electronic Countermeasures
FAC	Forward Air Controller
FAE	Fuel–Air Explosive (also FAX)
FAESHED	Fuel–Air Explosive Helicopter Delivered
FAX	Fuel–Air Explosive (also FAE)
FVG	Fixed Vehicle Gun
GP	General Purpose
HAR	Heavy Assault Rifle
HE	High Explosive
HEAT	High-Explosive Anti-Tank
HEI	High-Explosive Incendiary
ICRC	International Committee of the Red Cross
LASER	Light Amplification by Stimulated Emission of Radiation
LMG	Light Machine-Gun
LNG	Liquid Natural Gas
LORAN	Long Range Navigation
MAD	Mass Air Delivery *or* Massive Assured Destruction
MMG	Medium Machine-Gun
PE	Probable Error
PGM	Precision-Guided Munition
RII	Relative Incapacitation Index
RPV	Remotely Piloted Vehicle
SAR	Search and Rescue *or* Short Assault Rifle
SAWS	Squad Automatic Weapon System
SLUFAE	Surface Launched Fuel–Air Explosive
SPIW	Special Purpose Individual Weapon

SSB	Salvo Squeezebore
SSZ	Special Strike Zone
TEA	Triethyl Aluminium
WP	White Phosphorus

Conventions

..	Data not available
–	Negligible; not applicable

Contents

Tables and Figures

Chapter 6. Blast and blast weapons

Table

Chapter 7. Delayed-action weapons

Tables

Introduction and summary

Combatants have a legal obligation to care for the victims of war, and under the auspices of the International Committee of the Red Cross (ICRC), these obligations have been successively extended. From an early stage the Red Cross was concerned that unnecessary injuries to soldiers and civilians should be stopped. This would best be achieved by preventing war itself, but the Red Cross has not entered the field of war prevention; rather it has concentrated its efforts on the alleviation of suffering if war occurs. There can be little doubt that the greatest contribution to this would come from prohibiting or restricting the more inhumane and indiscriminate methods of warfare.

Modern conventional weapons have devastating effects and attention has been drawn to these during recent negotiations to modernize the 1949 Geneva Conventions. Proposals to prohibit or restrict the use of some of these weapons have been put forward, but all too often military considerations come before humanitarian concerns.

Several attempts have been made through the centuries to restrain legally the development of new weaponry. A few of these attempts have succeeded, only to be made obsolete by new technology. As will be seen in this book, an effort has been made in recent years to prohibit some of the more inhumane and indiscriminate weapons, and an examination of the legal, military and humanitarian issues raised by them is made.

Anti-personnel weapons may be defined as those weapons primarily intended to incapacitate *persons*. They may be distinguished from anti-matériel weapons, which are primarily intended to destroy or damage inanimate objects, although some munitions are referred to as 'general purpose' and may be used both against personnel and against matériel. Reference is made to general purpose munitions in so far as they are used against personnel.

Although nuclear, chemical, biological and incendiary weapons may be used as anti-personnel weapons, they are omitted from the present book since they are covered in other SIPRI publications (e.g., SIPRI, 1971, 1973, 1975a).

This book provides the background to the present international legal discussions of specific anti-personnel weapons.

Chapters 1 and 2 describe the rise of anti-personnel weapons from the earliest times until the present, showing the part they have played in history. At a time when there is a concerted effort to make the world a better place, we must not forget that the industrial powers produced devastating anti-personnel weapons in order to further colonialism. Modern anti-personnel weapons are more sophisticated than the sticks and clubs of the Stone Age, but they are still a very primitive way of tackling urgent social problems. They are unlikely to stop the trend towards a new order in the long run and they may greatly increase the human cost of progress.

Chapter 3 makes a brief review of the subject known as 'wound ballistics' –

that is, the study of the effects of projectiles in the human body. These are responsible for well over 90 per cent of casualties in modern warfare. In order to make an evaluation of weapons in the light of international humanitarian law, it is essential to understand something of what happens when, say, a man is shot.

Chapter 4 traces the trend towards smaller calibre and higher velocity military small arms. It is concluded that the full-power 7.62 mm ammunition similar to that used by most of the world's armies since the 1890s is unnecessarily powerful for present conditions and that for both military and humanitarian considerations the power of ammunition should be reduced. The modern tendency to capitalize on inflicting severe wounds by using very high velocity projectiles should be restrained by international law, and the proliferation of these new weapons calls for urgent measures. A further cause for concern is the trend in some countries for police forces to adopt more injurious weapons.

Chapter 5 describes the development of fragmentation weapons, which category includes most conventional weapons. As with small arms, the 'high velocity' effect is used to reduce progressively the size of the fragments. The modern tendency is to replace larger fragmentation warheads with a host of small grenades or bomblets. This improves the 'combat economy'. Rules are required to restrain the use of area fragmentation weapons in places where the civilian population may be affected. The US Rules of Engagement in Viet Nam (see appendix 9D) show that it is quite feasible to determine a 'safety zone' for each category of weapon. Such an approach could profitably be examined in the context of international law.

Chapter 6 describes the effects of blast weapons on the human body and their development. Fuel–air explosives and other concussion bombs should not be permitted for use as anti-personnel weapons.

In Chapter 7 the question of delayed-action weapons is examined. These should be severely restricted so as to reduce their indiscriminate effects. The new remotely delivered mines – which can be spread in large numbers far from the front lines – are a source of particular concern for humanitarian and environmental reasons. The users of delayed-action weapons should be required by international law to make sure that their weapons can be disposed of when they no longer serve a military purpose.

A number of attempts to devise weapons on the basis of other physical principles, such as sound waves, electric shocks, flashing lights and lasers, are described in Chapter 8. At present the laser appears to be the most likely candidate for new weapons. A number of other devices have also been tried out in internal security operations.

Chapter 9 reviews the development of international humanitarian law with respect to conventional anti-personnel weapons. There is no doubt that, in a period of history when the use of force is prohibited (other than for self-defence or collective security), it would have been better to have removed the hazard of anti-personnel weapons simply by disarmament. But as no such measures are being taken, there must be other civilizing steps: the two Additional Protocols to the four Geneva Conventions of 1949 are one such step. They could be appropriately supplemented by rules, such as those reviewed in appendix 9D, prohibiting or restricting the use of a number of the weapons described in this book.

1. The rise of anti-personnel weapons, from antiquity to 1900

Superior numerals, thus [5], refer to notes on page 16.

I. Early anti-personnel weapons

It is a sad fact that man's use of tools to kill or injure his fellow man is one of his most abiding characteristics and distinguishes him from nearly all of the animal kingdom. Even today, enormous amounts of time and energy are devoted to improving means of slaughter.

Most modern weapons, like primitive weapons, are designed to transfer a quantity of energy to the enemy's body in order to crush, penetrate or burn it. It takes no more energy now to incapacitate a man than it did in the Stone Age.

Man is a peculiar mammal in that he is little adapted to meet the hazards that surround him; he is not equipped with effective camouflage or long limbs, or with teeth, claws or horns to serve as weapons. At an early stage, man turned to the use of simple hand-held weapons, and projectiles made of wood and stone. Perhaps he lacked the innate inhibitions about attacking members of his own species which are found in other predatory animals (Lorenz, 1966; Hinde, 1966; Eibl-Eibesfeldt, 1975). Simple tools and hunting weapons became potential instruments of war.

The first aggressive weapons were 'anti-personnel' in that they were made to injure or kill other men. Only later as people built protective walls around themselves were more powerful weapons needed to breach these defences. Sticks and clubs for use in hand-to-hand fighting evolved into maces and axes with stone, bronze or iron heads. Some of the Egyptian Pharaohs are depicted with a mace, which appears to have been preferred to the sword. Before discovering metal, some primitive peoples had war clubs with edges of shark's teeth, ray's tails, or other sharp objects, such as obsidian (Turney-High, 1971). Axes were designed for cutting, for use against an unprotected foe, for piercing, or for use against an enemy wearing armour. When the easily wielded iron sword came, the club and the axe became obsolete (Oakeshott, 1960).

Swords of copper or bronze were short because of the weakness of the metal, and it was not until the Iron Age that the gradual transition to the sword as a major weapon took place. The Greeks, for instance, did not make use of iron swords until the Doric invasions of about 1100 BC.

The production of steel from iron, which was achieved during the first millennium BC, resulted in blades that could be honed to a fine edge (Derry & Williams, 1960). Sabres (swords primarily designed for slashing) remained a feature of warfare until the first decades of the twentieth century. They were used mainly in cavalry charges.

3

The spear also developed from the dagger of the Bronze Age, and later the pike gave the wielder a longer outreach. Javelins were spears designed to be thrown; a quiver of javelins was a common fixture on Greek and Roman chariots. Some Roman javelins were designed to break in two or bend at the tip to prevent their reuse by the enemy. A later development was the lance, designed to utilize the force exerted by a charging horse and rider.

The earliest projectiles were stones thrown by hand and later by sling (cf. Krause, 1905). Since the sling required considerable skill, some armies relied on mercenary slingers such as those from the Balearic Islands. In their hands, shot of stones or lead slugs had considerable accuracy and a range of about 200 m (Korfmann, 1973).

The bow marked the earliest use of mechanical energy to project a missile. It also is of prehistoric origin and was apparently used originally for hunting. Its development as a weapon of war is attributed to the Akkadians in their conquest of the Sumerians. It became the main weapon of war by about 1500 BC. The Greeks and the Romans did not favour the bow and for a time it went out of fashion. The most powerful bows had an effective range of 300–400 m, and a maximum range of twice that, which is similar to the ranges for which modern military rifles are designed. A trained man with a longbow could shoot about five arrows a minute. These arrows were often tipped with about 2 cm of steel and could penetrate chain-mail. In one recorded instance in 1182, such an arrow penetrated oak doors 10 cm thick (Oakeshott, 1960). In 1346, the Battle of Crécy demonstrated the effectiveness of the bow against soldiers wearing armour. The bow remained in service in European armies until about the end of the sixteenth century.

The crossbow, which uses a hand-crank to set the bow, probably entered Europe from China, and was inherited by the Romans from the Greeks and Carthaginians. The steel military crossbow of the fifteenth century had a range of some 380 m and a point-blank range of about 65 m (Hogg, 1970). Crossbows may have greater range and accuracy than conventional bows, but they are more complex and cumbersome and have a slower rate of fire. In the same way the heavier weapons which gave rise to early forms of artillery were slow. Examples of these are the catapult and the ballista. Some of these were designed to project small or large stones while others released arrows or iron-tipped darts weighing about 3 kg.

II. Early firearms

It was only many years after their appearance in the fourteenth century that the significance of firearms and explosives was appreciated. Firearms as we know them have their origins in the development of metallurgy and chemistry about AD 1200–1300 (Derry & Williams, 1960). The techniques of bell-founding appeared about AD 800, and by 1250 the Moors used cast-iron buckets to project stones using a powder charge. Gunpowder came into more general use about 1300 (Partington, 1960) and cannon by 1350 (Hogg, 1970).

The first firearms were developed while the crossbow and the ballista were still in use, and used similar projectiles, such as bolts or darts, usually made of iron. They had iron fins or feathers for stabilization and weighed about 200 g (about three times the weight of the normal crossbow bolt). The bolts were wrapped in leather so that they fitted tightly in the barrel of the gun. Later they gave way to small balls of about the same weight cast in lead. Stone, iron and bronze shot were used in heavier guns.

Early firearms were laboriously loaded at the muzzle and this restricted their rate of fire. Hand-guns were mainly used for sport, where time was not so vital. Rifled gun barrels were known as early as 1525 but they were not used in combat until the Thirty Years' War (1618–48); they permitted more accurate fire at longer ranges than smooth-bore guns.

The usefulness of the hand-held firearms improved considerably with the step-by-step evolution of the firing mechanism from match to matchlock to wheel-lock (originating in Italy between 1494 and 1559) and then to flintlock (originating in France about 1630). The flintlock was adopted by the French Army in 1660 and by the British in 1688 and it remained in use until the Battle of Waterloo in 1815. The addition of the bayonet in the 1600s led eventually to the obsolescence of the pike. The curved stock mitigated recoil and thereby improved the accuracy of fire.

Until the Napoleonic period, tactics were largely dictated by the effective range of the flintlock musket – about 200 m. The infantryman could carry about 60 rounds of ammunition and fire them at a rate of two per minute. The cavalry could cover 200 m in about 30 seconds. Once the musketeer had shot at the cavalryman, he had a good chance of being cut down by the cavalryman's sabre before being able to fire a second shot.

For many years artillery was used primarily to breach fortifications. Specialist gunners, sometimes hired for the occasion, operated the heavy pieces. Sometimes artillery was used for defence against besieging forces. About 1630 the Swedish king, Gustavus Adolphus, effectively introduced the use of concentrated fire from light artillery on to the battlefield to break up the 'Spanish square' of opposing infantry. By the time of Napoleon, the French Inspector General of Artillery, de Gribeauval, introduced new tactics and matériel which enabled the artillery to charge up close to the enemy and decimate the front lines (Manucy, 1949).

A great many kinds of shell and shot were developed to be fired by artillery. A shell[1] is a projectile containing an explosive or other chemical substance and is designed to detonate or disperse the active material on or over the target. Shot refers to solid projectiles designed to penetrate the target by means of kinetic energy; the 'cannon-ball', or round shot, was for many years the most common type.

Additional kinds of shot included:

(a) bar shot, shaped like a dumb-bell and intended to tumble in flight, so creating more injuries amongst a concentration of troops;

(b) chain shot, consisting of two balls linked by a chain and intended to destroy the masts and rigging of sailing-ships. It carried incendiary candles to set fire to the sails;

(*c*) *knife-blade shot*, which had hinged blades designed to open as the projectile left the muzzle; and

(*d*) *incandescent or hot shot*, which was simply iron shot heated until it was red-hot shortly before being loaded into the gun.

These projectiles were in the main intended for use against matériel targets, such as ships. Other kinds of ammunition were developed which were primarily anti-personnel. They included a quantity of small projectiles, such as pieces of iron, nails, stones or flints, which were loaded directly into the gun. Later, such missiles were enclosed in a container and became *case* or *canister* shot. Case shot is said to have been first used at the Siege of Constantinople in 1453 (Hogg, 1970), and a later version, filled with small iron balls, was known as *hail shot*. In 1573 a German gunner, Zimmerman, invented a shell with a powder charge which burst the lead jacket and dispersed the enclosed hail shot.

In 1784, following the siege of Gibraltar, a British lieutenant, Henry Shrapnel, proposed his *spherical case shot*. On 11 June 1852, ten years after Shrapnel's death, the British Government, which had by then adopted the shell into service, ordained that shells of this kind should be called *shrapnel shell*. In case shot, the shell opened at the muzzle, but the shrapnel shell could be fired to any distance up to about 1 200 m, before it opened to release the lead shot.

Another weapon which depended on the effects of gunpowder – though not as a propellant – was the hand-grenade. This consisted of a hollow iron sphere, about 5 cm in diameter, filled with powder. Although it was introduced during the seventeenth century, it was not widely used until the Russo–Japanese War of 1904, which foreshadowed the trench warfare of World War I.

III. The rifle

During the nineteenth century, percussion cartridges were invented which simplified the loading and firing of rifles. Conical bullets, such as the French Minié bullet (designed to fit the grooves in the barrel), improved the efficiency of the rifle. These innovations permitted the development of the breech-loading gun and the repeating rifle. The Minié bullet was widely used, not only by the French but also by the British, who paid the inventor the sum of £20 000 and modified it for use in the Crimean War (1853–56).

An account of wounds inflicted by the weapons of the time is given in the British official medical history of the Crimean War (Matthew, 1858). While sword and lance wounds were 'generally not of a grave nature', patients were categorized according to their most severe wound, which was 'almost invariably found to be that inflicted by the bullet' (ibid., p. 262).

> The conical bullets used so extensively in this campaign inflict a much
> more severe and dangerous wound than the old round. ... The worst
> and most dangerous wounds appeared to be inflicted by the British old-

fashioned Minié bullet with the iron cup. This sometimes had the effect of splaying out the ball on encountering an obstacle. (Matthew, 1858, p. 263)

The heaviest Russian conical ball (54 g) and the British Enfield bullet (37.5 g) caused more severe wounds, such as compound fractures of bones, than the older round balls, though these resulted in a more regular wound channel.

The Enfield version of the Minié bullet[2] was introduced into the British armies[3] in India by 1857. The paper cartridges were heavily lubricated with animal fat, and the ends were supposed to be bitten off by the user before loading the gun. However, since the cow is sacred to Hindus and the pig unclean to Muslims, the Indian troops refused to do this and were imprisoned by their British officers. This helped to precipitate a mutiny which developed into a major uprising against British rule.

According to Smith (1969), the Minié bullet also played a role in the history of the United States:

> It was the ball generally used in all the muzzle loaders used by both the North and the South during our Civil War; it was responsible in very large measure for the catastrophic loss of life in that terrible conflict. (Smith, 1969, p. 33)

Diffenbaugh (1965), summarizing the surgical history of the US Civil War, records that the Minié bullet 'produced marked destruction, shattering bone rather than piercing it, frequently emerging from the body in a transverse axis, producing horrible wounds' (p. 490).

Inspired by several earlier designs, a British Major Fosbery (1869) described how his own invention, an exploding bullet for use in the standard British rifle of the time, was first introduced in the summer of 1863 as an aid to judging the range of fire. The British were at the time engaged in 'pacification' operations in the North-West Frontier district of India. The steep mountains made it difficult to judge the distance to the enemy, and firing trial artillery rounds would remove any chance of surprise. The explosive bullets (the impact of which could be seen and heard) provided an effective alternative, enabling the artillery to be accordingly targeted.

It was not long before Fosbery's bullets were used 'on the enemy generally' when it became desirable to have a 'strong moral effect'. In this respect the exploding bullet seemed to be successful, for Fosbery records that the tribesmen 'were at pains of sending us a deputation, under a flag of truce, praying that their use might be discontinued' (Fosbery, 1869, p. 23).

Developments in small arms ammunition opened the way to breech-loading rifles of the modern type. By the 1860s the Spencer and Henry repeating rifles, and breech-loaders of many other types were in service in the United States. The Prussians used the Dreyse needle-gun in the Schleswig-Holstein War of 1864 and in the Seven Weeks' War of 1866 with Austria. The Austrians, who still used muzzle-loaders, suffered many more casualties. This impressed upon other European powers the advantages of breech-loading weapons. The breech-loading needle-gun could be reloaded lying-down, the loader thereby presenting a much smaller target to the enemy. These guns had a range of about 500 m. By the early 1870s nearly all the major powers had equipped their forces with breech-loading rifles. The Franco–Prussian War of 1870–71 was the first major war in which both sides used breech-loading rifles, with bayonets hardly being used at all.

The US Peabody rifle was purchased by Austria, Bavaria, Denmark, France, Mexico, Romania and Switzerland. In Switzerland, modifications were introduced by Martini, and this design was matched in England to the Henry rifling system to produce the 'Martini-Henry' rifle, adopted in 1871 with a calibre .45 inch (11.43 mm) cartridge. The Imperial Russian Government bought a rifle designed by Berdan (known as Berdan I) and then redesigned it to produce the Berdan II. Another US breech-loading rifle design, patented by Rider and developed by Remington, was adopted by Denmark, Sweden and Norway in 1867, Spain in 1871, Egypt in 1870 and Argentina in 1879, and was widely used in China, Austria, Italy and several South American countries (Smith, 1969).

After the success of the Turks against the Russians at Pleven in 1877, the value of the repeating rifle was generally recognized by the European powers (Smith, 1969). During this battle the Turks were able to use 30 000 Winchester repeating rifles purchased from the United States. This led the military authorities to adopt the repeating rifles being patented by designers such as Mauser, Mannlicher and Lebel in the following decade.

The Federal Assembly of the Swiss Confederation approved the adoption of a repeating rifle in 1866 and the gun chosen, the Vetterli, went into production the following year. Later, in 1870, the Früwurth bolt-action repeater was issued to the Austro-Hungarian gendarmerie.

'Smokeless powder' – a much more powerful propellant than the old black powder – was introduced at the same time and led to a further increase in the power of rifles, with a corresponding reduction in the calibre from 10–14 mm to about 7–8 mm. A smokeless powder for shot-guns had been demonstrated in 1864, following Schönbein's demonstration of gun-cotton (cotton treated with nitric and sulphuric acids to produce nitro-cellulose) in 1846, but it was not until the 1880s that the French *poudre B* and Nobel's ballistite made the production of more powerful explosive cartridges possible. Edouard Rubin, a Swiss Army officer, designed the copper-jacketed bullet, which did not melt in the added frictional heat. The rifles adopted for the new ammunition – such as Mausers, the British Lee-Metford and the US Krag – had a range of 1 000 m or more.

At that time experiments showed that at ranges of under 500 m these bullets could create remarkable 'explosive' effects on the head and other organs (see chapter 3). Conversely, some soldiers complained that at longer ranges they had insufficient 'stopping power' (see pp. 59–60).

IV. The machine-gun

Developments in ammunition and firing mechanisms paved the way for the introduction of automatic weapons. James Puckle patented a flintlock gun with a revolver chamber in 1718. The Duke of Montagu purchased two of them but there are no further records of their use (Hogg & Batchelor, 1976). In 1851 a Belgian, Captain Fafchamps, designed a weapon which was manufactured by Montigny and known as the mitrailleuse. The French Army was equipped with 156 of an improved version of these guns in time for the war against Prussia in 1870. The original model had 37 barrels, and the bullets were fired successively by turning a crank; the French Army model had 25 barrels. Here the bullets were set in a plate matching the barrels so that all barrels could be loaded simultaneously. All the barrels were fired in about one second and about 12 plates a minute could be loaded. The bullets had a range of about 1 800 m. In the war of 1870–71 the French used these guns as field artillery pieces, but they could not match the Prussian artillery, which had a range of about 2 500 m.

The Austrians purchased a 37-barrel version of the Montigny mitrailleuse of 11 mm calibre and used it for the defence of fortifications.

Meanwhile, the American inventor Dr R. J. Gatling had designed a competing weapon with revolving barrels, and was offering it to armies in several parts of the world. This gun was invented in 1861, improved in 1865 and adopted by the US War Department in 1866. Tests by the British Government in 1870 demonstrated its superiority over the mitrailleuse, over shrapnel rounds from artillery, and over six infantrymen firing rifles. As a result, production facilities were set up in England. At about the same time similar guns were acquired by the Russian Government and named Gorloff; they were used in the war against the Turks in 1877 and were still in service during the siege of Port Arthur in 1904–05. The British first used the Gatling guns in the Zulu War of 1879 and they remained in service until 1905.

The Gatling gun revolves six or more barrels, loading and firing each one at a time; the entire process is operated mechanically by a hand-crank. In 1883 a drum-feed system was introduced which increased the rate of fire to 1 200 rounds per minute (rpm) and in 1893 Gatling added an electric motor, increasing the rate of fire to 3 000 rpm. But by this time mechanical operating systems had become obsolete.

Many other designs for mechanically operated machine-guns were put forward during this period and some of them entered into service. A gun designed by an American, William Gardner, and produced by the then newly formed engineering company Pratt & Whitney, was adopted by the British Royal Navy in 1884 and widely used in operations ashore. The Gardner gun fired two barrels alternately at about 365 rpm.

A gun designed by a Swede, Helge Palmcrantz, fed a row of barrels, and was known as the Nordenfelt after the financier who marketed it. This gun was made in various calibres, had 2–10 barrels, and was in service with the British Royal Navy between 1880 and 1903. Benjamin Hotchkiss, an American, patented a 'revolver cannon' in Paris in 1874 and the company he established there sold about 10 000 of these guns to Belgium, France, Holland, Italy, Russia and the United States.

Gatling guns and many other designs of the period required an input of mechanical energy to carry out the functions of loading, firing, extracting the empty cartridge and then repeating the cycle. An American inventor, Hiram S. Maxim, living in Europe, considered using the energy produced by the exploding cartridge to perform these functions. Between 1882 and 1885 he took out patents on many lines of development, and by 1885 he produced and improved a working system using the recoil of the gun to load and fire a single barrel. With this model he arranged demonstrations in many European countries and established the Maxim Gun Company which used manufacturing facilities of the Vickers Company in England. By 1890 the gun had been supplied to the Austrian, British, German, Italian, Russian and Swiss governments.

The first use of the Maxim gun in war was against a tribe in Gambia on 21 November 1888 (Hogg & Batchelor, 1976). It became one of the most used weapons of World War I and has since been widely used all over the world. It was used by Russian forces in both World Wars and by Chinese forces in Korea. The modified Maxim, known as the .303 (7.70 mm) Vickers, was introduced in 1912 and remained in British service until 1968.

The original Maxim gun had a rate of fire of about 600 rpm although it could also fire single shots. It was chambered to the .45 in (11.43 mm) Martini-Henry rifle cartridge but was later chambered to the .303 in (7.70 mm) and other calibres. Larger calibres were also produced, such as the pom-pom (37 mm), which was used in the South African War of 1900. Maxim guns were usually water-cooled, though some versions were air-cooled. They were mounted on many forms of carriage, and on pack-saddles on horses and camels. In 1909 the German Army requested a lighter model for use from aircraft, and a design by Heinemann – known as the Parabellum – was produced in 1911, the first of a long line of aircraft guns.

Another American, John Browning, designed a machine-gun which channelled off some of the gas near the muzzle of the gun into a cylinder. Here the gas propelled a piston which then extracted the empty cartridge, loaded a new one and fired it. He offered his invention to the Colt Company in 1890 and, after testing in 1892–93, it became in 1895 the first automatic machine-gun in US service. Many current assault rifles and machine-guns operate on this principle. An Austrian, Captain Adolf Odkolek, sold a design for a gas-operated gun to the Hotchkiss Company in Paris in 1893. The French Army adopted it in 1897 but later modified it. The gun was bought by several countries, including the USA, Britain and Japan. The Japanese used it against the Russians in 1904 and acquired a licence to produce it, subsequently introducing their own modifications.

A third operating principle, known as delayed blowback, was introduced in 1888 by two Austrians, the Archduke Karl Salvator and Count Dormus. It was produced by the Skoda Company, after which it was named. It was adopted by the Austro-Hungarian Army in 1893 and improved models were introduced in 1902, 1909 and 1913.

Although the Maxim is the best-known recoil-operated gun, the Danish cavalry adopted a light recoil-operated machine-gun, the Madsen, in about 1902. Although it was not adopted by any major military power, it was so successful that it was produced almost unchanged for over 50 years and was used by 34 countries. It fired 7.62 mm bullets at a rate of 500–600 per minute but weighed only about 10 kg – less than half the weight of other machine-guns of the period.

The four operating principles – mechanical, recoil, gas and delayed blowback – continue to be applied in the design of modern automatic weapons.

V. Artillery

The development of artillery roughly parallelled the evolution of small arms, but artillery was faced with special problems. There was a temptation to increase the size of the weapons to give them longer range and demolishing power; on the other hand there was a need for mobility.

Early attempts to design exploding artillery shells were rarely successful because of the difficulty of constructing a safe but effective fuze. It was not until about the end of the eighteenth century that shells were reliable enough to be taken into general service.

In the 1860s rifled barrels were introduced, and this brought about the need for cylindrical or conical shells. New varieties of case and shrapnel shell were in-introduced. The shrapnel shell forms an intermediate category between the shot, which is solid and inert, and the shell, which is designed to break up into fragments under the influence of an explosive charge contained in it. Improvements in fuze design meant that shrapnel shells could be adjusted to burst at zero range, giving them a similar effect to that of case shells. As a result, the terms are sometimes used interchangeably; indeed, 'shrapnel' is now used to refer to projectile fragments in general.

The effects of the projectiles in use in the mid-nineteenth century are quite well described in the British medical history of the Crimean War. In this war most of the injuries were inflicted by round and grape shot at close range:

> Wounds by direct contact of round shot usually exhibited the limb either carried away or hopelessly mashed into a mass in which the various tissues were almost indistinguishable. . .When a shell explodes the wound produced by its fragments is usually much less severe than those inflicted by round shot . . . Grape differs from round shot only in degree; and canister has much the same effect as round musket balls, but generally produces less injury than is inflicted by the latter. (Matthew, 1858, p. 263)

'The Charge of the Light Brigade' during the Crimean War (1853–56)[4] showed the plight of cavalry in the face of a concentration of field guns. These had a range of about 1 500 m with round shot and 500 m with case shot.

The impact of these weapons was seen again at the Battle of Solferino in 1859 when in one day 22 500 men of the Austrian Army were slaughtered and the French and the Piedmontese lost 17 200 men (Fuller, 1932). In the war of 1870–71, the Prussians used artillery extensively, often stopping attacks at 2 000 m.

Between 1880 and 1890 steel began to replace iron in the body of shells, and in the mid-1890s gunpowder began to give way to high explosive (HE) fillers. At the same time the first specialized armour-piercing (AP) shells were developed.

The blast of HE shells makes them effective against buildings and other matériel targets, and the mass of small high-velocity fragments makes them lethal weapons against troops. As a result of this combination of properties, they have largely replaced case and shrapnel shells since World War I except for certain specific tasks.

At the end of the nineteenth century the French introduced the quick-firing 75 mm gun, having a mechanism designed to cope with the recoil and keep the carriage steady. This avoided the necessity to re-lay the gun before each shot. Vickers Sons & Maxim manufactured a gun of this kind which was introduced to British forces in the Ashanti campaign of 1900. It was said to be 'of a type superior to any then in use in the British Army' (Myatt, 1974, p. 61). Subsequently, similar weapons were generally adopted. The powerful propellants introduced in about 1890 gave field artillery a range of approximately 2 000 m and heavier projectiles could be fired. Smokeless powder decreased the chance of detecting concealed guns. By 1914 field guns had a range of about 6 000 m with shrapnel shells (Myatt, 1974).

VI. Rockets

The rocket has competed with artillery for hundreds of years, particularly in Asia. In Europe the use of rockets declined between the fifteenth and the eighteenth centuries, but in 1804 Sir William Congreve introduced new designs which were used by the British for nearly a century. They were first used against Boulogne in October 1806, and in 1807 they caused considerable damage in Copenhagen. Congreve's rockets, stabilized by a protruding stick, were made in several standard sizes, from 6 lb (2.7 kg) to 42 lb (19 kg), the 32 lb (15 kg) size being the most popular. These rockets could be fitted with incendiary, shrapnel or case warheads and had maximum ranges of up to 3 000 m.

After 1870, breech-loading rifled artillery largely superseded rockets, though they remained in service until World War I. The theoretical advantages of the rocket (cheapness and simplicity) continued to interest some weapon designers. The success of German designers in the 1930s greatly stimulated the development of rocketry, and from then on, rockets and guided missiles came to play an important role in warfare.

12

VII. The influence of weaponry on warfare

The high-powered rifle, the machine-gun and the quick-firing artillery which were developed during the nineteenth century significantly altered the way war was waged.

The British military historian Fuller (1932) calls the US Civil War the 'first of the modern wars . . . begotten by the industrial revolution' (p. 84). The period of the US Civil War saw the invention of the magazine-loading rifle and the machine-gun, the use of land-mines, booby traps, submarine mines, torpedoes, hand-grenades, rockets, explosive bullets, 'stink shells', and trench warfare, and the idea of bombarding a city (Richmond, Virginia) with incendiary shells (Fuller, 1932).

Writers, such as Havelock (1867), realized that the era of the cavalry charge and the lines of red- or blue-coated soldiers was drawing to a close. The cavalryman, let alone the infantryman, could no longer cross the danger zone separating the two lines of troops. The rifle and machine-gun, with their high-powered bullets, could easily hit the charging horse or its rider at 1 000 m and the cannon could do so at even longer range. On the other hand, the riflemen could pick off the artillerymen at longer ranges than they could reach with case shot.

But if neither side could get across no man's land and each was forced to dig trenches for protection, then 'the spade would be as indispensable to the soldier as his rifle' (Bloch, 1899).[5] Not only that, but the outcome of war would no longer be determined by the final cut and thrust of the sabre and bayonet but by the capacity of industrial society to pour out its resources:

> That is the future of war – not fighting, but famine, not the slaying of men but the bankruptcy of nations and the break-up of whole social organizations. (Bloch, 1899)

It was during the US Civil War that the prospect of replacing manpower with technology was stated by the Swedish inventor, John Ericsson, to President Lincoln:

> The time has come, Mr President, when our case will have to be sustained not by numbers, but by superior weapons . . . such is the inferiority of the Southern States in a mechanical point of view, that it is susceptible of demonstration that, if you apply our mechanical resources to the fullest extent you can destroy the enemy without enlisting another man. (Cited in Derry & Williams, 1960, p. 706)

This principle of pitting technology against numbers was applied in the following decades, particularly in putting much of the world under colonial domination. Fuller says:

> As regards aggression the years 1870–98 are only equalled by the age of Genghis Khan. Between 1870 and 1900 Great Britain acquired 4 754 000 square miles [12 200 000 km²] of territory, adding to her

population 88 000 000 people; between 1884 and 1900 France acquired 3 583 580 square miles [9 300 000 km²] and 36 553 000 people; and in the same years, Germany, a bad last, gained 1 026 220 square miles [2 700 000 km²] and 16 687 100 people. There were many other nations besides who acquired land; but these three examples will suffice to prove the stupendous and rapid progress of this crusade. (Fuller, 1932, p. 134)

New weapons and a superior technology enabled small bodies of men to conquer large territories and populations. They gave the Western soldier a fire-power which could no longer be matched by the muskets made for generations by village gunsmiths in Asia and Africa.

The Minié bullet was used against Africans in 1852, and introduced into British service in the following year. Myatt (1974) says, 'the heavy bullet inflicted terrible wounds at close ranges and often had sufficient velocity to pierce through three or four men' (p. 28). It was soon superseded by the Enfield rifle which in turn was used to suppress the Indian Mutiny in 1857. The Snider gun (mainly produced from converted Enfields) was the first breech-loader and 'proved effective in the Abyssinian Expedition of 1867–68 and in the Ashanti war of 1873–74' (Myatt, 1974). It became the weapon of the Indian Army almost until the end of the century, when it was replaced by the Lee-Metford.

At the same time similar weapons were important in the pacification of the Indian peoples in North America: the high-powered rifle was used not only against the people themselves but also for killing the buffalo on which many Indian people depended. In the meantime, other European armies, equipped with the French Lebel or the German Mauser rifles, were gaining control over much of the rest of the world.

In India, explosive bullets were introduced in the 1860s and used against mountain tribesmen (see p. 7). In the 1890s, 'it was found in Indian hill warfare that the Lee-Metford bullet did not adequately protect the troops using it . . .' (*The Lancet*, 10 June 1899, p. 1573). The colonial authorities accordingly commissioned the arsenal at Dum-Dum, near Calcutta, to design the more destructive bullet which came to bear its name.

> It is not an explosive bullet, in the sense of containing any explosive substance, but having a soft metal nose which expands when the bullet has once penetrated it has been found to possess a 'stopping' power which the Lee-Metford bullet did not. That this property should be present is the essential point, and the Government of India are still making experiments with a view of obtaining a rifle projectile which will prove adequate for their requirements in the mountain warfare with the semi-civilized tribes in which it has so often and so reluctantly to take part. (ibid.)

About the same time the US War Department Board 'considered that cup-pointed bullets such as the "man-stopper" might be offered to troops fighting savage tribes and fanatics in bush and jungle. The bullet shows great execution on live animals' (LaGarde, 1914).[6]

14

The machine-gun and the field gun were also used extensively in colonial wars. Myatt, for example, writes that:

> Successive improvements in firearms in the second half of the century began to tilt the balance in favour of the British, for although the tribesmen [in India] usually contrived to arm themselves with good rifles, they had not access to artillery or machine-guns. (Myatt, 1974, p. 188)

At Omdurman (Sudan) in 1898, British troops, armed with 20 Maxim machine-guns and 44 artillery pieces, killed 11 000 Sudanese in four and a half hours, losing only 48 of their own men (Derry & Williams, 1960). Gatling machine-guns, which came into use in the 1870s, were still used at the end of the century when US forces invaded Cuba (1898) and the Philippines (1899–1904). They violently suppressed local resistance to the new occupying power replacing Spain.

Myatt (1974) reports that the British used rockets at the battle of Arogee in Abyssinia in 1867–68, in the Sudan in 1897–98 and at Kumasi in the Ashanti War of 1900, and in various other expeditions along the West African coast.

In Europe this same period is remembered as an age of development of international humanitarian law, and it was suggested that some of these weapons should be banned. On the urging of successive Russian Tsars, the Powers agreed not to use certain of the new inventions such as explosive and expanding bullets against each other (see chapter 9).

VIII. Summary and conclusions

From the earliest times until the end of the nineteenth century, weapons suitable for hand-to-hand fighting have given way to projectile-firing devices. Technological development and mass production techniques made it possible to inundate the battlefield with huge quantities of projectiles while the increased range of high-powered rifles, machine-guns and artillery kept battle lines about 1 000 m apart. Face-to-face combat became rare and most battle injuries were due to projectiles.

The greatly increased fire-power of the industrial nations contributed to the rise of colonialism by enabling small forces of Europeans to overcome opposition from local forces equipped with hand-made muskets.

The period from 1860 to 1890 was one of rapid change in military small arms and ammunition. The magazine breech-loading, high-powered rifle was adopted by all the major powers and it remained, with very little change, the standard infantry weapon until after World War II.

In Europe, efforts were made to prohibit the use of the more destructive bullets by means of international legal agreements signed at St Petersburg in 1868 and The Hague in 1899.

Notes to Chapter 1

1. The English term 'shell' is said to derive from the German *Schale*, meaning 'outer rind or bark'. Earlier in English, and still in some languages, all explosive and incendiary shells were called 'grenades', which were mainly fired from mortars. English usage today confines the term grenade to small explosive projectiles propelled by hand or with the aid of a rifle shot, the term bomb or shell to projectiles fired by mortars, and the term shell to projectiles fired by cannons.
2. The Minié bullet was of .702 inch calibre and was introduced into British service in 1851. It proved unsatisfactory and in 1853 a new rifle of .577 inch calibre, made by the Royal Small Arms Factory at Enfield, was adopted. This was the first of the Enfield rifles.
3. Both the British government and the East India Company had their own armed forces.
4. In 20 minutes 247 men and 497 horses out of a total of 673 mounted soldiers were killed during a cavalry charge against Russian field artillery batteries (Dupuy & Dupuy, 1970).
5. Ivan S. Bloch was a Pole. His book, *The War of the Future in its Technical, Economic and Political Relations* (6 vols), was first published in Polish, Russian, French and German in 1897–1900. An abridged edition in English was published in England in 1899 and in the USA in 1902.
6. Bullets of a similar kind, known as hollow-point, have been issued to some US and other police forces in recent years, raising protests from civil rights organizations (*New York Times*, 26 September 1974; *Daily Telegraph*, 17 January 1975). In Britain several police forces purchased such bullets but were requested by the Home Secretary not to use them (*The Times*, 25 January 1975).

2. The rise of anti-personnel weapons, from World War I to the Viet Nam War

Superior numerals, thus [5], refer to notes on pages 49–52.

I. World War I

So far during the twentieth century, nearly 100 million people have died as a result of well over 100 wars. Four of these wars in particular have had a great impact on the development of anti-personnel weapons: the two World Wars, the Korean War and the Second Indo-China War.

World War I provided an opportunity to compare the optimism of some generals with the pessimism of I. S. Bloch, and to test the laws of war against the conduct of 'total war' between great industrial powers. As Bloch predicted in 1897, the opposing armies could not cross the no man's land between them without unacceptable losses. To break this deadlock, armies used illegal means of warfare, including gas and armed aircraft, and so destroyed some of the most important legal barriers to a new barbarism.[1] While more sophisticated weapons were used (such as the tank, submarine and aircraft), the special conditions of trench warfare led to a return to primitive hand weapons such as barbed clubs.[2]

The tank and the aircraft offered a means of breaking the deadlock of trench warfare imposed by earlier weapons. Chemical and incendiary weapons did not seem to prove decisive in this respect, although they were much discussed after the war.

All combatants were equipped with *high velocity rifles* of about 7.6 mm calibre and an effective range exceeding 1 000 m. In many cases the ammunition was of the pointed *Spitzer* type rather than the older round-nosed type, and most rifles were of the bolt-action type with a magazine containing about five bullets.

Machine-guns were available, but their significance was not appreciated by all parties in the early days of the war. French troops, equipped with a belief in *élan* and red trousers, proved easy targets for German machine-gunners in prepared positions at the beginning of the war. Machine-guns of the Maxim water-cooled type were used in large numbers by both sides. They were cumbersome to transport but were capable of continuous fire for long periods. These characteristics made them more suitable in defence than in attack, and possibly they determined the character of World War I, thus exposing basic fallacies in military doctrines.

Before World War I the French 75 mm artillery was successful and this contributed to some over-emphasis on this calibre on the French side. The British were equipped with the 13-pounder (5.9 kg) QF (quick-firing) gun adopted in

1904 following the South African War. It was originally intended to operate alongside cavalry, and fired a shrapnel shell containing 236 metal pellets at a muzzle velocity of 508 m/s to a range of nearly 6 000 m. The British 4.5 inch (114.3 mm) Howitzer, introduced in 1909, fired a shrapnel shell with 486 lead balls, and the German 77 mm gun fired case shot to about 300 m. The lighter artillery pieces were very important and probably caused more casualties than any other type of weapon.

The development of effective field artillery meant a more protected field and permanent fortifications, which then stimulated, particularly on the German side, the development of heavier artillery.

As the war degenerated into prolonged trench warfare, *indirect fire weapons* developed, such as rifle grenades and trench mortars. German forces profited from the experience of the Russo–Japanese War and were supplied with large quantities of percussion hand-grenades. At the beginning of the war, the British had only small numbers of their Percussion Hand Grenade No. 1, Mark I. In February 1915 the British .303 (7.70 mm) Rifle Grenade No. 3, Mark I was introduced, and later that year the grenade named after the inventor, William Mills, of Birmingham, England, was introduced. This grenade had a scored, cast-iron jacket and was intended to break into 48 pieces. Over 35 million of these grenades were produced. As the war progressed, more hand and rifle grenades were developed by the major powers. They were similar in design to hand-grenades but made to be projected from the end of a rifle using a special cartridge.

Mortars consisted of a simple steel tube attached at an adjustable angle to a base plate. They projected an explosive fragmentation bomb with the aid of a high explosive charge dropped into the tube before the bomb. A small mortar bomb has a similar effect to that of a large grenade, but it can be projected to a range of several hundred metres.

Aircraft were first used for reconnaissance, but later they were fitted with machine-guns and attacked each other as well as strafing ground troops. As they became more powerful they carried droppable munitions, such as fragmentation bombs and *flechettes* – steel darts about 10 cm long which, when dropped from a height, were able to pierce a man from head to foot. Flechettes were dropped by the British over enemy horse lines from canisters containing 250 flechettes attached to the underside of the aircraft as early as the Battle of the Aisne in September 1914. Larger exploding and incendiary cluster bombs were also used.

By 1915 both lighter-than-air and heavier-than-air aircraft were used to bomb towns as well as battlefields. These raids caused about 5 000 civilian deaths (Urlanis, 1971) and had a considerable initial psychological and political impact. This led to development of high explosive and incendiary bombs and also *fragmentation bombs* of some 10–15 kg. These were used against living and light matériel targets; examples are the 25 lb (11.3 kg) Hales bomb and the 20 lb (9.1 kg) Cooper Mk. 1 bomb. By end of the war it was possible to mount attacks involving hundreds of aircraft.

Although many new weapons emerged, the majority of them were designed to propel large numbers of small projectiles (bullets or fragments) in the direction of the enemy so as to make him 'keep his head down'. This restricted his mobility, but did not necessarily hit individual soldiers. The opportunities for aimed fire by the infantryman, let alone for bayonet fighting, were limited. Emphasis in the development of weapons shifted from aimed direct fire at a precise point to indirect fire designed to cover a given area for a given time, perhaps hours or even days, with a given concentration of injurious projectiles.

II. The inter-war period

The development of anti-personnel weapons during the inter-war period must be seen in the light of the political aftermath and the tactical lessons of World War I. The war dealt the final blow to the Ottoman Empire at a time when the increasing use of the internal combustion engine emphasized the strategic and economic importance of the Middle East oilfields and the Suez Canal area. When they sought to control these areas, the British and French found themselves confronted with a variety of armed nationalist and tribal resistance movements.

The Soviet Union needed to reconstruct its society and its armed forces. Germany was prohibited by the post-war treaties from re-establishing large armed forces and much of its capacity for military research, development and production was dismantled, and many of the older military doctrines were discarded. The United States withdrew its forces from Europe and demobilized much of its military organization.

Meanwhile analysts of World War I produced a number of influential books. The British military historians Liddell Hart and Fuller pointed to the importance of the tank in re-establishing battlefield mobility. Their books were translated, and apparently influenced Soviet and German planners operating a joint tank training and development area in Kazakhstan (Milsom, 1970). Extensive use of armour as 'bones' for infantry 'muscle' became – and remains – a fundamental German and Soviet tactic.

The Italian Douhet and the American Mitchell emphasized the use of air power and popularized the idea of air forces acting independently of ground forces and striking at the heart of enemy territory. Britain, however, was the only power at that time to establish an independent air force; it was under the control of Lord Trenchard. The strategic doctrines he developed were to play a prominent role in World War II.

Pacification of tribesmen in Western Asia and North East Africa with ground forces in 1920 cost the British Government large sums of money and Trenchard's proposal to substitute air forces for ground forces in these operations was accepted (Payne, 1966; Divine, 1966; Allen, 1972). From these beginnings arose the concept of 'pacification' by air which was to reach its zenith in Indo-China half a century later.

For these operations, aircraft equipped with machine-guns and fragmentation bombs were used. Slessor (1956)[3] gives a personal account of what was perhaps the first such operation as early as 1916 in the Sudan[4] – described as the largest

British military operation in that country since Omdurman (see p. 15) – where he dropped 20 lb (9.1 kg) Hales fragmentation bombs on Ali Dinar and his forces:

> The bombs used were all 20-lb Hales, which were very good little men-killing bombs, with instantaneous fuse and an excellent shattering effect. The targets bombed were mostly men in the open or in villages composed of *tukls*, or conical huts made of dhurra stocks, which of course were no protection against splinters. (Slessor, 1956, p. 655)

It is interesting that Slessor justifies what he calls the 'Air Method' on 'humanitarian grounds' since, he argued, the aim was not to kill as many as possible but to make normal conditions of life impossible:

> Turning now to the application of the Air Method, let me first define a little more clearly what we meant by 'interrupting the normal life of the people'. The aim was to deprive the offending tribe of their normal means of livelihood; to force them to abandon their grazing grounds, wells or villages when they had them – the desert Bedu, of course, did not, but lived in tents, moving from one grazing area or water point to another; to prevent the watering of cattle or camels, or at least to make it difficult or arduous; to prevent ploughing or harvesting or any form of cultivation of crops, date palms or fruit trees; to force the tribe to scatter itself and its flocks over cold uplands, to hide in caves or billet themselves and their flocks as unwelcome guests on the inhabitants of neighbouring villages where their hosts usually brought pressure to bear on them to submit to our terms, since the last thing they wanted was to get embroiled themselves; to deny to them any form of compensation which other forms of warfare might offer such as loot, the chance of capturing rifles and ammunition, and the sporting satisfaction of having a good fight on equal terms; and to go on doing all these things until they got so fed up with the hardship and inconvenience involved that they decided that submission to our terms was the lesser evil. (Slessor, 1956, pp. 61–62)

This philosophy was adapted to urban conditions during World War II when the Royal Air Force adopted a strategy of 'dehousing' the enemy population – a euphemism for mass area bombing of cities (SIPRI, 1975a). More recently, the application of a similar philosophy in Indo-China has given rise to the term 'ecocide' or environmental warfare (SIPRI, 1976b). The earlier applications were more significant in influencing the strategic thinking of future military leaders than the development of new anti-personnel weapons.

While the inter-war years saw considerable development of tanks and aircraft, and of the munitions pertaining to them, most armed forces kept the infantry weapons of World War I. This was due to the huge stocks available and also to conservative thinking. In 1936 the United States became the first country to adopt a self-loading rifle. Designed by John Garand, it accepted the .30-06 (7.64 mm) cartridge of World War I. A light machine-gun, the Browning Automatic Rifle (BAR), introduced in 1919, was also adopted as a standard weapon by the USA.

remaining in service throughout the Korean War, and still found in some armies.

The German Army, restricted by the Treaty of Versailles, turned to co-operation with foreign manufacturers. A Swiss company (said to be financially controlled by the German company Rheinmetall) developed an air-cooled machine-gun, the Solothurn MG-30, which served as the basis for the MG-34 adopted by the Wehrmacht in 1934. This weapon may be regarded as the first 'general-purpose machine-gun' (GPMG), a type which is by now in universal use. It fired a 7.92 mm Mauser round at the rate of 800–900 or even 1 000 rpm.

In the Soviet Union a light machine-gun, designed by V. A. Degtyaryov, was adopted in 1927 during the reorganization of the Red Army. Like the German weapons, it was used during the Spanish Civil War and became a major weapon in World War II (Yelshin, 1977).

Shortly before World War II, the British adopted a Czech-designed machine-gun produced at Brno, and manufactured it under licence at the Royal Small Arms Factory at Enfield; the weapon became known as the BREN (from BRno–ENfield). The Japanese also copied Czech designs and modified French and other weapons.

The sub-machine-gun (or machine-pistol) was introduced in limited numbers during this period and was to become typical of World War II. The German Schmeisser, Italian Beretta and US Thompson designs were introduced about 1918. The 'Tommy-gun', although said to be a police weapon, became identified with gangsters rather than organized military formations. Nevertheless, it was adopted by US armed forces in 1928 and used by the US Marines in Nicaragua.

Impressed by the use of sub-machine-guns in the Spanish Civil War, the German Army replaced the MP-18 with the MP-38; in Italy, Beretta also introduced a 1938 model sub-machine-gun.

While most of these weapons used 9 mm Parabellum pistol ammunition, the Soviet Union produced a military sub-machine-gun, the PPD-34, using 7.62 mm pistol ammunition (which is identical with the 7.63 mm Mauser round). The bullet is lighter than the 9 mm round, but the cartridge is about the same size. The bullet therefore has a higher initial velocity but loses momentum faster.

The mass slaughter of World War I did much to destroy old ideas of war and promoted public interest in peace, disarmament and international law. The League of Nations was established; international treaties, including a ban on chemical and bacteriological warfare, were signed; and the Disarmament Conference in Geneva got as far as producing a draft disarmament treaty in 1933.

But on a small scale, and often in remote places, the new weapons and tactics which were to characterize World War II were being developed. The treaties which concluded World War I failed to establish a world order. As a result, the stage was set for another war.

III. World War II

More than 20 million military personnel and an even greater number of civilians died during World War II (Urlanis, 1971). Of this number, over one million – the overwhelming majority of them civilians – died as a result of mass bombing raids which included the use of two atomic bombs (cf. SIPRI, 1975a). Most of the remaining civilian deaths resulted either from deliberate extermination policies or from disease, malnutrition and other incidental or deliberate effects of combat and blockade. The millions of battlefield casualties resulted more from the massive use of conventional weapons, most of them designed before the war, than from any dramatic new developments in anti-personnel weapon technology. Perhaps the only significantly different anti-personnel weapon to be developed during World War II was the napalm bomb (SIPRI, 1975a).

The most notable trend during World War II was not so much the development of new anti-personnel weapons as the tremendous increase in the density of armoured vehicles, artillery and aircraft deployed, particularly on the Eastern Front. Massive use of conventional weapons against huge armies meant many casualties. The German Army, for example, sometimes lost more than 50 000 troops per month.

The pressures of war accelerated the development of existing anti-personnel weapons, especially in the field of automatic infantry weapons. Most of the design changes adopted were aimed more at simplifying the manufacturing process than at improving the effectiveness of the weapons. This applied particularly to the production of machine-pistols or sub-machine-guns. Remarkably simple designs, such as the US M-3 and the British Sten gun, were produced in great numbers. Although they were not very accurate at the limits of range, they were light and handy and gave the infantryman a relatively high rate-of-fire weapon.

Similar considerations apply to such weapons as the German MG-42 machine-gun, which was introduced to supplement the highly effective MG-34. Modern versions of the MG-42 are still in use in the Federal German Army and in other countries.

All the combatants retained essentially the same ammunition in use since World War I, although Italy and Japan took steps to introduce somewhat larger calibre ammunition.

The only exceptions to this generalization were the German 7.92 mm Kurz bullet, which was followed by the development of the Soviet 7.62 mm M-43 round, and US M-1 .30 in (7.62 mm) carbine round. These rounds were designed for intermediate-power semi-automatic or automatic weapons of a type which assumed considerable significance after World War II.

The Germans appear to have been the first to appreciate the fact that the changing conditions of combat reduced the need for a full-powered rifle of the traditional type. They saw the possibility of replacing both the rifle and the sub-machine-gun with a single light-weight automatic rifle, firing an intermediate-power cartridge with an effective range of about 400 m. For some reason it appears that *Reichskanzler* Hitler had a personal objection to this idea which hindered its development. The first weapon of this kind to appear was therefore disguised by the developers as MP (machine-pistol)-43. Only later was the designation *Sturmgewehr* (assault rifle) given to the weapon. It was issued to some troops and put to use against the Soviet forces.

Soviet designers saw the value of this weapon and developed an intermediate-power version of their standard 7.62 mm ammunition in 1943. A number of weapons were designed to fire the round but it was not until after the war that a weapon of this kind – the Kalashnikov AK-47 – was adopted as a standard weapon (see chapter 4).

US forces were issued with the M-1 carbine (not to be confused with the M-1 rifle, a full-power semi-automatic weapon). It was a light-weight weapon with a special cartridge and was intermediate in power between pistol and rifle ammunition. It was originally intended as a substitute for pistols for officers and other special troops and it proved popular for a time. Over 6.3 million were produced (Smith, 1969) – more than any other US hand weapon.

Other anti-personnel weapons developed included the German S.Gr.W.42 8-cm mortar bomb, which was fitted with a device causing it to 'bounce' into the air before exploding. In theory, a fragmentation munition that explodes a metre or two above the ground is more effective against troops in the open than one which explodes only after hitting the ground, since in the latter case much of the effect is lost in the ground. The German 8 cm mortar, though not entirely successful,[5] represented an early attempt to tackle this problem, which is now more commonly solved by the use of a proximity fuze.[6]

Much effort was put into designing anti-personnel mines, some kinds of which could jump up into the air before exploding and projecting a large number of metal pellets or fragments. An example of this kind was the German 'S' mine, which when activated, was ejected about 2 m into the air before it exploded and projected both fragments and steel bearings about 30 m in all directions.

Another development in the field of anti-personnel mines was the use of plastics, such as Bakelite, to reduce the possibility of detection with magnetic mine-detectors. Mines of this kind – which are now in common use – rely primarily on blast rather than fragments for their casualty effects.

The rocket began to re-emerge as an important weapon. The German 15 and 30 cm Nebelwerfer rocket launchers were primarily intended for firing chemical and smoke rockets, but also fired high-explosive rockets. The most notable German developments were the much larger A-4 (V-2) rockets and other large long-distance designs which were to pave the way for post-war ballistic missiles.

Although these large German rockets received much publicity, it is probable that the 12 cm Soviet Katyusha rockets had more military use during the War. These were solid fuel rockets, fired *en masse* with devastating effect.

The Western powers also deployed a number of rockets. The British developed 2 in (50.8 mm) and 3 in (76.2 mm) rockets for use against aircraft. The 3 in rocket was modified for air-to-surface use. A six-tube 5 in (127.0 mm) rocket launcher was developed for use by both the Royal Navy and the British Army. The best-known tactical rocket launcher developed by the USA for use by the individual infantryman was the 'bazooka', which fired a small anti-tank rocket less than 2 kg in weight. The USA also developed a series of 4.5 in (114.3 mm) and 7 in (177.8 mm) rockets launched by multi-tube launchers, such as the 20-tube Whizz-Bang launcher, the 24-tube Grand Slam launcher and the 120-tube Woofus launcher. It seems that the Western powers placed less emphasis in their tactical doctrines on the use of rocket salvos than did Soviet forces, both during World War II and afterwards. (Recently there have been indications of increased Western interest in multiple rocket launchers; see chapter 5.)

Combat aircraft and their weapons were increasingly used in World War II. In addition to high explosive rockets and general purpose bombs, a variety of anti-personnel bombs were developed. These ranged from conventional fragmentation bombs to devices designed to explode after a time delay or when disturbed by a person or vehicle. It became a standard tactic to mix bombs of this kind with conventional bombs in raids on military and civilian targets in order to harass the defenders, rescue personnel, fire-fighters, and so on.

IV. The Korean War

The Korean War began five years after the end of World War II and during this period Korean forces in the north and south had largely been equipped with Soviet and US matériel of World War II vintage.[7]

Chinese forces were equipped mainly with a variety of weapons captured from Japanese, Kuomintang and US forces. An agreement with the Soviet Union in February 1950 made increasing numbers of Soviet weapons available and later China manufactured copies of Soviet weapons. The Chinese also manufactured copies or modifications of such weapons as the 1908 model Maxim machine-gun, the Czech ZB-26 light machine-gun, the US M-2 60 mm mortar, smaller Japanese artillery guns, and the US 4.5 in (114.3 mm) rocket.

Most of the ground fighting took place in the first nine months, although artillery and air attacks and occasional infantry offensives continued for two more years. The war was too short to permit much in the way of technical innovation other than a variety of improvisations in the field. But the combat conditions, and particularly US fears of being overrun by superior numbers of Asian enemy troops, promoted much research and development of anti-personnel weapons during the late 1950s and early 1960s. Some of these developments proved to be significant during the Viet Nam War.

Chinese and North Korean forces made extensive use of mortars, land-mines and grenades, owing to the simplicity of manufacture and to tactical conditions. Mines were often handmade from wooden boxes, glass bottles, oil drums, clay pots, bamboo and so on. Those which did not contain metal were particularly hard to detect and remove.

US and South Korean forces also made extensive use of mines, including field improvisations. One standard US improvisation was to suspend a drum of napalm in a tree and fit it with a high explosive detonator. The drum was sometimes wrapped in barbed wire which broke into pieces when the drum burst. Because of the great movements of forces in the early part of the war, many casualties resulted from 'friendly' mines (Beyer, 1962).

US forces made much use of the technique of 'close air support', developed during World War II. This technique involves the co-ordination of air attacks with ground forces already fighting the enemy. In this role, napalm bombs were often used because of their relatively clearly defined area of effect (SIPRI, 1975a). Where less precision was acceptable, or where 'friendly' ground forces were not involved, conventional bombs, rockets and aircraft cannons were used. US and allied air forces expended some 635 000 tonnes of air munitions (Futrell, 1961) and 1 915 000 tonnes of ground munitions (US Senate Committee on Foreign Relations, 1971) – that is, air munitions accounted for about 25 per cent of the total and probably a similar proportion of casualties on the North Korean side.

There is considerable evidence to suggest that the Korean War was particularly indiscriminate in its effects on the civilian population. Although the war was a United Nations operation, there is remarkably little consistent and reliable information available about the number of civilian casualties.[8]

V. The war in Indo-China, 1961–75

In the wake of the Korean War, US weapon designers set about the task of producing a range of new weapons for use against large concentrations of men (cf. Hitchman, 1952). These were ready by the early 1960s, at which time the USA escalated its involvement in Indo-China.

In early 1961 a programme of military, political, economic, psychological and covert actions was drawn up in the United States to 'prevent Communist domination of South Vietnam'.[9] Included in the military part of this programme were the following measures:

> Assist the G.V.N.[10] armed forces to increase their border patrol and insurgency suppression capabilities by . . . applying *modern technological area-denial techniques* to control the roads and trails along Vietnam's borders . . .
>
> Assist the G.V.N. to establish a Combat Development and Test Center in South Vietnam *to develop, with the help of modern technology, new techniques* for use against the Viet Cong forces. (US Senate Committee on Foreign Relations, 1972, p. 16; italics added)

In Annex 2 to the programme, 'CW, BW, light plastic, air-droppable landmines, fluorescent materials, etc.' are given as examples of 'technological area-denial techniques' (ibid., p. 23).

To the twin components of high technology and cloak-and-dagger tactics was added a third: the desire of the military establishments to try out new weaponry and tactics in combat.[11] These and other pressures led to the application of technology of a scale and sophistication which had never been seen before, and to the suppression of a peasant guerrilla army.

In addition to chemical weapons (SIPRI, 1971, 1973, 1976b) and incendiaries (SIPRI, 1975a), a range of new weapons, from small arms to mines and bombs, were introduced and used on an unprecedented scale. US and allied forces (supplied by the USA) used altogether some 15 million tonnes of ammunition (table 2.1), almost half of it dropped by air.

Table 2.1. US expenditure of munitions in Indo-China, 1965–73[a]

Tonnes = 10^3 kg

Year	Ground	Air	Sea	Total
1965	–	285 763	–	**285 763**
1966	535 400	458 418	4 536	**998 354**
1967	1 091 824	845 604	27 216	**1 964 644**
1968	1 346 628	1 303 960	45 813	**2 696 401**
1969	1 275 341	1 258 500	27 216	**2 561 057**
1970	1 071 870	886 724	11 793	**1 970 387**
1971	755 656	692 327	4 802	**1 452 785**
1972	776 430	983 707	32 114	**1 792 251**
1973	162 581	378 098	2 722	**543 401**
Total	**7 015 730**	**7 093 101**	**156 212**	**14 265 043**

[a] Includes munitions supplied by USA to its allies; total does not include munitions expended prior to 1965, ground or sea munitions for 1965, air munitions expended after July 1973, or ground munitions expended after June 1973.

Sources: US Senate Committee on Foreign Relations (1971); US Department of Defense release, 17 August 1973; US Department of Defense, *personal communication*, 2 November 1973.

Conventional high explosive munitions

Some two-thirds of these munitions were expended in South Viet Nam where the military targets mostly consisted of suspected troop concentrations and the social infrastructure of the guerrilla-occupied areas. An estimated 98 per cent of the seven million tonnes of ground munitions expended by US and allied forces were fired in South Viet Nam. Fighter-bombers and B-52 heavy bombers each expended nearly 1.5 million tonnes of munitions. Munition expenditures by the liberation forces are not known but probably reached several hundred thousand tonnes during the war. In all, over 10 million tonnes of ammunition were expended in South Viet Nam alone – equivalent to nearly 600 kg/ha or 600 kg per capita (SIPRI, 1976b). (This is approximately 10 times the density of munitions dropped on North Viet Nam.)

Most of the ammunition used consisted of conventional general purpose artillery shells and aircraft bombs. The USA and its allies alone used some estimated 250 million 105 mm artillery shells[12] and 23 million 500-lb (230-kg) aircraft bombs (SIPRI, 1976b). A high proportion of these munitions were fired or dropped unobserved against areas reportedly containing enemy positions or troop concentrations but where precise targets could not be identified.[13] Much unobserved fire was referred to as 'H & I' (harassment and interdiction), the military purpose of which was to make it more difficult for enemy forces to move through or concentrate in an area. This method is extremely costly, and since the effects are generally not observed, its military effectiveness is difficult to evaluate. The US Air Force provided the information that field surveys had shown that the B-52s (table 2.2), each one of them dropping on a typical raid of the order of 100 500-lb

Table 2.2. Tonnage of munitions dropped in Indo-China by B-52 heavy bombers

Tonnes = 10^3 kg

Year	North Viet Nam	South Viet Nam	Laos	Cambodia	**Total**
1965	0	28 607	425	0	**29 038**
1966	5 179	76 397	11 853	0	**93 447**
1967	37 754	157 790	40 918	0	**236 511**
1968	17 971	428 379	85 787	0	**531 485**
1969	0	293 349	144 655	62 475	**500 585**
1970	0	100 612	210 227	59 250	**370 384**
1971	0	55 894	208 755	30 565	**295 143**
1972	88 797	320 491	55 682	33 934	**499 007**
1973[a]	10 064	25 314	38 810	26 454	**100 664**
Total	**159 765**	**1 486 833**	**797 112**	**212 678**	**2 656 264**
Per cent	*6.0*	*56.0*	*30.0*	*8.0*	*100.0*

[a] January–March only.

Source: US Department of Defense release, 18 July 1973.

bombs, or about 23 tonnes, killed from 0.7 to 3.5 enemy soldiers per bomb load (*US Congressional Record*, Vol. 118, 10–11 May 1972, pp. 16748–16836).

H & I fire is highly indiscriminate and forces the civilian population to leave the area, which in turn has severe social and economic consequences. Damage to the environment is long-term, widespread and severe (SIPRI, 1976b).

The US air war in Laos was described as the 'support of and participation in a large-scale air war over Laos to destroy the physical and social infrastructure of the Pathet Lao held areas and to interdict North Vietnamese infiltration' (US Senate Committee on the Judiciary, 1970, p. 19).

The destruction of villages with the aid of fragmentation bombs and other munitions has been a basic technique of 'pacification' at least since World War I (see above, p. 19), and in spite of the official veil of secrecy and denial, considerable evidence has been produced before the US Senate Foreign Relations Committee and the Subcommittee on Refugees to show that this technique was vigorously used in Laos. A survey conducted among refugees in 1970, for example, concluded that 'the bombing is clearly the most compelling reason for moving' (cited in US Senate Committee on the Judiciary, 1970, pp. 44 ff.).

Four phases in the escalation of US bombing of Laos are indicated:

> 1. The first phase ran from approximately May 1964 until October 1966. Bombing during this period was rather sporadic, carried out mainly by Laotian T-28's and directed largely against enemy troop concentrations in jungle areas.

> 2. The second phase ... from fall 1966 to early 1968 ... began to include enemy held or threatened villages or towns. American aircraft became increasingly prominent ...

> 3. The third bombing phase began in 1968, shortly after the partial bombing halt over North Vietnam in March, with American aircraft outnumbering Laotian T-28's for the first time ... directed increasingly against populated areas.

> 4. In the fourth and current [1970] phase, which began very early in 1969, the most significant bombing increase has occurred. It followed the complete bombing halt over North Vietnam in November 1968. Refugees say, according to one source, that during some of this bombing phase, jets have come daily – dropping napalm, phosphorus, and anti-personnel bombs. 'They say the jets bombed both villages and forests, that they spent most of their time in holes or caves, and that they suffered numerous civilian casualties. They say that everything was fired on, buffaloes, cows, cornfields, schools, temples, tiny shelters outside the village, in addition to, of course, people.' (ibid. p. 29)

The Subcommittee report goes on to say:

> Just how extensive this 'support bombing' was is revealed in reports from the field and in testimony before congressional committees. Estimates of the number of bombing sorties conducted during the peak periods of last year [1969] range as high as from 400 to 800 sorties per day. (p. 29)

According to another source:

> By 1968 the intensity of the bombings was such that no organized life was possible in the villages. The villagers moved to the outskirts and then deeper and deeper into the forest as the bombing climax reached its peak in 1969 when jet planes came daily and destroyed all stationary structures. Nothing was left standing. The villagers lived in trenches and holes or in caves. They only farmed at night. All the informants without any exception had his village completely destroyed. In the last phase, bombings were aimed at the systematic destruction of

the material basis of the civilian society. (Chapelier & Van Malderghem, 1971, pp. 18–19)

This account is difficult to reconcile with the Rules of Engagement for US aircraft, some of which have been published (appendix 9D). Several areas were not covered by the rules, which were primarily intended to avoid civilian casualties in areas where support for the Vientiane government might be won. The rules did not apply to the Royal Lao Air Force. They were complicated and difficult to apply and pilots did not always abide by them. Finally, it has been claimed that after 1969 the rules 'appear to have been discarded and are only cited to placate Congressmen in Washington'.[14]

It should be noted that the increase in the bombing of Laos occurred following the 'bombing halt' over North Viet Nam. A similar shift in the pattern of bombing occurred in 1973 following the Paris Agreements. In southern Laos the major part of the US air effort was directed at stopping the flow of supplies from North to South Viet Nam.

Towards the end of the 1960s Cambodian territory was used increasingly for the transit of men and supplies to the liberation armies in South Viet Nam. The United States responded by bombing Cambodia[15] in areas believed to be used as a 'sanctuary' by these forces. B-52 heavy bombers, following the bombing halt in North Viet Nam, dropped over 66 000 tonnes of bombs in Cambodia in 1969 alone, even before the overthrow of Prince Sihanouk in March 1970.

The Cambodian Air Force was equipped with T-28 trainers fitted out as light attack aircraft. US Spooky and Shadow gunships (see p. 33) and other attack aircraft engaged in close support and ground attack operations in Cambodia. At the same time other US aircraft operating in South Viet Nam freed South Vietnamese aircraft for operations in Cambodia.

In addition to the massive use of general purpose high explosive munitions, the United States introduced many new weapon systems into the Indo-China War.

Bomblet dispenser systems and cluster bombs

New cluster bomb units (CBUs) and bomblet dispenser systems were developed (chapter 5) and procured (table 2.3). Various forms of dispenser were placed in or under an aircraft. These were designed to disperse hundreds of small bomblets over an area of perhaps 1–20 ha. The bomblets (BLUs) were of the fragmentation type or contained chemical, incendiary or smoke agents. A typical bomblet is fluted, causing it to spin in the air, arming the fuze and imparting a lateral motion, thereby broadening the impact pattern. The bomblets explode in the air or on the ground immediately or after a delay.

As the war progressed, CBUs of increasing sophistication were developed. The BLU-77 for example, is a dual-purpose bomblet able to *penetrate* a hard target but *bounce* from a soft landing (i.e., the reverse of what would normally be expected), before exploding in the air, thereby maximizing effectiveness against either armoured vehicles or personnel.

Table 2.3. US procurement of fragmentation cluster bombs, fiscal years 1964–73

Number of units

Type	1964	1965	1966	1967	1968	1969	1970	1971	1972	1973	Total
ADU-253	–	–	–	38 515	–	–	–	–	–	–	38 515
ADU-272	–	–	–	17 712	–	–	41 480	–	–	–	59 192
Canister with BLU-3	–	18 072	148 464	–	–	–	–	–	–	–	166 536
CBU-1	3 800	–	–	–	–	–	–	–	–	–	3 800
CBU-2	10 964	–	200	15 700	10 386	–	–	–	–	–	37 250
CBU-3	2 573	3 441	1 087	–	–	–	–	–	–	–	7 101
CBU-7	–	3 026	4 800	–	–	–	–	–	–	–	7 826
CBU-9	–	–	527	–	–	–	–	–	–	–	527
CBU-14	–	30 965	38 200	25 200	–	15 700	27 203	8 000	–	–	145 268
CBU-24/29/49	–	–	–	60 936	67 865	103 329	133 490	58 158	–	–	423 778
CBU-25	–	–	10 255	19 000	781	25 500	32 075	14 213	45 459	39 500	186 783
CBU-38	–	–	–	–	–	99	1 580	1 475	11 100	–	14 254
CBU-46	–	–	–	–	9 265	4 805	–	–	–	–	14 070
CBU-58	–	–	–	–	–	–	6 000	37 483	33 000	43 200	119 683
CBU-59	–	–	–	–	–	–	–	327	–	–	327
M1A2/4	–	21 150	–	9 700	29 800	58 263	12 900	9 400	–	–	141 213
Mk-15	3 400	2 300	4 500	–	–	–	–	–	–	–	10 200
Mk-20	–	–	535	1 400	2 870	8 650	16 600	13 458	34 753	51 900	130 166
Total	**20 737**	**78 954**	**208 568**	**188 163**	**120 967**	**216 346**	**271 328**	**142 514**	**124 312**	**134 600**	**1 506 489**

Source: US Department of Defense (unpublished procurement records).

According to some US Army commanders, CBUs were the ordnance preferred for attacks on enemy forces in the open which were in close combat with US ground troops. In what appears to have been a fairly typical example of such an attack, 'aircraft dropped cluster bomb units followed by napalm and 500-pound bombs on the attackers', and the CBUs 'could be delivered very close to friendly units and were a highly lethal weapon' (Rogers, 1974, pp. 114, 134).

> Cluster bomb units ... were the most effective ordnance for the situation which existed: enemy troops in the open, echeloned in depth, and in contact with our own troops. Since the pilot can release the small bomb units from their canister at low level, he can drop them within thirty meters of our own troops, and, when they explode on contact, our troops are unharmed, since the lethal radius of the ordnance is slightly less than that distance. (Rogers, 1974, p. 46 *fn*.)[16]

Although there was essentially no ground fighting in North Viet Nam, US aircraft did drop large quantities of munitions designed for use against personnel and light matériel – CBUs, napalm, phosphorus and even CS gas. According to US military authorities, major targets for CBU attacks were anti-aircraft defences – an operation referred to as 'defence suppression'. Aircraft dropping CBUs would normally precede aircraft engaged on other missions. Since these attacks were frequently in populated areas, area fragmentation bombs obviously would result in a large number of civilian as well as military casualties. While it was not possible to obtain precise numbers,[17] Gestewitz (1968) succeeded in obtaining a percentage distribution of the sources of injury of casualties in the Democratic Republic of Viet Nam for the years 1965–67. These figures show a marked increase in the proportion due to CBU bombs of the 'pellet' kind (table 2.4).

A relatively high proportion of bomblets apparently failed to detonate as intended and remained a continuing hazard in the ground (US Senate Committee on the Judiciary, 1974, pp. 22–24). Such malfunctioning may not necessarily be a

Table 2.4. Distribution of casualties by weapon in the Democratic Republic of Viet Nam, 1965–67

Per cent

Source of injury	1965	1966	1967
Small arms ammunition (including strafing by aircraft)	16	3	1
High explosive shells and bombs	60	29	28
Pellet bombs	11	28	50
Rockets	11	28	12
Incendiary munitions (including napalm bombs)	2	12	9
Total	**100**	**100**	**100**

Source: Gestewitz (1968).

Table 2.5. US aircraft with predominantly anti-personnel applications developed for use in the war in Indo-China

Aircraft designation	Type	Description of armament	Entry into service
Bell AH-1 *Huey Cobra*	Helicopter	1. XM-28 system: 2 7.62-mm Miniguns each with 4 000 rounds; 2 XM-129 44-mm grenade launchers, with 300 rounds; 1 Minigun + 1 × M-129	Prototype delivered December 1965; deployment to Viet Nam early autumn 1967; over 1 000 produced
		2. External: 76 2.75-inch rockets *or* 28 2.75-inch rockets *or* 2 XM-18E1 Minigun pods *or* XM-35 20-mm gun kit	
		3. XM-35 20-mm cannon kit (6-barrel weapon)	1969
		4. SMASH (South-East Asia Multi-sensor Armament System for *Huey Cobra*): passive infra-red and moving target indicator fire-control system for day/night use	1970 (prototypes)
Bell AH-1J *Sea Cobra*	Helicopter	Twin engine version of above for US Marine Corps; XM-197 3-barrel 20-mm gun system + external 7.62-mm Minigun pods or 2.75-inch rockets	Delivery to USMC began in 1970; 202 ordered by US Army, 1972 for sale to Iran
Bell AH-1Q *Huey Cobra*	Helicopter	Gunship version of AH-1G, equipped to fire TOW anti-tank missiles	Experimental versions used against armour in Viet Nam 1972; deployed with US forces in Europe 1974 –
A-37 (Cessna Model 318)	Fixed wing jet trainer	Development of T-37 jet trainer for armed COIN operations; GAU-2B/A 7.62-mm Minigun in fuselage; *External Weapons options*: SUU-20 bomb and rocket pod; MK-81 or MK-82 bomb; BLU-32/B napalm bomb; SUU-11/A gun pod; CBU-24/B or CBU-25/A dispenser and bomb; M-117 demolition bomb; LAU-3/A rocket pod; CBU-12/A, CBU-14/A or CBU-22/A dispenser and bomb; BLU-1C/B napalm bomb; LAU-32/A or LAU-59/A rocket pod; CBU-19/A canister cluster	Prototype 1963; evaluation of A-37A in Viet Nam 1967; A-37B designed 1967; 410 delivered by early 1973, of which 164 supplied to GVN

Table 2.5 (*continued*)

Aircraft designation	Type	Description of armament	Entry into service
Fairchild AC-119G *Shadow*	Fixed wing cargo	Gunship from converted 2 piston-engine transport aircraft; fitted with 4 side-firing 7.62-mm Miniguns plus illumination and light-intensifying night observation systems	. .
Fairchild AC-119K *Stinger*	Fixed wing cargo	As above but with 2 auxiliary jet engines and 2 20-mm cannons	. .
Lockheed AC-130 Gunship II	Fixed wing cargo	Gunship version of C-130A *Hercules* transport; fitted with 4 20-mm multi-barrel cannon + 4 7.62-mm Miniguns and infra-red night observation equipment; *or* 2 40-mm grenade launchers + 2 20-mm guns and digital fire-control computer	Evaluated 1967; in service in Viet Nam 1968–69
Lockheed AC-130E	Fixed wing cargo	Gunship version of C-130E extended range aircraft; similar to above but with heavier armour and more ammunition and advanced electronics	. .
Lockheed AC-130H	Fixed wing cargo	Converted from above after service in Viet Nam; new engines; one 40-mm gun replaced by 105-mm howitzer	. .
Canberra B-57	Fixed wing bomber	Converted to gunship version	20 deployed from 1 October 1970

Source: Pretty & Archer (1974).

disadvantage from the military point of view in a war where 'area denial' is a primary strategy. But the problem of unexploded weapons after a war is of considerable concern and there is little doubt that certain kinds of cluster bomb have proved a particular hazard. (This problem is discussed further in chapter 7.)

Gunships

A notable feature of US tactics in Indo-China was the extensive use of aircraft for offensive operations. As well as conventional attack aircraft, aircraft armed with rockets, cannons, bombs and napalm tanks, both helicopters and fixed wing aircraft were converted to 'gunships' (table 2.5). This was achieved by the addition of automatic grenade launchers and high rate-of-fire machine-guns (table 2.6) and

33

Table 2.6. US aircraft armament systems with predominantly anti-personnel applications developed for use in the war in Indo-China

Systems designation	Description
General Electric M-61A1 *Vulcan*	20-mm aircraft gun, 6 barrels, electrically or hydraulically operated; high rate of fire, normally 6 000 rpm
General Electric GAU-4	Similar to above, but gas-operated
General Electric SUU-16/A	Pod for external mounting of M-61A1 20-mm aircraft gun
General Electric SUU-23/A	Pod for external mounting of GAU-4 20-mm aircraft gun
General Electric XM35	Mounting for modified M-61A1 20-mm aircraft gun on AH-1G helicopter
Hughes MK 4 Mod 0	Gun pod for twin-barrelled 20-mm MK 11 Mod 5 gun; fitted to A-4, F-4, A-6, A-7, or A-10, F-100 and UH-1 aircraft
General Electric XM-197	Light-weight 3-barrel version of M-61A1 20-mm aircraft gun; 400–1 500 rpm; used in AH-1J attack helicopter and OV-10A aircraft
Emerson Electric XM-21	System made up of 2 7.62-mm M-134 machine-guns and 2 XM-158 pods with 7 rockets each; fires 4 800 bullets per minute or 6 pairs of rockets per second
Emerson Electric XM-28 (SM-28E1)	System made up of 2 7.62-mm M-134 machine guns *or* 2 40-mm grenade launchers, *or* one each; fitted to AH-1G *Huey Cobra* helicopter; rate of fire: 4 000 rpm for each gun and 300 rpm for each grenade launcher
Emerson Electric XM-93	GAU-2B/A machine-gun system (rate of fire: 2 000–4 000 rpm) for mounting in cargo compartment of UH-1N helicopter
Emerson Electric XM-94	XM-129 40-mm grenade launcher system (rate of fire: 400 rpm) for mounting in UH-1N helicopter
Emerson Electric XM-18E1	M-134 7.62-mm machine-gun (rate of fire: 2 000–4 000 rpm) for mounting under weapon sponsons of AH-1G helicopter; 1 500 round drum with standard NATO 7.62-mm ammunition type M-59, M-80 or M60
Hughes XM-27E1	Similar to above for mounting on OH-6A *Cayuse* helicopter
General Electric SUU-11B/A	Similar to above for mounting on standard bomb lugs of a wide range of tactical aircraft up to Mach 1.2

Source: Pretty & Archer (1974).

34

they were made additionally versatile through devices such as night vision equipment. Later, specially designed attack helicopters were deployed on a large scale for the first time.

The first gunships were elderly C-47 cargo planes equipped with newly developed machine-guns operating on the Gatling multi-barrel principle. The 20 mm Vulcan gun (now standard for US combat aircraft) normally fires at a rate of 6 000 rpm. A scaled down 7.62 mm version firing standard NATO ammunition normally fires at a rate of 4 000–6 000 rpm. A three-barrelled, light-weight version of the 20 mm gun was produced for use in helicopters. The advantage of cargo aircraft is that they can carry much greater quantities of ammunition than conventional attack aircraft.

The AC-47 gunships were usually equipped with three 7.62 mm Gatling-type guns, each capable of firing at rates of up to 6 000 rpm. Later, B-57 *Canberra* bombers and C-119 *Provider* and C-130 *Hercules* cargo aircraft were equipped as gunships (designated AC-119 and AC-130 respectively). It has been said that weapon systems such as these could place several bullets per square metre on an area the size of a football pitch in a few seconds. For the automatic grenade launchers a new family of 40 mm grenades was developed (see chapter 5) that can fire some 300–450 grenades per minute.

Gunships frequently operated at night and were equipped with increasingly sophisticated equipment, ranging from high intensity searchlights and flare systems to infra-red, low light level television, and image intensifying systems.

According to US Director of Defense Research and Engineering John S. Foster, Jr., gunships proved to be 'the most effective air interdiction system in Southeast Asia' (US Senate Appropriations Committee, 1971, part 1, p. 406).

Scatterable mines

From the earliest phases of the War, US forces placed emphasis on 'area denial' – an attempt to prevent the use of large tracts of territory by the resistance forces. Small anti-personnel mines, some resembling a large tea-bag, were developed and over 100 million were procured for use in Laos and elsewhere in Indo-China (table 2.7). These mines could be scattered in thousands from aircraft and led to a whole new area of military technology and tactics. Whereas, previously, emplaced mines were often kept under the control of the emplacer, the new scatterable mines can be dropped from the air deep behind enemy lines. This prospect is an enticing one from some military points of view but a highly disturbing one for civilians (see chapter 7).

Land-mines were used extensively by all sides in South Viet Nam. Typically they cause amputation of one or both legs or cause such injuries that surgical amputation is necessary. By 1973 it was estimated that there were over 80 000 amputees in South Viet Nam, perhaps 50 per cent of them injured by land-mines. (By comparison, there were some 20 000 US amputees by the end of World War II; Dr A. Swanson, in US Senate Committee on the Judiciary, 1968.)

Table 2.7. US procurement of anti-personnel area denial mines, fiscal years 1965–73

Number of units

Type	1965	1966	1967	1968	1969	1970	1971	1972	1973	Total
XM-48 'Button bomblets'[a]	–	–	13 625 000	31 700 000	–	–	–	–	–	**45 325 000**
Mines in CBU 28/37[b]	–	2 222 400	17 664 000	11 587 000	–	–	–	–	–	**31 473 400**
XM-41E1 'Gravel mines'[c]	–	–	11 250 000	26 150 000	–	–	–	–	–	**37 400 000**
Total mines	–	**2 222 400**	**42 539 000**	**69 437 000**	–	–	–	–	–	**114 198 400**

[a] 'Button bomblets' are small anti-personnel mines containing 116 g composition B explosive; normally dispersed by means of a 10-tube SUU-41 Tactical Fighter Dispenser.
[b] CBU-28 and CBU-37 are designations given to SUU-13 dispensers filled with 4 800 BLU-43 'Short Dragontooth' and BLU-44 'Long Dragontooth' anti-personnel mines respectively.
[c] A small canvas-covered charge of lead azide normally dispersed in a 10-tube SUU-41 Tactical Fighter Dispenser, from helicopters or by ground forces.

Source: US Department of Defense (unpublished procurement data).

Table 2.8. US procurement of 2.75 inch rockets, fiscal years 1965–73

Thousands of units[a]

Type	1965	1966	1967	1968	1969	1970	1971	1972	1973	Total
US Air Force										
Fragmentation	412	843	1 056	1 237	960	110	120	410	600	5 748
Phosphorus	–	80	288	375	779	848	289	395	114	3 168
Flechette	–	40	263	–	–	–	43	–	–	346
Armour piercing	–	–	–	–	–	–	–	–	252	252
US Navy										
All types	–	917	1 091	821	166	236	–	–	–	3 231
US Army										
All types	–	–	–	–	–	–	2 073	1 120	–	3 193
Total	412	1 880	2 698	2 433	1 905	1 194	2 525	1 925	966	15 938

[a] Rounded off to nearest thousand.

Source: US Department of Defense (unpublished procurement data).

Table 2.9. US procurement of 105 mm anti-personnel flechette artillery ammunition, fiscal years 1965–73

Thousands of rounds

Type	1965	1966	1967	1968	1969	1970	1971	1972	1973	Total
US Army										
XM-546	–	10 000	63 000	–	–	–	–	–	–	73 000
XM-494	–	–	–	20 000	–	–	–	–	–	20 000
US Marine Corps										
XM-546	–	15	40	20	60	–	–	–	–	135
Total	–	10 015	63 040	20 020	60	–	–	–	–	93 135

Source: US Department of Defense (unpublished procurement data).

Flechette munitions

The USA introduced a category of weapons which made use of small, nail-like, fin-stabilized projectiles, or *flechettes*. Flechettes were mainly fired from aircraft rockets (table 2.8)[18] and 105 mm and 106 mm artillery (Beehive rounds) (table 2.9). Other variations were tested, including flechette-firing smooth-bore shot-guns (see chapter 4).

Fuel–air explosives

The *fuel–air explosive* was another new weapon. The principle of detonating a cloud of vapour or particles was tried out during World War II but it was only during the Viet Nam War that successful fuel–air explosive (FAE) bombs were introduced. Bombs of this kind were reportedly used against personnel on several occasions where they were believed to cause death by blast or asphyxiation. In fact, death can occur from *physical* asphyxiation, due to the rupture of the lungs by blast, rather than from *chemical* asphyxiation. This raises the fine legal point of whether or not FAE constitutes a 'deleterious or asphyxiating gas' in the sense of the Hague Conventions (see chapter 6). On one occasion, it is reported that five C-130 transport aircraft each dropped 24 CBU-55 FAE bombs on troop positions, leaving 'hundreds and perhaps thousands of corpses over zones of several acres' (*The Times*, 24 April 1975).

Small calibre, high velocity assault rifles

One of the earliest of the new US weapons to be sent to Viet Nam for trials was a new light-weight rifle, the AR-15, later redesignated the M-16. This rifle fires a smaller calibre bullet than conventional military rifles, but at short ranges the bullet may cause a more severe wound owing to its high velocity and propensity to yaw upon hitting the target (see chapters 3 and 4). Subsequently, large-scale orders were placed for the weapon, and over four million have been produced. Priority was given to supplying the RVN forces and US combat forces. Later the US Army adopted it as its standard assault rifle and several other countries have purchased them for their own forces.

Initially the guerrilla forces were largely equipped with captured US weapons and afterwards mainly with Soviet or Chinese weapons of the AK 7.62 mm intermediate power type. Some authors (e.g., Whelan, Burkhalter & Gomez, 1968) imply that there is no great difference in the wounding effects of these weapons, whereas others disagree. The M-16 tended to cause an exit wound with 'a gaping, devastated area of soft tissue and even bone, often with loss of large amounts of tissue' (Dimond & Rich, 1967, p. 620). Further X-ray examination showed a 'typical minute lead splatter . . . not found in other missile categories in our series of 750 missile wounds' (ibid.). This suggests a tendency for the bullet to break up in the wound, releasing all or part of the lead core. These reports led to the suggestion that bullets such as these may be comparable to the prohibited dumdum bullet.

The 'electronic battlefield'

Accompanying the new technologies for incapacitating troops, there was also development of devices for detecting movements of personnel (table 2.10) and transmitting signals to remote fire-control centres or air bases. These devices are promoted by the concept of the 'automated' or 'electronic' battlefield (*SIPRI Yearbook 1974*, chapter 11). In 1967 it became clear to US Secretary of Defense McNamara that the US air attacks on North Viet Nam itself were not succeeding in stopping the flow of men and supplies to South Viet Nam.[19] Some of these supplies came south by boat, others arrived through the port of Sihanoukville (Kompong Som) in Cambodia (until the *coup* in Cambodia in 1970). The greater part, however, was transported by porters, on bicycles and by trucks through a complex of difficult mountain jungle trails through south-eastern Laos.

To prevent this flow of men and matériel, the US initiated a programme known as 'Igloo White'. The trail area was extensively seeded with the new scatterable anti-personnel mines, and cluster bombs were used on a large scale to hit men and vehicles. Transport aircraft and B-57 bombers converted to gunships were also used, especially at night.

To help these attacks the whole paraphernalia known as the 'electronic battlefield' was deployed. Signals from electronic sensors planted in the ground or in trees were relayed to computers in Thailand by overflying aircraft. The computers were used to analyse the 'patterns of activity' and determine the most 'lucrative' target areas for attack.

The Igloo White programme did not prevent the launching of a major offensive in South Viet Nam in 1972. Clearly, in the conditions prevailing, the deployment of the new anti-personnel weaponry increased the cost of transporting men and supplies through Laos, but it did not prove decisive.

Improvised munitions

The liberation forces in Indo-China were supplied with munitions by the Soviet Union, China and other socialist countries, and, inadvertently, by the United States. Soviet and Chinese weapons – small arms, grenades, mines, mortars, artillery and rockets – were conventional in design but usually well-tried and effective. The 130 mm Soviet gun was particularly effective because of its range and accuracy. In many cases these munitions were reported to have a much higher reliability than comparable US munitions as the fuzes of US munitions were not waterproof and frequently failed to function in the monsoon rains. As many as 50 per cent of the US hand-grenades and 30 per cent of the mortar rounds failed to function during the monsoon. In the case of hand-grenades and M-72 anti-tank rockets, more rounds were destroyed each month as unusable than were used against the enemy. It has been estimated that Soviet artillery round fuzes had a reliability approaching 99 per cent whereas those of the USA had a reliability of about 90 per cent (Swearington, 1969).

The liberation forces were adept at recovering dud US munitions, renovating

Table 2.10. Characteristics of some personnel sensors used by US forces in Indo-China [a]

| Name of sensor | Type | Method of delivery | | Detecting range for men
m | Size
cm |
		Hand-emplaced	Air-dropped		
Anti-intrusion Alarm Unit (AAU)	Acoustic	Yes	—	—	43.5 × 7.6 (incl batt)
Commandable microphone (Commike)	Acoustic	—	Parachute	30	94 × 12.1 (diam)
RCA prototype	Acoustic	(Yes)	—	30	As packet of cigarettes
SPIKEBUOY	Acoustic	—	Free fall	(30)	167.6 × 12.7 (diam)
Air-delivered Seismic Intrusion Detector (ADSID) phase I	Seismic	—	Free fall	30	78.7 × 7.6 (diam)
Air-delivered Seismic Intrusion Detector (ADSID) phase III	Seismic	Yes	Free fall	30	50.8 × 7.6 (diam)
Ground-emplaced Seismic Intrusion Detector (GSID)	Seismic	Yes	—	30	23 × 11 × 13
Micro Seismic Intrusion Detector (MICROSID)	Seismic	Yes	—	30	(Very small)
Miniature Seismic Intrusion Detector (MINISID)	Seismic	Yes	—	30	20.6 × 20.6 × 7.6
Acoustic Seismic Intrusion Detector (ACOUSID)	Seismic/ acoustic	—	Parachute	30	134.6 × 7.6 (diam)
Seismic Hand-emplaced Acoustic Intrusion Detector (SHAID)	Seismic/ acoustic	Yes	—	20	79 × 13
Balanced Pressure System (BPS)	Pressure	Yes	—	(100)	—
Wire Intrusion Detector (WID)	Pressure	Yes	—	Length of wire	—
Electromagnetic Intrusion Detector (EMID)	Electro-magnetic field	Yes	—	20	18 × 18 × 8
Noiseless Button Bomblet (NBB)	Radio-frequency	Yes	—	Direct contact	<2.5 cm³
Infra-red Intrusion Detector (IID)	Active infra-red	Yes	—	100–120	—
Passive Infra-red Intrusion Detector (PIRID)	Passive infra-red	Yes	—	Line of sight	Sensor: 8 × 2 Processor: 11 × 13 × 16
XM3 personnel detector	Chemical	(Yes)	b	—	—
Magnetic Intrusion Detector (MAGID) phase III	Magnetic	Yes	—	3–4	31.7 × 6.4 (diam)

[a] This table is by no means a complete list of automated battlefield sensors: the intention here is only to give a few typical examples of the different types.
[b] May also be dangled by cable from a helicopter.

Source: 'The automated battlefield', chapter 11, *SIPRI Yearbook 1974*.

Weight kg	Lifetime (of batteries) days	Transmitter range	Remarks
4 (incl batt)	30–45	No own transmitter	Uses transmitter contained in MINISID III
11.8	20–30	Line of sight	Suspended, commandable
—	—	Line of sight	Able to discriminate footsteps
18.2	(30–45)	Line of sight	Buried
11.4	<90	Line of sight	Cost: $1 900
5.9	100	Line of sight	Cost: $975
2.7	45	—	
2	<90	Line of sight	
3.6	30–45	Line of sight	
18.1	45	Line of sight	Suspended, commandable. Cost: $3 500
9	45	Line of sight	
—	12–18 months	(8 km)	
—	30	—	Wire-connected, for local use by patrols
7	45	—	
30×10^{-3}	2 000 activations	100 m	Emits radio-frequency when moved; signals picked up by Automatic Radio Frequency Buoy (ARFBUOY) receiver/transmitter
43.6	1 year	—	Wire-connected
1.6	45	No own transmitter	Uses transmitter contained in MINISID
—	—	—	Detects ammonia; also known as 'People Sniffer'
1.8	45	No own transmitter	Uses transmitter contained in MINISID; cost: $280

them and converting them into booby traps, or they would salvage the explosive and other materials and construct improvised munitions of various kinds. A special organization was set up in each operational district for this purpose and underground workshops were established. Booby traps using bullets or shot-gun cartridges have been described by Rich (1968). Land-mines were made out of mortar or artillery shells, and unexploded BLU-3 anti-personnel fragmentation bomblets were extensively reused as grenades (Swearington, 1969).

In some areas, a variety of handmade weapons of primitive design were employed, such as spears, bows and arrows, and sharpened bamboo stakes (*punji* stakes). These weapons were quite capable of putting a man out of action for several weeks but the wounding effects are not to be compared with those of high explosives or high velocity missiles (Kovaric *et al.*, 1969; Rich, Johnson & Dimond, 1967).

VI. The impact of the Viet Nam War on the arms race[20]

The Indo-China War has had a substantial impact on the arms race by promoting two kinds of proliferation. Firstly, there has been the technological proliferation of new kinds of weapon systems.

The United States spent hundreds of millions of dollars on research and development of new weapon technology for use in Indo-China. In the fiscal year 1972 alone, 12 per cent – about $800 million – of the total US military research and development budget was devoted to Indo-China War-related technology (statement of Director of Defense Research and Engineering, John S. Foster, Jr., in the US Senate Committee on Appropriations, 1971, part 1, p. 345). The US Air Force alone spent $665 million on research and development related to the Indo-China War between 1965 and 1973 (US House of Representatives Committee on Appropriations, 1973, part 7, p. 961).

A leading trade journal gave the following evaluation of the impact of this investment:

> The Vietnam war's contribution to aerospace development has been formidable. It has transformed the helicopter from the slow, noisy, vibrating and unreliable vehicle of the fifties to the fast, quiet, smooth and reliable machine it is today. Gen. Westmoreland demanded these qualities for stable weapon-aiming . . . The rigid motor was born on the field in Vietnam. So was the infrared sensor, to see convoys taking advantage of the night . . . So was the laser-targeting . . . So was the RPV, or remotely piloted vehicle, to wage war without losing any pilots at all, and to get 100 times the kill or intelligence per dollar. The C-5A, whence sprang the civil jumbo jets, is the result of Vietnam thinking. So are the light fighter and the A-X, in response to the battle cry . . . for plain combat aircraft . . . The ceasefire will hit US production – bleakly in some areas. But the major part of America's military aerospace R&D is unlikely to be affected. (*Flight International*, 1 February 1973)

There can be little doubt that this investment in limited war and counter-insurgency technology by the world's major supplier of arms will have a significant effect on military doctrines and procurement policies throughout the world, and the impact will be seen for many years to come.

Among the new developments was the collection of sensor devices which led to the concept of the 'automated battlefield' (see *SIPRI Yearbook 1974*, chapter 11) and the emergence of remotely piloted vehicles (RPVs) as potential battlefield attack weapons (see *SIPRI Yearbook 1975*, chapter 12). There was also the increasing sophistication of electronic devices, such as infra-red detectors and low light level television cameras sensitive enough to detect men at night, and portable infantry radars able to detect men at ranges of 50–10 000 m (Senkus, 1967).

The second kind of proliferation is the spread of the new weapons and technologies to other countries, for example:

1. Cluster bomb munitions have been developed in France (the *Giboulée*) and the UK (BL755) and reportedly supplied to several other countries, such as Kenya (*Sunday Times*, 18 July 1976). US-made munitions of this type were used by Israel in the 1973 War and in Lebanon.

2. The technique of casting metal balls in a plastic shell, used in some US cluster bombs instead of the traditional fragmentation principle, has been adopted in the West German Diehl-DN-51 hand-grenade.

3. The notched steel wire which breaks into small pieces, used in the US M-26 hand-grenade and 40 mm grenade, is used in the Belgian PRB-423 hand-grenade and in a new Swedish Bofors 40 mm grenade, which also contains metal balls.

4. The widespread use of the 40 mm grenade in Viet Nam has led to the development of 40 mm grenade launchers for all the 5.56 mm rifles, and a number of larger automatic launchers for aircraft.

5. M-16 rifles, using the very high velocity 5.56 mm ammunition, have been reported in many armed forces, including those of Lebanon, Israel, the Philippines, Portugal (in Angola), Thailand, Malaysia, Indonesia, and the UK (in Aden and Indonesia). Many similar weapons are now being produced by other manufacturers (chapter 4). Israel has adopted its own 5.56 mm calibre rifle, the *Galil*.

The end of the war in Indo-China may have increased the rate of proliferation of new weapons in several ways, such as:

1. Fewer supplies for US forces have stimulated US manufacturers to look for other markets.

2. A considerable amount of surplus matériel from Indo-China has been given as military assistance or sold (at one-third cost) to other governments.[21]

3. The USA has focused its attention on other areas, such as Europe, seeking to adapt the new technologies.[22]

4. Other armed forces are likely to seek to acquire the new technologies, and other manufacturers to supply them.

These processes are in turn likely to stimulate the development and spread of weapons manufactured by the Soviet Union and other suppliers.

New Soviet weapons did not appear in Viet Nam in anything like the same profusion. The 'Grail' heat-seeking anti-aircraft missile and the 'Sagger' wire-guided anti-tank weapon appeared in Viet Nam only in 1972. The Vietnamese never acquired missiles fully able to defeat the B-52 bomber.[23]

The Styx anti-ship missile, which sank the Israeli ship *Eilat* in 1967, and which might have threatened the ships of the US Seventh Fleet, first appeared in Viet Nam in 1972 although it had been supplied to other countries many years before.

The Soviet weapons appearing in Viet Nam illustrated the conservative Soviet design philosophy: improvements to simple, rugged, existing weapons, using proven, off-the-shelf components where possible (Mounter, 1973). There was little evidence during the war itself that the combat in Indo-China had had a significant impact on the Soviet weapon technology. The new technologies known to have emerged from the Viet Nam War came from the United States.

But Soviet designers must have studied the lessons of the war. They probably concluded that the Soviet philosophy of simple, rugged, conventional weapons, produced in large numbers, proved to be a sound one; but that, on the other hand, aircraft can be expected to play an increasing role in the attack. It has been reported in Western technical journals that the Soviet Air Force has increased its attack capability in the past few years and is now equipped with a comprehensive range of cluster bombs (*International Defense Review*, April 1976).

Light-weight weapons designed for jungle warfare may also be suitable for urban guerrilla warfare. For example, rifles of the US 5.56 mm calibre have been reported in Northern Ireland, while 'tea-bag-type' mines have been adapted as 'letter bombs'.

VII. The influence of weaponry on warfare

The development of the high-powered rifle, the machine-gun and quick-firing artillery in the nineteenth century contributed much to the evolution of warfare from a contest between groups of armed men to a contest between manned arms. This process has continued in the twentieth century with military aircraft, armoured vehicles, self-propelled guns, rockets and missiles on the battlefield.

The production of weapons passed from the hands of craftsmen to large-scale industries towards the end of the nineteenth century. Increases in population and the introduction of conscription, coupled with mass production of matériel, enabled huge armies to be deployed in the field, and the length and depth of front lines greatly increased. At the time of the Napoleonic Wars a battlefield stretched to perhaps 10 km in length. In the early part of the twentieth century the Russo–Japanese War was fought on front lines of about 100 km. Front lines on the Eastern Front during World War II sometimes exceeded 2 000 km (Sidorenko, 1970).

At the same time there was an enormous increase in the fire-power available to combat troops. During the nineteenth century, armies engaged in front line assaults typically deployed about 10 artillery guns per kilometre of front. During

World War I this figure rose to about 150 guns/km and during World War II the quantity sometimes exceeded 300 guns/km (ibid.).

During the Napoleonic Wars an infantry battalion could fire about 200 bullets per minute; by World War II, a battalion could fire about 30 000 bullets per minute. Between 1923 and 1968 the amount of metal which could be fired in a single salvo by a Soviet rifle division increased exponentially from 336 kg to 53 000 kg (ibid.); from 1945 to 1968 alone, *fire-power increased 25 times* (see plate 12).

The quantity of munitions expended per man-year by US forces increased from 0.2 tonnes during World War II to 1.3 tonnes during the war in Indo-China (White, 1974). This development is partly due to increased use of aircraft and mechanized vehicles. If the amount of munitions expended is considered only in relation to combat troops, it has been calculated that US troops in Indo-China dispensed *26 times more munitions per man* than comparable US troops in World War II (White, 1974). In brief, technological developments promoted the evolution of mass means of attack.

During the twentieth century, military thinking turned from the requirements of attacks on limited concentrations of men (which could for the most part be visually observed) to calculations of the quantities of ordnance required to cover systematically a given area to a given density for a given period of time, the intention being to 'neutralize' any forces supposed to be within that area.

Once such methods of areal destruction are adopted, it would seem to be a simple step − to the military mind − to resort to the use of tactical nuclear weapons.

For military purposes the casualty radius of conventional artillery munitions against personnel in the open might be estimated at 5, 10 or 50 m. But it is estimated that a 5 kt nuclear bomb surface burst has an effective casualty radius against personnel in the open of up to about 775 m; a 10 kt bomb a radius of about 1 000 m; and a 20 kt bomb a radius of about 1 500 m (Sidorenko, 1970). (For personnel in foxholes or trenches the distances are reduced by about one-half.)

Thus nuclear weapons could be seen as being much more efficient than conventional munitions. Though the tactical use of nuclear weapons is a shocking prospect, the fact is that the mass use of conventional weapons can also be highly destructive to the civilian population and habitat, as well as to agricultural areas and the natural environment (Lumsden, 1975; SIPRI, 1976b).

A major effect of the development of weapon technology in the nineteenth century was to bring about a continuous decline in the proportion of casualties caused by swords, pikes, bayonets and the like, and an increase to almost 100 per cent in the proportion of casualties due to firearms. Of the casualties resulting from the use of firearms at the end of the nineteenth century, nearly 90 per cent were due to small arms. The twentieth century has seen a continuous decline in the proportion of casualties due to small arms and an increase in the proportion due to fragmentation weapons, the latter now typically accounting for about 70 per cent of battle casualties.

In the twentieth century there has also been an increasing use of aircraft in warfare, both as battlefield attack weapons and for attacks behind the lines. Aircraft

Table 2.11. The increasing use of air power: US forces in World War II, Korea and Indo-China[a]

Thousand metric tons

	Munitions expended			
	Air	Ground	**Total**	Air/total *per cent*
World War II	1 957[b]	3 572	**5 529**	*35.4*
Korea	634[c]	1 913	**2 547**	*24.8*
Indo-China				
1966	449	535	**948**	*47.4*
1967	844	1 091	**1 935**	*43.1*
1968	1 302	1 345	**2 647**	*49.2*
1969	1 257	1 274	**2 531**	*49.7*
1970	885	1 071	**1 956**	*45.2*
1971	691	755	**1 446**	*47.8*
1972	982	776	**1 758**	*55.8*
Total **Indo-China**[d]	**6 410**	**6 847**	**13 221**	*48.5*

[a] Although these are the best official figures available they are not always complete or strictly comparable; for example, World War II air munitions figures do not include rockets and aircraft cannon ammunition. Indo-China figures include allied expenditures.

[b] Includes approximately 1 179 000 tonnes of bombs dropped on German and Japanese area targets. If this quantity is disregarded, the remainder (778 000 tonnes) amounts to 17.9 per cent of tactical munitions expenditure.

[c] Includes an unknown quantity of bombs dropped during missions referred to as 'interdiction' but which are difficult to distinguish from World War II strategic area bombing.

[d] Does not include munitions expended before 1966 and 377 310 tonnes of air munitions and 162 550 tonnes of ground munitions expended in 1973.

Sources: *US Senate Committee on Foreign Relations* (1971); Office of the Assistant Secretary of Defense for Public Affairs (*personal communication*, 15 September 1975).

delivery accounts for an ever increasing proportion of the munitions expended in war (table 2.11).

By World War II, hundreds – and in some cases more than one thousand – aircraft were dispatched to attack target areas simultaneously. But, since then, the major air forces have been reduced although the weapon-carrying capacity of the individual aircraft has been greatly increased. For strategic area attacks, nuclear weapons would presumably be substituted for the 'thousand bomber' attacks of World War II.

Aircraft may be equipped with a variety of anti-personnel weapons, including machine-guns, rockets and fragmentation bombs. Since World War II, air-dropped anti-personnel fragmentation cluster bombs have come into increasing prominence, a trend which may be further promoted by the recent development of infantry guided missiles, laser range-finders and so on, which have added to the

Table 2.12. The technological substitution of fire-power for manpower: decline in ratio of casualties to manpower deployed, US forces, 1941–71

	Rate per thousand man-years of war effort		
	World War II (1941–45)	Korea (1950–53)	Indo-China (1966–71)[a]
Battle deaths[b]	9.3	5.6	4.5
Wounded[c]	21.4	17.2	15.2
Total casualties per thousand	**30.7**	**22.8**	**19.7**

[a] US fiscal years, not calendar years.

[b] Includes those who died of wounds.

[c] Includes only non-fatal wounds requiring hospital treatment.

Source: US Bureau of the Census, 1971, from White (1974).

capabilities of the infantryman – and consequently added to the interest in means, to combat him.

While the importance of manpower may sometimes have been obscured by the rise of sophisticated military technology, several major twentieth century conflicts have emphasized that sophisticated weaponry, like advanced technology generally, is not evenly distributed. 'Capital-intensive' forces have on many occasions been confronted by 'manpower-intensive' forces. 'Asymmetric' conflicts of this kind have stimulated the development of anti-personnel weaponry and tactics.

For soldiers of capital-intensive armies, increased fire-power per combat soldier has decreased the proportion of casualties sustained (table 2.12), while protective measures, rapid evacuation of the wounded and advanced medical treatment have greatly reduced the chances of death (table 2.13).

The use of the helicopter to evacuate rapidly the wounded from the battlefield has been a major factor in reducing battle deaths for these armies. This and modern medical facilities have enabled US forces to reduce the proportion of living wounded who die after hospitalization, from some 4 per cent in World War II to about 2 per cent in the Viet Nam War.[24] Israeli forces during the war of 1973 also showed how modern military services could reduce the number of those killed.[25]

It is obvious that facilities of this kind must be regarded as exceptional and that for most countries combat deaths are probably on a level with those typical of World War II, where the rule of thumb was *one-third dead, one-third seriously wounded and one-third lightly wounded*.[26] The effect of discrepancies in the medical and evacuation facilities available in underdeveloped countries must be taken into account in considering the effects of anti-personnel weapons. These weapons must be seen in the general context of the uneven distribution of power, wealth and technology.

Table 2.13. Improvement in the prognosis for battle casualties due to advances in medical treatment and evacuation procedures: decline in the ratio of battle deaths to surviving wounded, US forces, 1941–71

Thousands

	World War II (1941–45)	Korea (1950–53)	Indo-China (1966–71)[a]
Battle deaths [b]	291.6	33.6	44.0
Wounded [c]	670.8	103.3	147.2
Total casualties	**962.4**	**136.9**	**191.2**
Ratio of dead to wounded	*1:2.3*	*1:3.1*	*1:3.5*

[a] US fiscal years, not calendar years.
[b] Includes those who died of wounds.
[c] Includes only non-fatal wounds requiring hospital treatment.

Source: US Bureau of the Census, 1971, from White (1974).

In spite of the increasing sophistication of anti-personnel weapons they remain remarkably primitive means of tackling political tasks of global significance. There is little to distinguish between throwing pebbles and projecting small pieces of metal. It is hard to believe that in the long run such means can stand in the way of necessary social change – all they can do is greatly to increase the human cost of social change. For this reason, much stands to be gained by any measures adopted by the international community to restrict the use of anti-personnel weapons.

VIII. Summary and conclusions

In the two World Wars the inventive and industrial resources of nearly all the major powers were put into the war effort. The Korean War was not long enough to lead to major developments in weaponry; but the experience of the confrontation between the forces of the major Western industrial power and a potentially more numerous Asian enemy stimulated considerable research into anti-personnel weapons. Some of these new weapons were put to use during the Second Indo-China War – a war which lasted so long that many further weapon developments were fielded before its conclusion.

Warfare during the twentieth century has been dominated by the development of area weapons and means of delivery, and military thinking has turned from the problems of defeating groups of men whose presence on the battlefield could be observed from a commanding position to the needs of covering large areas of territory with a lethal concentration of projectiles. Though the tank and the air-craft re-established battlefield mobility, they also led to the dispersal of enemy troop formations and increased the need for area weapons.

The importance of area weapons is shown by the fact that battle casualties due to small arms ammunition have decreased from over 90 per cent at the end of the last century to about 20–30 per cent in recent armed conflicts. Conventional area weapons mainly depend upon dispersing small fragments or pellets of iron or steel at high velocity. The fire-power available to front-line combat troops of the major powers has increased by as much as 26 times since World War II.

The USA has been the primary motor in the development of anti-personnel weapons since World War II. But other nations are quick to adopt the new technologies and the present period is threatened by the rapid proliferation of dangerous new anti-personnel weapons.

The quality of medical treatment available to the wounded determines very much the mortality due to various weapons. Where medical treatment is up-to-date, death rates can be substantially reduced. This factor must be taken into ac-count in comparing the effects of weapons used in various parts of the world.

Notes to Chapter 2

1. The term is that of Schwarzenberger (1974) who raises the question of whether the laws of war are not merely a 'civilized interlude' between pre-industrial and advanced industrial barbarism.
2. The Imperial War Museum in London displays a collection of such weapons.
3. Sir John Slessor, a young officer in the 1920s, rose to be Marshal of the [British] Royal Air Force after World War II.
4. The British engaged in such operations at least as late as 1943, in Ethiopia (Hender-son, 1974).
5. A number of other 'jumping' or 'bounding' munitions have been reported in recent years, including the US XM54 white phosphorus anti-personnel mine and a Belgian 40 mm grenade.
6. A proximity fuze matches the outgoing radio signal from the fuze with the incoming reflection from the ground and detonates the munition at a predetermined distance from the target.
7. Beyer (1962) reports that throughout the period of the Korean War, Soviet weapons captured by US forces were manufactured in or prior to 1950.
8. President Eisenhower announced to the US Congress that more than 1 million South Koreans had been killed (*Keesing's Contemporary Archives*, 1953, p. 13080). Ober-dorfer (1975) cites 1.3 million civilian dead in North Korea and 1.4 million dead in South Korea, while Huntingdon (1968) refers to 2–3 million civilian dead. Born (1964) refers to a total (civilian and military) of 9 million dead but it seems likely that Born has confused 'war victims' (including dead, wounded, missing, homeless, refugees, orphans, and so on), with war dead.
9. The *Program of Action to Prevent Communist Domination of South Vietnam* was drawn up by the inter-departmental Task Force on Vietnam and circulated under the name of Brig. Gen. Edward G. Lansdale, US Air Force – an officer who organized sabotage and psychological warfare activities in Viet Nam in 1954 (Sheehan, 1971). It

may be assumed that the US Central Intelligence Agency (CIA), with which General Lansdale was believed to be long associated, was largely responsible for drawing up the *Program of Action*. The plan was approved in substance by President Kennedy on 11 May 1961 (letter by McGeorge Bundy, The White House, to the Secretary of State, entitled *National Security Action Memorandum No. 52*; in US Senate Committee on Foreign Relations, 1972).

10. GVN, Government of (the Republic of) Viet Nam.

11. General David M. Shoup, Commandant of the US Marine Corps from 1959 to 1963, writes: 'There were also top-ranking Army officers who wanted to project Army ground combat units into the Vietnam struggle . . . to test plans and new equipment, to test new air-mobile theories and tactics, to try the tactics and techniques of counter-insurgency, and to gain combat experience for young officers and non-commissioned officers . . . The Marines had somewhat similar motivations, the least of which was any real concern about the political and social problems of the Vietnamese people' (Shoup, 1969).

12. Around 1967–68 US forces were firing about 150 000 artillery shells per month, at a cost of about $2 000 million per year (John S. Foster, Jr., in US Senate Committee on Appropriations, 1971, part 1, p. 465).

13. Senator Edward M. Kennedy, for many years chairman of a US Senate subcommittee to investigate problems connected with refugees and civilian casualties, stated in 1967: 'As I understand it, about 85 per cent of the shelling which is done, the bombing and shelling is what is called unobserved shelling' (US Senate Committee on the Judiciary 1968, p. 145).

14. This statement, cited by Littauer & Uphoff (1972), is attributed to a former US Air Force photo-reconnaissance expert attached to the US Embassy in Vientiane, as quoted in *Bi-Weekly Asian Release*, Dispatch News Service International, 22 November 1971.

15. The name of Cambodia was changed to the Khmer Republic in 1970 and to Democratic Kampuchea in 1976.

16. This evaluation by a field commander seems to contradict the calculations of a US technical expert arguing for napalm, presented at the Lugano Conference (ICRC, 1976), where, it was claimed, CBU fragmentation munitions caused more casualties to 'friendly' forces than napalm bombs when used in close air support. Perhaps the reason for the discrepancy is that different munitions are referred to – bomblets dropped at tree-top level from a fixed dispenser attached to the aircraft might be more accurately placed than, say, those dispensed from free-fall cluster bombs which open in mid-air. Some support for this explanation is provided by eyewitness reports of large numbers of the 'pea-pod' cases from free-fall CBUs in North Viet Nam and Laos (where US ground forces were not involved) but not in South Viet Nam (where US ground forces were involved).

17. Such numbers, even if they exist, often remain classified for security reasons. Ben-Hur & Soroff (1975), for example, writing on Israeli burn casualties in the Arab–Israeli October 1973 War, also present the data in the form of percentages for security reasons.

18. Table 2.8 also shows a remarkable increase in the proportion of white phosphorus (WP) rockets procured for the use of the US Army. WP rockets are said to be used for 'marking' targets which are then attacked by other munitions, such as high-explosive rockets or bombs. Beller (1969), however, reports that WP rockets were used for attacking targets – to the extent of emptying HE rockets and refilling them with WP. Schell (1968) gives an eyewitness account of an attack by a US helicopter

which fired WP rockets on a group of thatch-roof houses. (For a full account of white phosphorus munitions and their medical and toxic effects, see SIPRI, 1975*a*.)

19. An account of McNamara's doubts as to the effectiveness of the bombing of North Viet Nam, his statement on 25 August 1967 before the US Senate Committee on Armed Services in which he argued against a policy of increased bombing, and the opposition that his views roused amongst supporters of the bombing campaign, is given by Hoopes (1969), former US Under Secretary of the Air Force. Support for some of McNamara's views is given by Biles (1972), in a study for the US Senate Committee on Foreign Relations, where he analysed the effectiveness of the bombing in Indo-China on the basis of the documents published in the *Pentagon Papers* (Sheehan, 1971; Gravel, 1971).

20. A version of this section appeared in the *SIPRI Yearbook 1974*, pp. 17–21.

21. For example, the South Korean forces evacuated from South Viet Nam took with them 90 993 tonnes of matériel. Usable items worth $50 million were available for sale on the open market (*Japan Times*, 14 March 1973). The Philippines received 120 single-engine Beaver aircraft formerly used for target spotting in Viet Nam (*International Herald Tribune*, 6 October 1973).

22. As early as 12 December 1970, the US Secretary of Defense assigned the Defense Special Projects Group – which was involved in the development of sensor technology and other projects – a 'new mission which recognized our withdrawal from support of the Southeast Asia systems and focused on our expanding the sensor technology to provide the worldwide capability in both tactical combat applications and installation security' (statement of Maj. Gen. John R. Deane, Director, Defense Special Projects Group, in US Senate Appropriations Committee, 1971, part 1, p. 745). The United States invited 14 NATO countries to a two-week demonstration by 30 US manufacturers of 'automated battlefield' equipment at Hohenfels in West Germany in May 1972. The objective was to 'sell the equipment to NATO members' (*International Herald Tribune*, 27 March 1972) and to 'interest the Atlantic allies in what remote sensors can do to improve the combat efficiency of their forces, in hopes that the allies will decide to manufacture and employ them' (*Aviation Week & Space Technology*, 8 May 1972). It was also reported that large-scale troop exercises with US and German battalions were planned to 'determine which devices work best in the relatively congested areas of Europe' (*International Herald Tribune*, 27 March 1972).

23. US sources report that during the 11-day concentrated bombing attacks in December 1972 on the Hanoi–Haiphong area, when over 700 B-52 sorties were flown (a sortie is one mission by one plane), 15 B-52s were shot down and six or seven damaged. One B-52 was lost previously and one subsequently. Since about 200 B-52s were operating over Indo-China, this represents about 7.5 per cent of the fleet. All are said to have been shot down by SA-2 'Guideline' missiles, although the Democratic Republic of Viet Nam claimed that one was shot down by a MiG-21 interceptor aircraft. The USA estimated that on average 60–62 missile firings were required to shoot down each B-52 (US House of Representatives Committee on Appropriations, 1973, part 1, p. 265; *Aviation Week & Space Technology*, 8 January 1973; Baldwin, 1973).

24. For US soldiers the time between wounding and evacuation to treatment facilities was 10.5 hours in World War II, 6.3 hours in Korea and 2.8 hours in Viet Nam (up to 1967), the decrease being mainly due to the use of helicopters (Whelan, Burkhalter & Gomez, 1968). Between 1965 and 1967, 1.6 per cent of the wounded who reached US Army hospitals died within 24 hours, a high proportion of whom would have died on the battlefield (and thereby been counted among the killed-in-action, rather than among the died-of-wounds) without the rapid evacuation. Only a further 0.9 per cent

51

died of wounds 24 hours or more after hospitalization – a truly remarkable figure. In addition to field hospitals in Viet Nam, US soldiers had available specially equipped medical transportation aircraft to take them to hospitals in the Philippines, Guam, Okinawa, Japan, Hawaii or the continental United States.

25. Although Israeli forces resorted to rapid evacuation techniques – including the use of armoured vehicles – they were also able to assign surgeons to every field unit, thus offering the troops immediate medical emergency care on the battlefield under fire (Ben-Hur & Soroff, 1975). This method proved highly effective but resulted in a considerable loss of medical personnel.

26. The Viet Nam War offers some examples of the discrepancies in medical treatment facilities typical of the present world. The Army of the Republic of Viet Nam had available a series of field hospitals, in which some 700 of the approximately 1 000 medically trained RVN doctors worked. Of the remaining doctors, some 150 were available to treat the civilian population on a part-time basis, while others were involved in administration or other occupations. The standard of hospitals available to the civilian population was often deplorable and it was common for patients to share a bed or lie on the floor. Some hospitals did not have running water or sanitary facilities (US Senate Committee on the Judiciary, 1968).

The Liberation forces attempted to provide basic treatment facilities near to the theatres of operation. Some personnel were trained in first aid and basic medical skills, and some underground treatment facilities were built. These facilities, however, were also subject to attack. The result is that, although in some aspects the medical services provided were impressive, in other aspects the standard was once suggested to have been 'parallel with American medicine during the [US] Civil War' of a century ago (Ahearn, 1966).

3. Projectile wounds and wound ballistics

Superior numerals, thus[5], refer to notes on page 76.

I. The study of wound ballistics

Since it is impossible in peace-time to study scientifically the effects of bullets on live human subjects, a number of standard procedures have been developed for simulating the effects of bullets on the human body. One method is to shoot at cadavers, usually preserved by the injection of formalin solutions. This has the advantage of making the tissues firm enough to enable sectioning for subsequent microscopic examination but limits the applicability of the findings to living tissue.

A second method is to take a skull or an organ, such as the stomach of a dead person or animal, and fill it with a substance of similar consistency to that of its *in vivo* contents before firing a bullet into it. A third method is to fire directly into a block of a material with a density similar to that of the soft tissue of the body. Gelatin, soap or clay are often used for this purpose. Bullets may also be fired into live animals under anaesthesia.

The effects of wounds in muscle and soft tissue, wounds involving bones, and wounds where the bullet passes through a compartment or cavity containing a fluid substance or air may conveniently be studied with the aid of these methods.

More recently, certain aspects of wound ballistics have been studied by means of computer simulation. A computer is programmed with a general formula describing the ballistic characteristics of a bullet. The computer then calculates values on the basis of variations in the parameters – for example, the distance travelled in the wound by a bullet before it tumbles (Janzon, 1974).

Each of these methods has its limitations. But so, too, has the clinical study of actual war wounds. Rarely is it possible to obtain precise details about the source of injury, the range, and so on. Further, the human body is so complex that bullet injuries vary greatly.

It is reasons such as these that make precise comparisons of different bullets impossible, since a definitive scientific study would require shooting bullets into live human beings under a great variety of standard conditions. It is therefore difficult for experts to agree on whether a projectile is 'inhumane'.

II. Early clinical reports

Numerous and vivid reports of projectile wounds caused by lead musket balls appeared in medical literature for hundreds of years. Early accounts were published by De Vigo in 1514 and Paré in 1582. More systematic observations were made by, for example, Clowes (1588), Wiseman (1705) and Guthrie (1815). A recent review of this literature concludes:

> ... it would seem that musket balls frequently caused large wounds and that they usually lodged in the body. They were capable of shattering limbs to such an extent that amputation was required to prevent infection developing in the damaged tissues. They frequently carried clothing and protective armour into the wounds. (Scott, 1974, p. 6)

Lead musket and shrapnel balls were heavy (over 30 g) and were fired at relatively low velocity. At close ranges they deformed on impact to form flattened lumps, 20–30 mm in diameter. Consequently the transfer of energy to the body was efficient.

Conical bullets of the Minié type, of which there were an enormous variety (Lewis, 1956), also exceeded 30 g but had longer range and greater accuracy owing to the higher velocity and the spin caused by the rifling. The higher velocity resulted in more severe wounds than those caused by the older, round balls (Matthew, 1858; Otis, 1876).

One authoritative account describes these effects as follows:

> If a modern rifle bullet, armed with its full force, strikes a hard and powerful long bone, like the femur for example, near the middle of its shaft, it is broken up into fragments of various shapes and dimensions, often too numerous to be counted. A large proportion of these fragments are driven violently in various directions, and thus are converted into secondary missiles. They exert much the same kind of action among the surrounding tissues, as a charge of irregularly shaped projectiles from a grape-shot or canister. A huge hollow is formed inside the limb, which, when it is fully laid open and the effused blood sponged away, offers to view a mass of lacerated muscle intimately mixed with sharp-pointed and jagged-edge splinters of bone ... With all this extensive destruction within the limb, the external aspect of the wound through which the bullet first entered may exhibit nothing more to view than a small opening into which the top of the little finger enters with difficulty. (Longmore, 1877)

Exploding bullets were used during the US Civil War (Lewis, 1956) and by the British in India in the 1860s (Fosbery, 1869). Their use between the forces of the major powers was prohibited by the St Petersburg Declaration of 1868 and there are only few reports of their clinical effects; an example is found in a letter to *The Times* on 10 December 1868 where it was stated that 'in one instance the bullet had entered the back of the neck, and then exploding, had entirely blown away the face' (cit. Scott, 1974). The US General Ulysses S. Grant records in his memoirs: 'The enemy used in their defense explosive musket balls ... Where they hit and the ball exploded, the wound was terrible' (Grant, 1885, p. 538).

III. Early experimental studies

The period from 1870 to 1900 was noteworthy for the development of weapon technology and for experimental studies of projectile wounds (Bruns, 1889; Delorme & Chavasse, 1892; Horsley, 1894; Kocher, 1875, 1880).

Mach & Salcher (1887) published the first photographs of bullets in flight, a technique developed by Boys (1893). Horsley (1894) described experiments by many different researchers and concluded that the velocity of the projectile and the hydrodynamic effects it creates in the tissues were the main factors in wounding. The Prussian War Ministry commissioned an extensive series of studies, shooting at cadavers with full-power ammunition at ranges from 25 to 2 000 m. One thousand preparations from these experiments are on record as having been preserved at the Friedrick Wilhelm Institute in Berlin (MacCormac, 1895).

The principal advantage of the new high-powered small calibre (6.5–8 mm) ammunition being introduced was the much greater range of the bullets. It was soon discovered that at short ranges (under 500 m) the high velocity of this ammunition was capable of causing 'explosive' effects in such targets as cans filled with water and skulls filled with soft plaster of Paris. In blocks of soap the lack of elasticity served to 'fix' the temporary cavity formed by the rapid discharge of energy by the projectile (Keith & Rigby, 1899).

At the longer ranges at which the ammunition was often used, however, this 'explosive' effect did not occur and the wounds were often milder than those of older bullets (Bruns, 1889; MacCormac, 1900). Indeed, Stevenson (1897) wrote: 'The severity of the explosive effect is, if anything greater with the older rifle bullets than it is with the new.' The British military authorities, concerned by reports about the lack of 'stopping power' of the Lee-Metford bullets being used by troops in India, began studies to increase the wounding power. A number of bullets were tested, including one produced at the British arsenal at Dum-Dum which had an approximately 1 mm diameter circle at the tip unjacketed. The dum-dum bullet had a greater wounding effect than the fully jacketed bullet, but not such a great effect as the hunting bullet used by von Bruns (1898; 1915) which had about 5 mm of the tip uncovered (Keith & Rigby, 1899).

Von Bruns presented his results at the Congress of German Surgeons in 1898 and they did much to promote the ban on expanding bullets, which was accepted the following year at the Hague Peace Conference.

But experts at this conference pointed out that designing the bullet to expand on impact was only one way of increasing the wounding effects (see pp. 214–15). In the years following the conference many of the major powers replaced round-nosed bullets with pointed, or *Spitzer*, bullets. In 1908 (the year after the British acceded to the prohibition on expanding bullets), tests at the Royal Arsenal, Woolwich, England, demonstrated that the pointed bullets had a greater wounding effect than the round-nosed bullets (Scott, 1974). A similar conclusion was arrived at by LaGarde in the United States, and by the official medical histories published after World War I. Garner (1920) attributes to this effect the origin of unfounded allegations during the war that expanding bullets had been employed (see chapter 9).

Knowledge of the effects of high velocity bullets accumulated from experimental studies before World War I was supplemented by the casualty data of that war. The state of knowledge existing at the end of the war was summarized as follows:

> The wounding effects of a bullet depend on (*a*) the amount of energy it transmits to the tissues, (*b*) the velocity of the transmission, (*c*) the direction of the transmitted energy, and (*d*) the density of the tissues. The first three of these factors depend almost entirely on the energy, velocity and shape of the bullet. (Wilson, 1921)

After World War I further experiments were performed. Callender & French (1935) reported the results of experiments carried out for the US Army Ordnance and Medical Departments where they shot at goats, pigs, clay, and tin cans filled with water. For the first time an attempt was made to measure the loss in velocity as a projectile passed through the target, and to find out the amount of energy used in producing the wound. In later experiments they attempted to measure the *rate* of loss of energy, or, in other words, the power used to cause the wound.

Where bullets were fired at pigs at 300, 600 and 1 000 yards (274, 548 and 914 m), it was noted that the worst wounds resulted at 274 m but that at 914 m some of the wounds were worse than those caused by the same bullets at 548 m. It was also noted that the smallest bullets used (6.5 mm) caused the worst wounds at all ranges.

In another series of experiments reported by Callender & French it was found that round-nosed bullets tended to break up at the tip when striking bone at velocities in excess of 730 m/s, while pointed bullets broke up at the base when striking bone at 790 m/s or more, with effects similar to those of soft-nosed hunting bullets. Bullets fired at fluid-filled cans at less than 610 m/s tended to cause a clean perforation, whereas smaller bullets fired at velocities of 824 m/s caused the can to burst – an effect similar to that of the high velocity bullet when it hits the head (Horsley, 1894; Keith & Rigby, 1899; Clemedson *et al.*, 1973). The behaviour of bullets after they strike a dense medium was studied using modelling clay. These studies showed that the yaw of the bullet is greatly increased, sometimes to 140° or more, but that the gyroscopic forces exerted by the spin continue to act on the projectile, causing the yaw to diminish again. This mechanism explains the finding that some wounds have small entrance and exit openings which hide the internal destruction. When the yaw is increased, the retardation forces are much greater and much more energy is therefore expended in the wound.

Callender & French also found that the physical disturbance started by a projectile in the body lasts longer than the time that the bullet is there. Further, the forces transmitted by a bullet when hitting a fluid-filled container or organ (such as the stomach or head), are transmitted equally in all directions, according to the laws of hydraulics. These forces may be sufficient to rupture the organ or blow the skull to pieces.

Callender & French also pointed out that the high rate of energy delivery may explain the very destructive wounds caused by small fragments from high explosive shells which had been noted during World War I. They compared high velocity bullets with soft-nosed hunting bullets, of the kind which are prohibited for use in war by the Hague Declaration:

> Soft nosed hunting bullets show a dispersion of the lead core beginning at the impact point on the skin and disseminate practically all their energy as the result of the break-up of the bullet. With the higher velocities it is not necessary for the bullet to break up, for the particles of the medium hit acquire sufficient velocities to produce destructive action similar to that produced by the hunting bullet. (Callender & French, 1935, p. 201)

During World War II a number of published studies confirmed and refined the conclusions of earlier studies. Black, Burns & Zuckerman (1941) fired small steel spheres into blocks of gelatin at velocities between 500 feet/s (153 m/s) and 5 000 feet/s (1 530 m/s) and studied the effects using photographic methods. They showed that as the ball emerged from the block of gelatin, the gelatin increased to three to four times its original volume for a brief instant before returning to its original shape. A similar rapid expansion was shown in shadowgraphs of the hind leg of a rabbit when it was hit by a high velocity projectile. It was suggested that this was due to the formation of a temporary cavity with explosive violence within the medium.

Experiments performed in the United States during World War II, where high-speed X-ray photography was used, confirmed the relationship between the cavitation effect and the energy of the projectile (Harvey *et al.*, 1962). It was calculated that for every joule of energy lost by a projectile in muscle, a temporary cavity with a volume of 0.801 cm³ is formed. These studies were again supplemented with clinical experience gained during World War II and the Korean War (Beyer, 1962). Although it remains difficult to compare precisely the effects of different bullets in combat conditions, most of the parameters that might define the wounds caused by penetrating missiles have been thoroughly investigated and it is possible to draw some general conclusions.

IV. The wounding power of small projectiles

The wounding power of missiles depends largely on the kinetic energy:

$$KE = \frac{mv^2}{2}$$

where KE = kinetic energy in joules, m = mass in grams, v = velocity in metres per second. Obviously, there is a minimum energy at which the missile can be expected to penetrate the body. According to Bircher (1899), a Swiss shrapnel lead ball 12.5 g in weight and 12.5 mm in diameter requires a velocity of 100 m/s, a kinetic energy of 62 joules, in order to produce a human casualty in every case. At 50 m/s, a kinetic energy of 15 J, the lead ball produces a contusion of the skin in an area not covering bone but does not penetrate, due to the elasticity of the skin. At the same velocity a bone may be perforated. As a result of such calculations, 'casualty criteria' (that is, the amount of kinetic energy required of a particular missile to put a man out of action) were adopted by many armies at the end of the last century. In France the criterion was 39 J, in Switzerland 62 J, in Germany and the United States 78 J, and in Russia 235 J.

According to Rohne (1894), the German casualty criterion of 78 J means that a soft lead ball of 13 g requires a velocity of 110 m/s, whereas one of 11 g requires a velocity of 120 m/s to put a man out of action. Köhler (1897), using the French criterion of 39 J, calculated that the 11 g French shrapnel ball, 120–160 of which were contained in a shell, required a velocity of 81 m/s, whereas the much smaller Russian shrapnel ball, 340 of which were contained in a shell, required a velocity of 210 m/s (cit. Finck, 1965).

Although casualty criteria such as these are arbitrary they proved better indicators of wounding power than measures such as the penetration of pine boards (Beyer, 1962). According to Gurney (1944), the figure of 78 J was valid for fragments ranging from 50 mg to 30 g. This is equivalent to a velocity of approximately 570 m/s for a 50 mg fragment, and approximately 73 m/s for a 30 g fragment. Nowadays more complex tables have been produced to help the weapon designer, taking into account different times to incapacitation, and different areas of the body hit. Such tables take account of actual casualty data.

An even more sophisticated approach has been developed at the US Army Ballistic Research Laboratory, Aberdeen Proving Ground, Maryland, USA. There an elaborate, three-dimensional computer model, the Computer Man, has been developed. This model encodes the entire body of a man into sections 5 x 5 x 25 mm. The tissue types are classified within each of these small blocks. This model is then matched with information regarding the probable distribution of impact points and trajectories of bullets, their ballistic properties, and so on, enabling various bullets to be compared in terms of a Relative Incapacitation Index (RII).

The size of the temporary cavity which the bullet generates as it enters the body has been indentified as the feature which contributes most to instantaneous incapacitation, since the larger the temporary cavity, the greater the probability of injuring one of the centres of vital activity necessary for the continued performance of the individual (Dobbyn, Bruchey & Shubin, 1975). The size of the temporary cavity is taken to be largely a function of the impact velocity of the projectile and other physical characteristics of the bullet.

With the invention of high explosives during the second half of the nineteenth century, the velocity of projectiles increased dramatically. This increase in velocity served to emphasize the importance of the kinetic energy equation, for whereas energy increases linearly with mass, it increases quadratically with velocity.

This relationship is demonstrated in table 3.1, which shows the size of missiles required to match a casualty criterion of 78 J at various velocities.

Table 3.1. Weight and velocity of missiles required to produce a kinetic energy, or casualty criterion, of 78 joules[a]

Weight of missile g	Velocity of missile m/s
10.0	110
5.0	180
1.0	400
0.5	585
0.1	1 200
0.05	1 650

[a] Seventy-eight joules was adopted as a casualty criterion by the German Army at the end of the last century and was still used by the United States Army during World War II. The equivalent French criterion was 39 J, the Swiss 62 J, and the Russian 235 J.

Source: Beyer (1962).

The figures in this table may be compared with the standard military bullet of some 9–10 g and an initial velocity of some 850 m/s. Such missiles have an initial kinetic energy of some 3 500 J, which is about 45 times the casualty criterion. Even at 400 m, which is the maximum range at which small arms have been found to have any major tactical application in modern warfare, the energy is still some 20 times the casualty criterion.

V. Lethality and 'stopping power'

Lethality, or the probability of a 'kill', $P(K)$, is an important military consideration, though the term is somewhat ambiguous for the non-military person. A 'kill' here means that the target (whether person, weapon system, or otherwise) is put out of action. It is remarkably difficult to achieve absolute incapacitation without literally killing; and even more difficult to achieve this result within, say, five seconds.

Users of weapons often talk in terms of the 'stopping power' of the weapon (*Lancet*, 10 June 1899; Goddard, 1935; Dobbyn, Bruchey & Shubin, 1975). Dumdum bullets, for example, or hollow-point pistol bullets are believed to have greater 'stopping power' then non-expanding bullets. Stopping power, therefore, also refers to the probability that a given projectile will cause incapacitation immediately or within five seconds.

Studies carried out in the United States during and after World War II concluded that immediate incapacitation could only be achieved by severe injury to the spinal column above the second or third thoracic vertebra, or to parts of the brain. Thus, rapid incapacitation is harder to achieve than the fatal or severe injury which results from injury to major organs or blood-vessels.

Experiments were carried out where projectiles were fired at live animals (goats) and the animals examined by medical officers asked to judge the comparable impact on soldiers:

> ... the experiments ... showed that a moribund animal, which had suffered wounds that would eventually lead to its death, was by no means invariably incapacitated soon after wounding, to anything like the extent that would be necessary to prevent a human soldier from continuing to offer effective resistance for periods of many minutes or hours. (Dunn & Sterne, 1952)

It was estimated that the probability that a hit by a given projectile would result in rapid incapacitation varied between 0.00 and 0.01 for various fragments and velocities, while the probability that the same fragment would result in fatal or severe injury varied between 0.00 and 0.36. In other words, even for the most effective projectile, the probability of death or severe injury is three to four times greater than the probability of immediate incapacitation.

Put in another way, this means that the increment in the likelihood of superfluous injury due to changes in projectile design is three to four times greater than the likelihood of any increment in military effectiveness.

The notion that certain projectiles have more 'stopping power' than others, in the sense of having a noticeably higher probability of incapacitation within seconds, is largely a myth. Some bullets may have greater wounding power, but wounding power and stopping power are not the same thing although they are frequently confused.

VI. The definition of 'high velocity' projectiles

As it is known that the wounding power of a missile is related to its velocity, and as this fact has been prominent in the recent legal examination of various kinds of ammunition (ICRC, 1973, 1975), it is important to adopt a clear position with regard to the term 'high velocity'.

We must distinguish between *initial velocity, impact velocity* and *residual velocity*. The initial velocity of a missile is the velocity first imparted to it by the propellant; in the case of ammunition fired by a gun it is synonymous with the term 'muzzle velocity'. Impact velocity is the velocity of the projectile as it hits the target. Residual velocity is the velocity of a projectile if and when it emerges from the target. The difference between the impact velocity and the residual velocity provides a measure of the energy deposited in the wound. Studies have shown that the amount of tissue devitalized by a projectile is directly correlated to the energy deposited (Berlin *et al.,* 1976).

It is possible that a few wounds are caused by missiles with impact velocities of less than some 150 m/s (Beyer, 1962), but many battlefield casualties from rifle and machine-gun ammunition, as well as from high explosive shell fragments and other anti-personnel weapons, are the result of impact velocities of some three to eight times that velocity.

Beyer (1962), 'for simplicity in discussion', chose to consider velocities of less than 1 200 feet per second (364 m/s) as low; velocities of 1 200–2 500 ft/s (364–758 m/s) as medium; and velocities over 2 500 ft/s (758 m/s) as high. Finck (1966), following Beyer, states that high velocity is 'usually considered' as being more than 750 m/s.

Few military rifle bullets have an *impact* velocity, as opposed to an initial velocity, of more than 750 m/s. But the severe wounding effects characteristic of military rifle ammunition, clearly distinguish it from pistol and sub-machine-gun ammunition, which has low initial and impact velocities.

For this reason it seems appropriate to adopt the approach of, for example, Byrnes et al. (1974), who state that 'a high velocity bullet travels faster than the speed of sound' in air (i.e., about 350 m/s). This criterion has two major advantages: (a) the speed of sound in air is a standard criterion of measurement, and (b) it falls conveniently between the impact velocities of the two major classes of military small arms ammunition. This makes pistol and machine pistol ammunition of low velocity while rifle and machine-gun ammunition is of high velocity.

All contemporary military rifles and machine-guns fall into the high velocity category. It may be that the introduction of new generations of military small arms with initial velocities approaching 1 000 m/s would justify the term 'hypervelocity'.

A projectile travelling at twice the speed of sound in air (Mach 2.0)[1] retards four times more rapidly than the same projectile travelling at the same speed as sound, that is, the amount of retardation depends upon the velocity. This offers a further explanation of the fact that very high velocity projectiles which have severe wounding effects at close range have reduced effects at longer ranges.

The speed of sound in tissue is usually estimated to be about the same as the speed of sound in water (about 1 450 m/s). This has the effect of reducing the significance of this factor in explaining the rate of retardation in tissue as opposed to air. In tissue, the absolute velocity squared, the density of the medium and the ratio of the cross-sectional area to the mass are of greater significance in determining the rate of retardation.[2]

It will be seen from the formula for retardation that velocity, being a square function, has the effect of greatly multiplying all other causes of retardation, and therefore wounding effect. Beyer (1962) concludes: 'Of all factors to be considered in the missile casualty as a physical phenomenon, impact velocity is decidedly the most important' (p. 116).

Although current small arms bullets do not approach the speed of sound in tissue, fragments from high explosive munitions may do so. Recently, Charters & Charters (1976) predicted that in the next decade, projectile velocities will increase, and reported experiments showing that small steel spheres at impact velocities of the order of 2 000 m/s could be expected to have significantly different wounding effects than larger spheres, with approximately the same energy, impacting at about 750 m/s. The smaller spheres showed less depth of penetration in gelatin blocks but greater lateral damage. A very high velocity sphere impacting on a human thigh might, it was suggested, cause massive tissue damage on the side of impact but fail to perforate the limb. 'This type of wound would be particularly disabling and may require new approaches to debridement and wound closure' (Charters & Charters, 1976).

VII. The wounding mechanism of high velocity projectiles

Hydrodynamic pressure wave

When the speed of a projectile exceeds about 600 m/s, hydraulic shock waves precede and extend from the path of the bullet. The exact velocity at which this occurs depends upon a variety of factors, such as the calibre and bullet type, and the type of tissue. The total effect depends on the size and condition of the victim.

In muscles, bones or other tissues of a consistent density the high pressure wave may have little effect. But in organs such as the head or liver containing incompressible tissue of relatively fluid consistency, the pressure wave may result in the rupture or shattering of the organ. Even in 1899, Keith & Rigby pointed out that 'the momentum of any of the modern military bullets in the first hundred yards of their course is sufficient to burst the skull open were it five times its normal strength'. The bullet must enter the skull with an energy of some 70 J in order to achieve this effect. These effects constitute one reason why high velocity projectiles are sometimes described as causing 'explosive-type wounds'.

Cavitation

As a projectile passes through soft tissue it forms a wound channel, the size of which depends upon the diameter and velocity of the projectile, and upon other factors. At low velocity, the wound channel is of the same size as the missile, or insignificantly larger. Indeed, owing to the elasticity of the skin, an entry wound may appear slightly smaller than the projectile. At high velocity, a conical wound cavity is formed behind the projectile which may expand to as much as 30 times the diameter of the projectile. The elasticity of the tissues may reduce the size of this temporary cavity, but the diameter of the permanent cavity may nevertheless be many times that of the projectile.

This effect is easily demonstrated by firing at blocks of soap (Keith & Rigby, 1899). Soap has the advantage that it retains the maximum cavity, which can therefore be easily observed, measured or photographed. This rapid expansion of the wound cavity in the space of some microseconds may be misinterpreted as resulting from explosive bullets, particularly when the bullet itself disintegrates (Snellman, 1966; Austria, Sweden & Switzerland, 1977).

The pressure exerted by the rapidly expanding wound cavity causes much damage to the soft tissue even far from the actual wound cavity. Muscle may be severely torn, and nerves and blood-vessels in the neighbourhood of the shot passage can be seriously dislocated. The pressure on blood-vessels may give rise to thromboses, and damaged nerves may lead to paralysis.

The extensive pulping of soft tissue in the area of the wound is an ideal site for infection, and this may kill unless adequately treated (see below, p. 73).

These effects are clearly related to the amount of energy deposited by the projectile. Fears expressed in the 1890s, that the high velocity bullets then coming into service would result in exceptionally severe wounds, generally proved unfounded in the combat conditions of that time because most hits were at ranges of over 500 m. But in the close combat typical of some more recent conflicts, massive soft tissue wounds resulting from high velocity bullets have been reported (e.g., Beyer, 1962; Dimond & Rich, 1967).

Pressure changes in gas pockets

As the temporary cavity collapses, it sets up pressure changes in gas pockets in neighbouring organs of the body, such as the intestines or lungs. The rapid decrease in pressure in the tissues surrounding the air pocket will probably cause further damage to the tissues. This may result in perforation of the intestines and haemorrhage in the lungs (Snellman, 1966). Though this is an important additional consideration in the wounding power of high velocity rifles, it is never as serious as the primary damage caused by the temporary cavity (Harvey *et al.*, 1962).

The shape of the projectile

The shape of a projectile helps to determine its ability to overcome the resistance of a surrounding medium, whether air or tissue. In general, the power to overcome resistance is directly proportional to the mass and inversely proportional to the cross-section. An elongated bullet, travelling head on, has greater powers of penetration than a round one; this indeed is one reason for the reduction in calibre of military rifles which took place at the end of the last century (Treves, 1900). The elongated bullet, being more able to overcome the resistance of the air, maintains its velocity better than a spherical bullet and thus is able to convey more potential energy to the target. It is also better able to penetrate the target.

Again, the steel spheres used in some modern anti-personnel munitions may be more capable of maintaining their velocity than irregularly shaped fragments or the deformed lead balls typical of the older shrapnel munitions. Conversely, an irregular fragment from a high-explosive munition, by retarding more rapidly in the body than a sphere of the same mass and velocity, may penetrate less deeply but cause a larger surface wound than the sphere (figure 3.1).

At the end of the nineteenth century, bullets with an ogival form at the head were the most common, with the curvature of the head made up of that part of a

Figure 3.1. Comparison of the mean cross-sectional areas of wound tracts in the thighs of goats caused by high velocity spheres (A), high velocity fragments (B), low velocity fragments (C) and low velocity spheres (D)

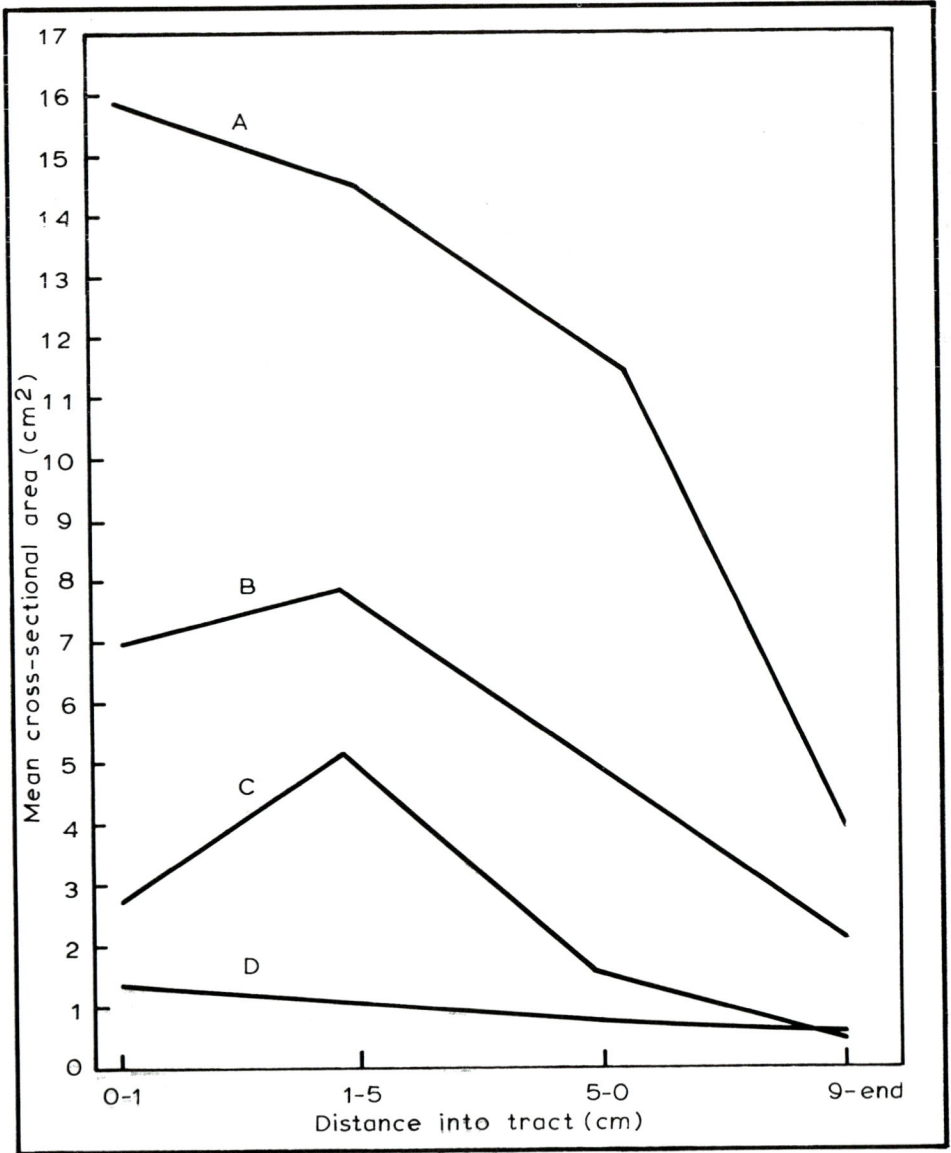

Source: Mendelson & Glover (1967).

circle, the radius of which is equal to two diameters of the base of the bullet. This shape offers a low resistance and provides the bullet with a high power of penetration.

However, a bullet with a high power of penetration is also more likely to pass right through the body, causing a clean wound. Reports in the medical literature of 1895–1900 frequently included accounts of soldiers wounded at long range by Mauser or Lee-Metford ogival bullets with relatively little effect (e.g., Treves, 1900; MacCormac, 1895; Küttner, 1900).

Perhaps for this reason most of the military powers adopted *Spitzer,* or pointed, bullets during the first decade of the twentieth century. Bullets with this shape maintain their velocity well in air but are more inclined to 'tumble' after impact with human tissue, causing a more severe wound. Most current military bullets are of the *Spitzer* kind. For shot-guns and pistols for police use there is a greater variety of projectile forms, including round-nosed, flat-nosed and hollow-point, some of them designed to deform on impact (see chapter 4).

The stability of the projectile

During the past century, bullets evolved from the round ball to an elongated form, at first with a round nose, later with a pointed nose. At the same time barrels were rifled, so as to impart a spin to the bullet as it emerged from the gun. The reason for both these developments was to improve the stability of the bullet's flight in air and thereby increase the range and accuracy. An alternative means of stabilizing the flight of a missile is to fit it with fins, as in arrows, flechettes and rockets.

The spinning effect of a bullet can be likened to that of a top. At first the gyrations are large and the bullet 'wobbles' as it emerges from the barrel. This initial instability contributes to the increased severity of wounds which is common at short ranges of up to some 30–50 m. The spin becomes increasingly more controlled for a period until the momentum decreases below a certain level, whereupon the projectile starts to wobble again.

When the spinning projectile hits a denser medium, such as human tissue, the 'wobble' is greatly magnified but it continues to spin. So if a bullet passes through a sufficient depth of tissue it may leave only a small exit hole, but, because of the wobbling effect in the wound, internal damage is much more severe than is apparent from the surface appearance. The rate of spin of the military rifle is usually high and may be of the order of some 3 500 revolutions per second. However, this spin is only adequate to stabilize the bullet in air (Beyer, 1962).

Thus, a further factor determining the wounding power of a bullet, which does not apply to a spherical projectile, is the tendency for an elongated projectile to deviate along its longitudinal axis from the line of flight (to yaw). Normally the yaw of a bullet in flight in air is only about 3° (Beyer, 1962), but when an elongated bullet hits a medium denser than air — such as body tissue — the gyrations and yaw are multiplied proportionately to the increase in density. A bullet that hits the body point first will frequently turn through 90° or more.

The relationship between the angle of yaw and the retardation in a medium of given density has been calculated. Theoretically the angle of yaw can be of any value up to nearly 180°, and yaws of more than 170° have been observed in bullets passing through water.

A yaw of 170° increases the retardation factors 172 times and a yaw of 179°, 190 times. This readily explains why a superspeed bullet is stopped in a very few feet of a homogenous medium such as water.

This also explains why a supervelocity bullet is retarded so greatly in producing a casualty. The extreme retardation of such bullets can result in a wound with comparatively enormous destruction, tissue pulping, bone shattering, and other extreme manifestations only possible with the modern fast-moving military bullet. (Beyer, 1962, p. 132)

All bullets tumble sooner or later. But whether they tumble within, say, 50, 150 or 300 mm of their passage through the body depends upon such design factors as the amount of spin imparted by the rifling of the gun, the form, the placing of the centre of gravity in the bullet and the yaw transmitted to the bullet. Computer simulation (Janzon, 1974) is a useful means of analysing this phenomenon.

The average length of a bullet wound tract in the human body is about 140 mm. A bullet which attains its maximum yaw after the passage of 150 mm of tissue will on average cause less severe wounds than one which yaws most at 50 or 100 mm. This has been clearly demonstrated in a number of experiments reported at the Lugano Conference of Government Experts (ICRC, 1976). In one experiment a variety of current standard military bullets were fired at blocks of soap moulded into the size and shape of the human thigh. A standard 5.56 mm bullet caused a much larger cavity than either a full-power or an intermediate power 7.62 mm bullet. The 5.56 mm bullets reached their maximum yaw and broke up within the block of soap, which was about 150 mm thick. The 7.62 mm bullets had only begun to yaw significantly as they left the block and the cavity they left in the block was smaller.

In other experiments, bullets were fired into blocks of soap 280 mm and 500 mm thick, giving all the bullets the opportunity to reach their maximum deviation from the line of flight before exiting from the block. In this case the cavities formed by the full-power 7.62 mm bullets had a greater total volume than those of the 5.56 mm bullets. Thus, the question of which class of bullet is the most 'severe' might appear to depend to a large degree upon the thickness of the target.

But the point at which bullets tumble is not determined by the calibre (diameter) but by other design factors, such as the positioning of the centre of gravity; bullets can be designed to tumble early or late. Since it is known that the average length of wound tracts in the human body is 140 mm rather than 280 mm or 500 mm, it follows that a bullet that is designed to tumble at less than 140 mm can be expected to cause severe wounds more often than a bullet designed to tumble after 140 mm.

Projectile deformation and break-up

High velocity military bullets are jacketed with steel or copper alloy so as to withstand the force of propulsion by a high explosive charge. This jacket is not necessarily strong enough to withstand the forces exerted by the rapid deceleration of the bullet in the body, particularly when it 'tumbles', or when it comes in contact with a hard material, such as bone or steel car-bodywork. Some bullets are deliberately designed to deform or break up on impact (chapter 4), though in principle such bullets are prohibited for military use by the Hague Declaration of 1899.

Some types of modern military bullets appear to break up more readily than others, suggesting a design factor (Austria, Sweden & Switzerland, 1977). In the soap-block experiments reported above (p. 66) standard 5.56 mm bullets broke up in nearly every case, although they did not hit any harder substance than the soap (which is chosen because its density is similar to that of human muscle). Clinical reports also indicate that the 5.56 mm bullets currently in use frequently break up (Dudley *et al.*, 1968; Rich, 1968).

Experiments have indicated that where a bullet passes through a soft steel plate, or even through vegetation, before hitting the target, the wounding effect may be greatly enhanced. In this case, the greater energy of a full-power 7.62 mm bullet may cause it to inflict a worse wound than a 5.56 mm bullet (Scott, 1974).

Flechettes may deform on impact, bending into a hook-like projectile, and the fins may break off to form additional missiles (Hobart, 1973a). The likelihood that flechettes will behave in this way depends upon the impact velocity; it appears more likely with high velocity flechettes fired from rifles or shot-guns (chapter 4) than by those projected by artillery or rocket canister munitions (chapter 5).

Clearly, a projectile that hits a living target at a velocity sufficient to cause the break-up of a hard metal jacket contains energy greatly in excess of the traditional casualty criteria. Deformation or break-up means excess energy and this means a more serious wound. A bullet that does not deform or break up, and which travels on a straight path through the body will carry much of the excess energy with it on exit, causing a much less severe wound.

Secondary missiles

A high velocity projectile enters the body with such force that it impels particles of tissue radially from its path, which then act as secondary missiles. Fragments of bone are an important source of secondary missiles in the body, and cases are recorded, for example, of a coin in a soldier's pocket being hit by a bullet and breaking up into pieces, which then act as secondary missiles. A high proportion of the injuries from blast weapons are due to secondary missiles such as stones, earth, splinters of wood or pieces of glass.

VIII. The 'explosive-type' wound

Projectile wounds caused by high velocity missiles have been observed and investigated for about one hundred years. The formation in the course of microseconds of a temporary cavity up to 30 times the diameter of the projectile, the pulping of tissues, the shattering of bones, the bursting of organs, and so on, have frequently been likened to the effects of a tiny explosion in the tissues. The term 'explosive-type' wound is often used to describe the typical effects of a high velocity missile.

All current military rifle and machine-gun bullets are of high velocity type, and all are capable of causing explosive-type wounds. But the higher the velocity at 100 m (the sort of range at which the average bullet wound actually occurs) and the greater the likelihood of the bullet attaining its maximum yaw or of deforming or of breaking up within 140 mm of human flesh, the greater the probability that an explosive-type wound will occur in combat conditions.

According to Hobart (1971a), a bullet produces an explosive-type wound when the following conditions are fulfilled:

1. the bullet has a high striking energy;
2. the bullet gives up all its energy to the target; and
3. the energy is given up to as small an area of the human target as possible.

Also important are the physical characteristics of the projectile which determine its ballistic properties, both in flight and on impact. The destruction of tissue by a high velocity missile also depends upon several other factors, such as:

1. the stability of the bullet after penetration;
2. the density or compressibility of the tissue;
3. the number of secondary missiles, particularly bone fragments, and the velocity imparted to them; and
4. the fragmentation of the primary missile in the tissue.

The implications of these factors for the weapon designer have led to the development of smaller diameter rounds with higher velocity and ballistic instability, so that they tumble early in the wound, causing a larger cavity. The military justification for such wounds is stated by a leading authority as follows:

> To incapacitate is to render a man incapable of carrying out his task (i.e., to continue forwards in the assault or to use his weapon either in an assault or defensive role). The ideal incapacitation is obviously to kill but this is not always possible. The vulnerable parts of a standing man lie in only 15% of the presented area, so there is an 85% chance that a hit with a conventional round will not kill immediately. It follows, therefore, that the selected round must have a much greater chance of incapacitation, regardless of whether a vulnerable point is hit or not, and *this requires that the bullet should produce an explosive type wound* . . . (Hobart, 1971, p. 68; italics added)[3]

Clearly in this type of argument military efficiency is diametrically opposed to the humanitarian principles of international law, an antithesis which is difficult to resolve, except at the expense of one or the other.

IX. Local effects on the parts of the body

The human body is obviously more vulnerable to projectile wounds in some areas than in others. The actual distribution of hits on the body has remained very

Table 3.2. Location of wounds in battle casualties

Per cent

| | Crimean War [a] | | Prussian–Danish War [a] | | | World War II [b] | Korea [b] | Viet Nam [b] | |
	French	British	Danes I	Danes II	Prussians	USA	USA	USA	Body surface area
Head, neck	16.7	21.5	14.6	21.1	16.0	17	17	14	6
Thorax	}16.5	15.5	16.3	23.5	16.9{	7	7	7	}38
Abdomen						8	7	5	
Upper extremities	31.5	30.0	33.4	26.4	31.0	25	30	18	18
Lower extremities	35.3	32.3	38.1	38.1	36.4	40	37	36	38
Other, multiple	–	–	–	–	–	3	2	20	–

[a] Data for the Crimean War (1853–56) and the Prussian–Danish War of 1864 are taken from Berndt (1897); figures are not available for multiple wounds but most injuries at that period were due to single small arms projectiles.

[b] Data obtained from various US military sources and published by Neel (1973). The data for World War II and Korea do not include multiple injuries whereas those for the Viet Nam War do; for this and other reasons the figures are not strictly comparable but are adequate to demonstrate the general distribution of wounds.

similar for 100 years at least (table 3.2) and is approximately proportional to the actual surface area of the various regions of the body presented in combat. The head is more likely to be hit relative to its surface area, than the abdomen, thorax and limbs.

The body as a whole is more vulnerable to a wound of the head, neck, thorax or abdomen than it is to wounds of the arms and legs. This is shown by the relative lethality of wounds in the different regions. Multiple wounds, especially in the abdomen, play an important role in increasing the mortality.

The limbs

The limbs make up 56 per cent of the body surface area but often account for more than 60 per cent of battle casualties (table 3.2).

Tissue in the path of the projectile is severely damaged, being reduced to pulp and flung from the wound; also surrounding the permanent cavity there is an area of damaged tissue. In experimental studies, severely damaged muscle fibres have been detected 10–15 mm from the wound tract and less severely damaged fibres up to 35 mm away. Local haemorrhage is noted 20–30 mm and in some cases up to 55 mm from the walls of the permanent cavity (Hopkinson & Watts, 1963). High velocity bullets and fragments may cause multiple fractures to long bones, even when they are not directly in the path of the missile, and nerves and blood-vessels some distance from the wound tract may also be damaged.

Generally, high velocity missile injuries to the lower extremities have more severe effects than do upper extremity injuries, perhaps because they contain larger blood-vessels and also because the wounding effect may be compounded by the weight of the body bearing down on the limb as it fractures.

It is now possible to avoid amputation in many cases of severely damaged limbs. But this requires advanced surgical techniques. Gorman (1969), for example, reported that an average of 6–8 cm of damaged artery must be excised following high velocity missile wounds. This was too much to allow rejoining by simply stretching together the two ends remaining and therefore a piece of a suitable blood-vessel had to be taken from elsewhere in the body and grafted on (recent practice emphasizes more conservative excision.)

By means of advanced surgical methods US battle deaths from extremity wounds decreased from about 13 per cent of total battle deaths in World War II (Beebe & DeBakey, 1952) to about 7.4 per cent of total battle deaths in Viet Nam (Maughon, 1970).

The head

The head and neck make up about 6 per cent of the body surface area but account for some 15–20 per cent of battle casualties and 47 per cent of battle deaths (Beebe & DeBakey, 1952; Maughon, 1970).

The effect of the passage of a bullet or other missile through the brain is similar to the passage through other soft tissues. However, the brain is enclosed in the skull, which prevents the full expansion of the temporary cavity caused by high velocity missiles. This expansion is sufficient to shatter the skull, mainly along the suture lines (Keith & Rigby, 1899; Harvey *et al.*, 1962).

If, by comparison, an empty skull is shot at, a high velocity bullet will normally penetrate the skull, leaving only small holes without shattering the bone.

Rifle bullets almost invariably cause extensive destruction of the brain and skull. In many cases severe damage to one hemisphere of the brain has been noted even though the bullet track lay entirely in the other hemisphere. Even apparently superficial, tangential high velocity projectile wounds may cause severe internal injury to the head.

If a bullet traverses the head, the defect on exit is usually larger than that on entry. High velocity bullets frequently disintegrate and fragments of the bullet as well as of bone are impelled radially from the missile path into the brain tissue (Moritz, 1943); battlefield mortality is high (Martin & Cambell, 1946; Maughon, 1970).

The abdomen and thorax

The abdomen and thorax account for about 38 per cent of the body surface area, about 15 per cent of battle casualties and about 40–45 per cent of battle deaths.

Passage of a high velocity missile through the abdomen causes violent movements due to the formation of a large temporary cavity and the succeeding pulsations. The negative pressure in the collapsing temporary cavity causes an expansion of the gas in the intestines, which may rupture their walls, cause large tears in organs such as the pancreas and spleen, and break mesenteric blood-vessels, causing severe haemorrhage (Harvey *et al.*, 1962; Jones, Peters & Gasior, 1968; Snellman, 1966).

A permanent cavity is less noticeable in the lungs owing to their spongy character, and the movements of the thorax are restrained by the rib-cage. Harvey *et al.*, (1962) reported that all the lungs they shot at collapsed more severely than is usual from pneumothorax. Studies of war casualties show that the temporary cavity resulting from bullet wounds of the thorax may be sufficient to fracture four or five ribs and extensively damage the lungs, causing severe haemorrhage (Virgilo, 1970). Combat casualties with abdominal wounds from small arms ammunition frequently include fractured vertebrae, sacrum, lacerations of the intestines and a 'shattering' of the solid organs, such as the liver and kidneys. Experimental studies with pigs have shown that high velocity projectiles that hit the abdomen tangentially without penetrating into the abdominal cavity may nevertheless cause severe internal injuries (Jernberg, 1971).

Intestinal injuries resulting from fragment injuries frequently take the form of multiple small perforations, while high velocity injuries more often produce extensive damage involving long segments of the bowel (Jones *et al.*, 1968).

Multiple wounds

Modern high rate-of-fire automatic weapons and fragmentation munitions result in multiple wounds in about 16–18 per cent of battle casualties and 25–40 per cent of battle deaths (US World War II data; from Beyer, 1962). The high lethality of machine-guns compared with rifles is attributed to the greater likelihood of multiple hits (Beyer, 1962). Multiple wounds may also result from the break-up of a single bullet. During World War II it was noted that the more abdominal organs were injured, the greater was the probability of death; this was attributed to a 'multiplicity factor' (Wolff *et al.*, 1955; Artz *et al.*, 1955). Whelan, Burkhalter & Gomez (1968) suggest a similar factor in Viet Nam.

Experimental studies have shown that combining sources of trauma – such as mechanical injury, burns or radiation injury – greatly increases the mortality (Schildt, 1972).

X. General physiological effects

Local effects of the severity described above have potential repercussions for the body system as a whole, the most important of which is the syndrome usually referred to as 'shock'.

Although 'shock' is a term which is somewhat loosely used to cover a number of conditions (Simeone, 1963), in the context of war wounds it refers to the syndrome resulting from the loss of body fluids. Massive tissue wounds or injuries of major blood-vessels can lead to rapid death from haemorrhage. Where the loss of fluid is less severe, shock may set in.

Hypovolemic shock (shock resulting from an inadequate volume of body fluids) results in the loss of function of the kidneys and may lead to heart failure. Beyond a certain stage it becomes irreversible because the inadequate blood supply leads to the death of the tissues or vital organs (Hardaway, 1969). It is therefore of the greatest importance that the wounded person be supplied with liquids intravenously as soon as possible after wounding. Rapid evacuation from the battlefield or site of injury is therefore of great significance in improving the chances of recovery for the wounded person. Fluid requirements for patients with typical vascular injuries of the extremities average about 8.6 units of blood (Hughes, 1971).

An injury to the body, such a projectile wound, stimulates the autonomic nervous system and causes a release of hormones into the bloodstream. These hormones affect the flow of blood in the peripheral areas of the body, in effect giving important organs higher priority. Blood clots forming in the vicinity of the wound may further restrict the flow of blood.

Rybeck (1974) demonstrated that missiles with an impact velocity of about 500 m/s and impact energy of 80 J did not cause significant haemodynamic changes following wounding of the thighs of anaesthetized dogs. Missiles with impact velocities of about 1 000 m/s and 1 400 m/s (with impact energies of 260 J and 441 J respectively) caused an immediate increase in the blood flow, local resistance to flow and decreased oxygen consumption in the injured leg and the opposite effects in the uninjured leg. When blood was transfused from an injured dog, similar haemodynamic effects were noted in the recipient.

The implication of this study is that low velocity projectiles have essentially local effects whereas high velocity projectiles (over about 800 m/s) have significant physiological effects on the body system as a whole.

Collins *et al.* (1968) reported an appreciable incidence of hypoxaemia in battle casualties, most commonly in cases of fractured femurs caused by high velocity missile wounds. They attributed this to pulmonary embolism, resulting in reduced oxygen intake in the lungs.

XI. Wound infection

It has been widely believed that the heat generated by the friction of the bullet in the barrel of the gun is sufficient to sterilize it (Spencer, 1908; Ogilvie, 1944), but LaGarde (1914) reviewed experiments and showed that this was not the case. This conclusion is also supported by the work of Thoresby & Darlow (1967). They contaminated high velocity bullets with a test organism, *Serratia marcescens*, and showed that it grew in the target material. They also showed that infective particles from contaminated clothing or an aerosol in the surrounding atmosphere could be sucked into the wound from either end by the collapsing pulsating temporary cavity.

In subsequent experiments, Thoresby & Watts (1967) demonstrated experimentally the infection of high velocity bullet wounds with *Clostridium welchii, Cl. oedematiens* and *Cl. septicum*, causing the condition popularly known as 'gas gangrene'.

As these writers point out, the likelihood of infection is closely related to battlefield conditions. Clean clothes and a shower before a battle reduce the probability of wound infection. So does rapid evacuation and treatment.

The likelihood of infection is related to the extent of wounding. A through-and-through wound by a missile with a low impact velocity is less likely to become infected than a wound from a high velocity missile, which sucks in infective particles and provides a considerable quantity of an excellent growth medium for bacteria in the form of tens or even hundreds of grams of devitalized tissues.[4]

In addition to high and low velocity spheres and fragments, Mendelson & Glover (1967) reported the effects of low velocity .22 in (5.56 mm) bullet wounds, and wounds from a small explosive charge in the thighs of goats. None of the goats wounded by the low velocity bullets died from infection in the untreated wound, whereas 100 per cent of those sustaining the explosive wound died of infection. The wounds from spheres and fragments were intermediate in lethality

73

Table 3.3. Comparative mortality of various wounding agents in the thighs of goats [a]

Wounding agent	Weight g	Number of cases	Mortality per cent
Low velocity bullets	2.6	?	*0*
Low velocity spheres	2.7	27	*18*
Low velocity fragments	2.6	47	*34*
High velocity fragments	2.6	15 (20)	*40 (70)*
High velocity spheres	2.7	25 (18)	*80 (50)*
High velocity bullets	2.6	..	..
Blast	–	..	*100*

[a] These incomplete data, resulting from several experiments, are taken from Mendelson & Glover (1967). Figures in parentheses refer to slightly different results in a further experiment noted by the authors.

(table 3.3). Though no data were provided on the effects of high velocity .22 inch (5.56 mm) bullets, it is likely that such data would indicate lethality intermediate between that from high velocity spheres and that due to explosive wounds.

XII. Medical treatment of projectile wounds

The most important principle in first aid is to stop the loss of blood and ensure that the injured person is able to breathe. Intravenous infusion of blood or a plasma substitute may be necessary to prevent shock from loss of fluids.

The surgical treatment of projectile wounds has been the subject of intensive study over hundreds of years. The wound is usually excised to permit debridement (removal of devitalized tissue), as recommended by Pierre Joseph Desault (1744–1795), and is then washed with a copious supply of saline. Modern practice emphasizes *delayed primary suture* (Porritt, 1953). Because of the difficulty of fully removing the devitalized tissue soon after wounding, the wound is cleaned and debrided but not closed for four to seven days, when further inspection confirms complete removal of necrotic tissue (Jones, Peters & Gasior, 1968).

It is believed that this procedure reduces the chance of infection and leads to more rapid wound healing. It rather assumes, however, that the wounded man can be rapidly evacuated to safe and adequate treatment facilities, which is not always possible in combat conditions.

Further treatment, of course, depends upon the nature of the wound. Simple flesh wounds may heal in a few weeks without much in the way of additional treatment. Fractures of the long bones of the leg require traction equipment to prevent shortening of the limb and consequent handicap (Ganzoni, 1975).

Vascular wounds, injuries to specific organs or damage to the brain or central nervous system, may all require specialist treatment, which may not be readily available in wartime conditions.

XIII. Summary and conclusions

Projectile wounds result from the transfer of a large amount of kinetic energy in a short space of time, usually to a small area of the body. In general, the larger the amount of energy transferred relative to the area and the shorter the time, the larger the resulting wound.

Wound ballistics is the study of the effects of projectiles in the human body. It is therefore basic to the understanding of the wounding effects of both bullets and fragments, which between them cause over 90 per cent of combat casualties in conventional warfare.

In the case of high velocity missiles, the effect of the rapid transfer of energy is to create a temporary cavity behind the projectile which may attain a diameter up to 30 times that of the projectile; the cavity collapses in a series of pulsations as the projectile passes. These violent changes in the tissues are sufficient to fracture bones, rupture organs and blood-vessels and damage nerves even outside the immediate path of the missile.

As more efficient explosives and projectile systems have developed, the size of projectiles has been reduced and their velocity increased. In order to make the maximum use of kinetic energy in inflicting a wound, steps have been taken to ensure that the projectile retards as much as possible in the target medium. This has sometimes been achieved by designing a projectile which deforms or disintegrates on impact. Failing this, in the case of an elongated projectile, such as a rifle bullet or flechette, the amount of energy deposited can be increased by ensuring that the projectile deviates substantially from its line of flight when it hits the target (that is, it yaws or 'tumbles'). In broadside position it retards much more rapidly than in point-on position.

Since the average length of the wound channel in a human projectile casualty has been estimated at 140 mm, bullets – such as some 5.56 mm bullets – designed to tumble in about 100 mm will more frequently cause severe wounds than those caused by bullets which tumble later.

Rapid first aid, medical evacuation and modern surgery, where they are available, can greatly reduce the mortality from wounds of the extremities, but are less able to affect the prognosis in the case of penetrating bullet wounds of the head.

Notes to Chapter 3

1. The 'Mach' is a particularly appropriate unit to use in referring to the speed of projectiles in flight. It is named in honour of the Austrian physicist Ernst Mach (1838–1916), who first photographed bullets in flight (Mach & Salcher, 1887).
2. Retardation (r) may be described by the formula

$$r = \frac{k\rho\delta d^2 v^2 f(v/a)}{M}$$

   where k is a constant determined by the shape of the projectile; $\rho =$ density of the medium; δ is a constant to allow for the effect of wobble or yaw or other deviation from true flight; d is the diameter; $f(v/a)$ is a drag coefficient where v is the velocity of the projectile and a the velocity of sound in the medium and M is the mass of the projectile. This means that: (a) as d^2 increases (as when a bullet tumbles), so does the retardation; (b) doubling the velocity (v) increases the rate of retardation by 4 (v^2); (c) ρ is considered to be unity in air but 800 or more in water or tissue. (Beyer, 1962, p. 121)
3. Estimates as to how much of the anterior aspect of the human body represents a vulnerable area are somewhat contradictory. Black, Burns & Zuckerman (1941) calculated that 67 per cent of the body surface of a standing person was vulnerable to small high velocity fragments, whereas McMillen & Gregg (1945) estimated the vulnerable area to be 43 per cent, where 'vulnerable regions included the organs, cavities, canals and those nerves and blood vessels which have a diameter greater than 0.25 centimetre. Hands and feet were not included in the survey' (Beyer, 1962, p. 232). Vital organs account for 10–15 per cent of the area of the standing figure. These figures vary considerably when the person kneels, lies prone or assumes other positions.
4. In the study reported by Berlin *et al.* (1976), amounts of debrided tissue ranged from 2.4 g to 650 g from high velocity bullet wounds in the thighs of pigs, with the mode for various ranges and bullets at about 60 g. They obtained a correlation coefficient of 0.67 between the energy deposited by the projectile and the amount of tissue debrided.

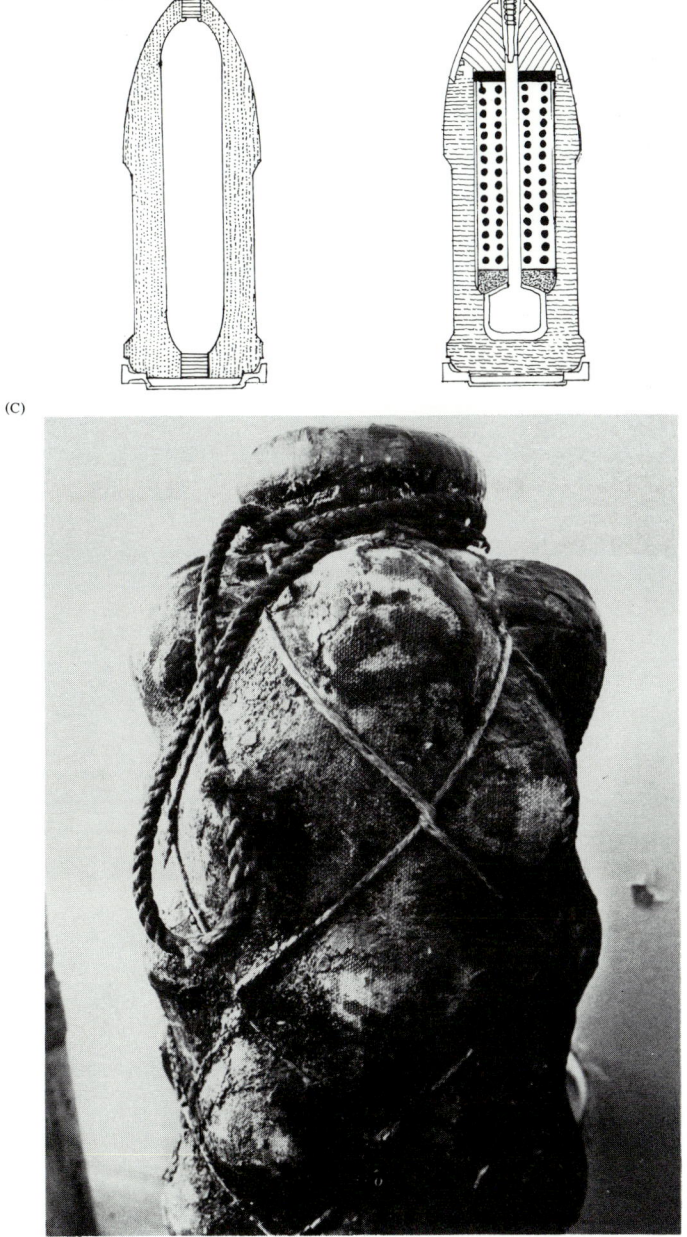

(A) (B)

(C)

Photo: M. Lumsden

Plate 1. 'A great many kinds of shell and shot were developed to be fired by artillery ...
the shrapnel shell could be fired to any distance up to about 1 200 m, before it opened to
release the lead shot' (pp. 5, 6). '... an early form [of cluster bomb] was in use over a century ago' (p. 146). Pictures show (A) early common shell for rifled gun; (B) shrapnel shell
containing lead musket balls; and (C) Swedish 'cluster bomb' from the 1840s made up of a
bundle of grenades.

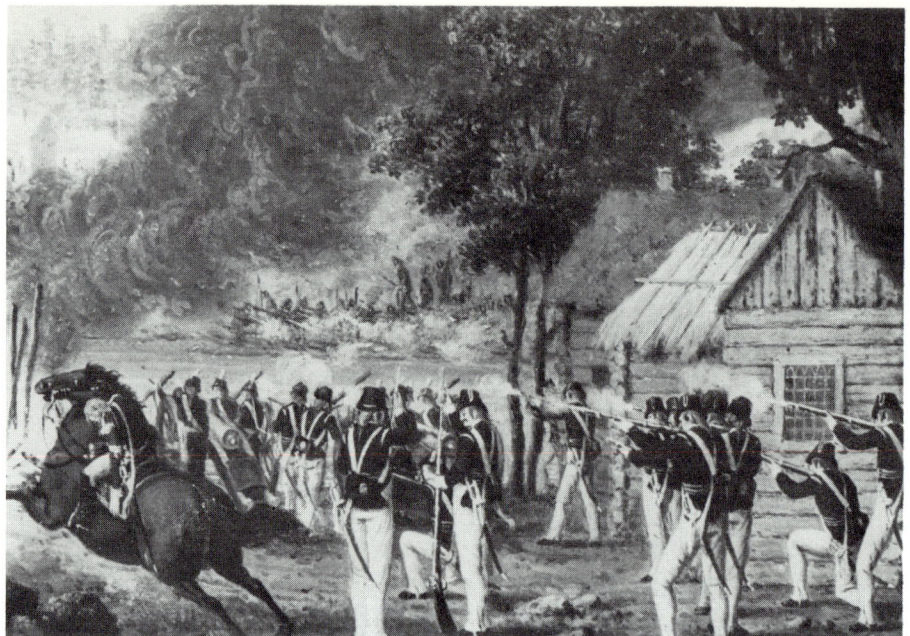

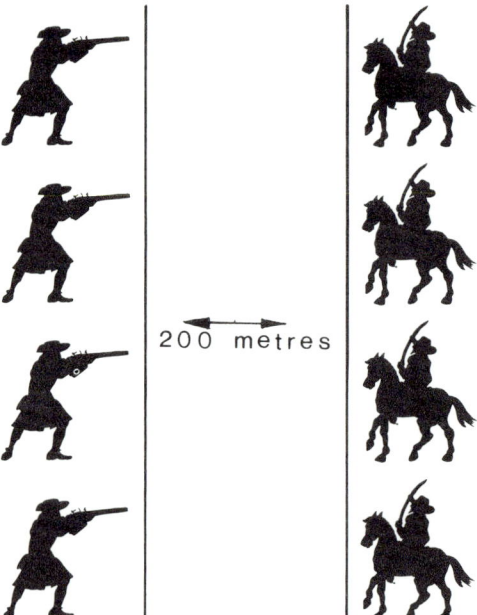

200 metres

Plate 2. 'Until the Napoleonic period, tactics were largely dictated by the effective range of the flintlock musket – about 200 m. The infantryman could carry about 60 rounds of ammunition and fire them at a rate of two per minute. The cavalry could cover 200 m in about 30 seconds. Once the musketeer had shot at the cavalryman, he had a good chance of being cut down by the cavalryman's sabre before being able to fire a second shot' (p. 5).

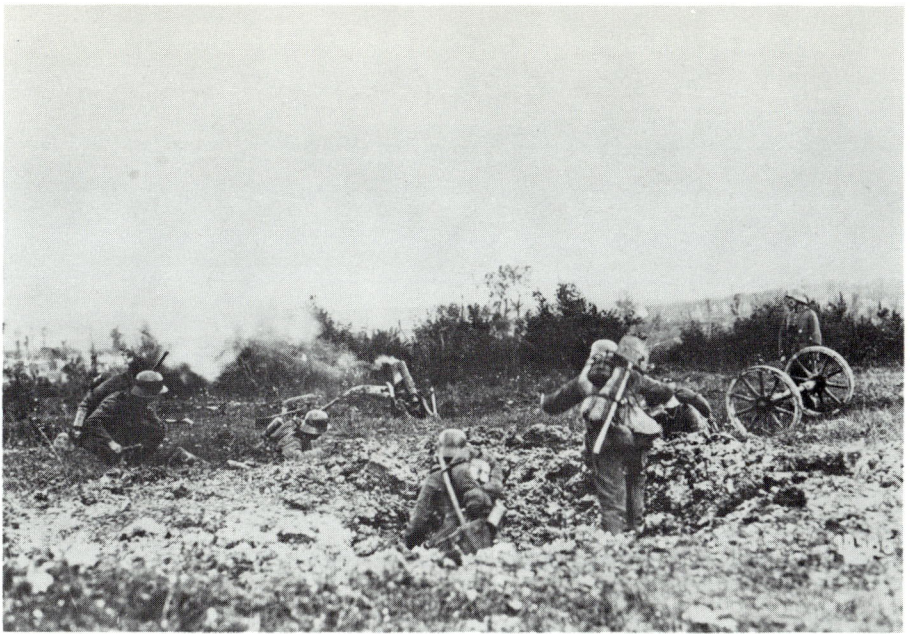

Photo: Armémuseum, Stockholm

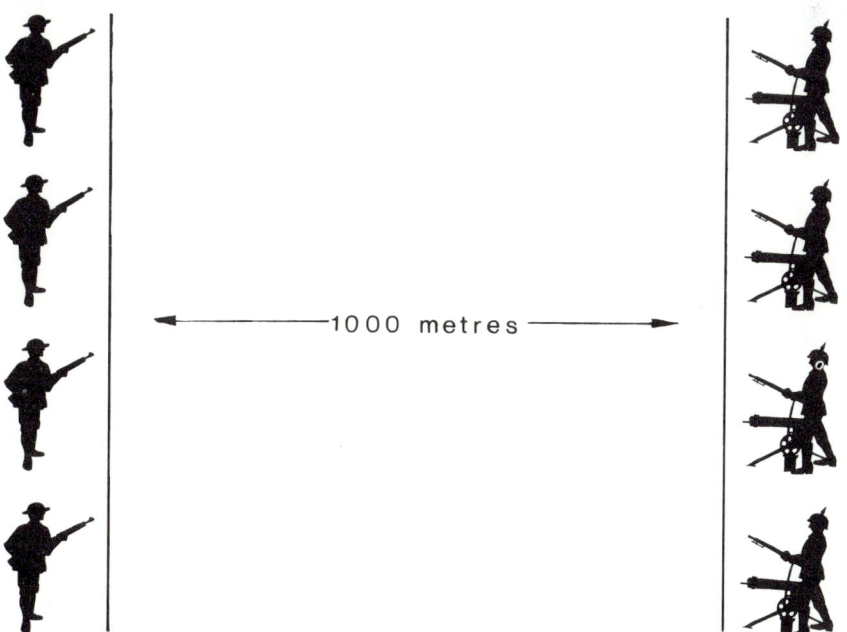

←——— 1000 metres ———→

Plate 3. 'The rifle and machine-gun, with their high-powered bullets, could easily hit the charging horse or its rider at 1 000 m and the cannon could do so at even longer range . . . . if neither side could get across no man's land and each was forced to dig trenches for protection, then "the spade would be as indispensable to the soldier as his rifle" . . . the outcome of war would no longer be determined by the final cut and thrust of the sabre and bayonet but by the capacity of industrial society to pour out its resources' (p. 13). Photograph shows German troops during World War I.

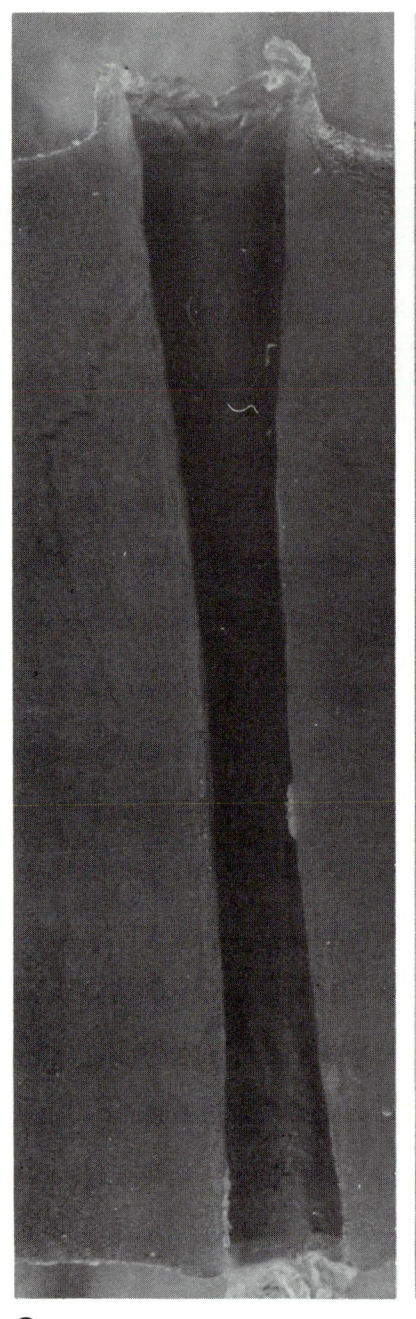

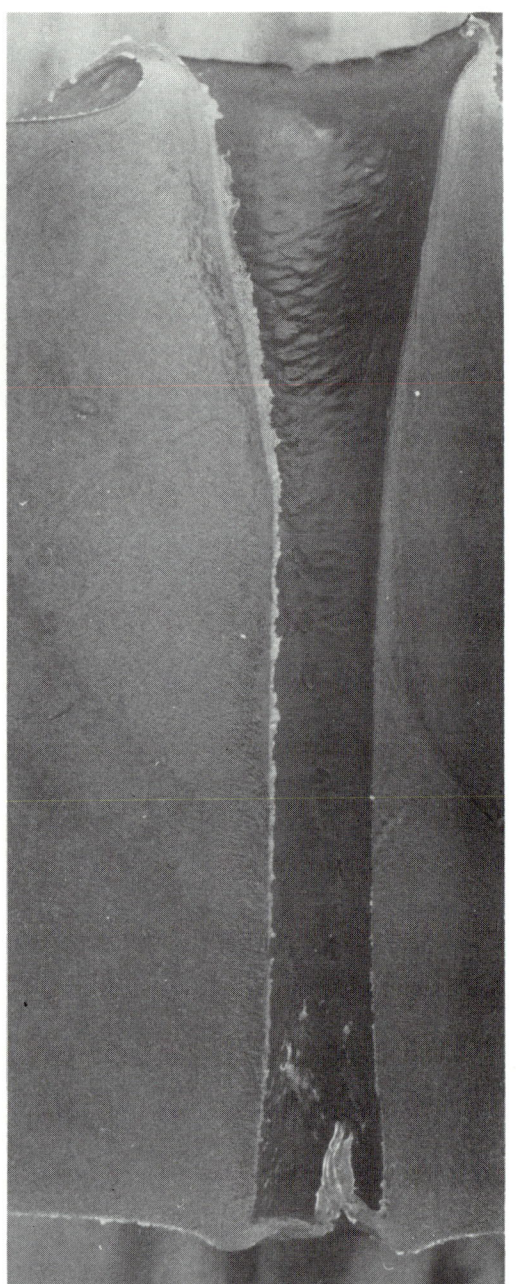

(A)

(B)

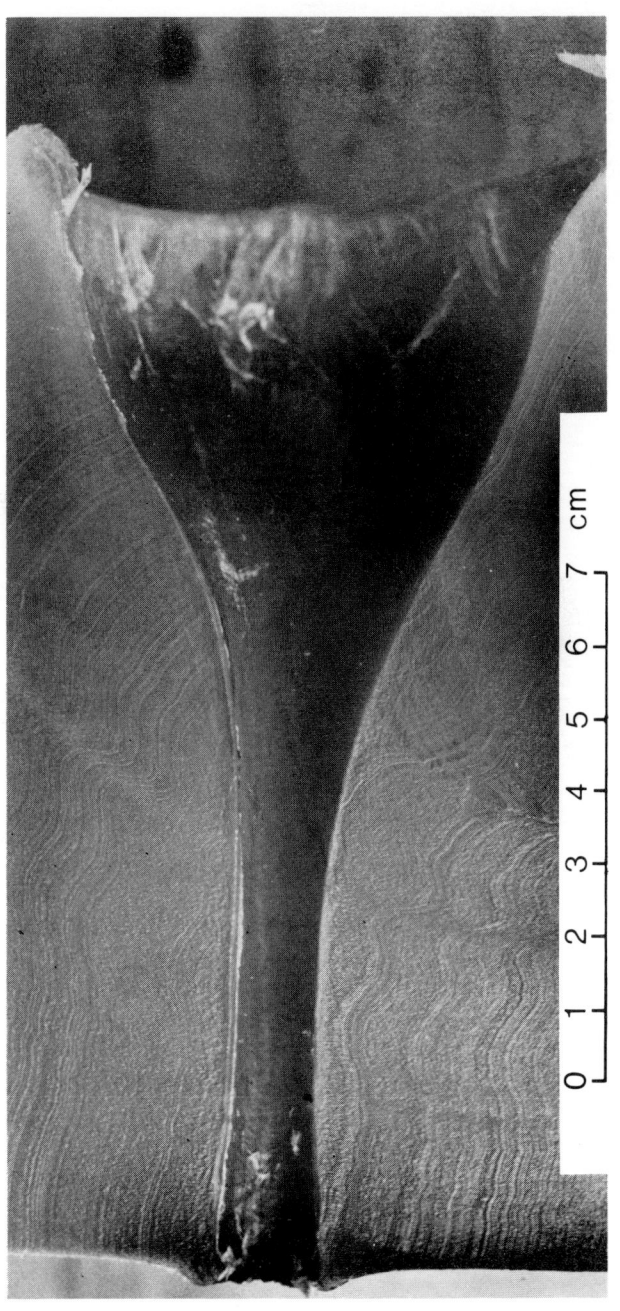

(C)

0 1 2 3 4 5 6 7 cm

Plate 4. '. . . the higher the velocity at 100 m (the sort of range at which the average bullet wound actually occurs) and the greater the likelihood of the bullet attaining its maximum yaw or of deforming or of breaking up within 140 mm of human flesh, the greater the probability that an explosive-type wound will occur in combat conditions' (p. 68). Pictures show 'wound tracts' in 150 mm blocks of soap of the consistency of human muscle at 100 m range caused by (A) Soviet 7.62 × 39 mm, (B) NATO 7.62 × 51 mm, and (C) US 5.56 × 45 mm ammunition.

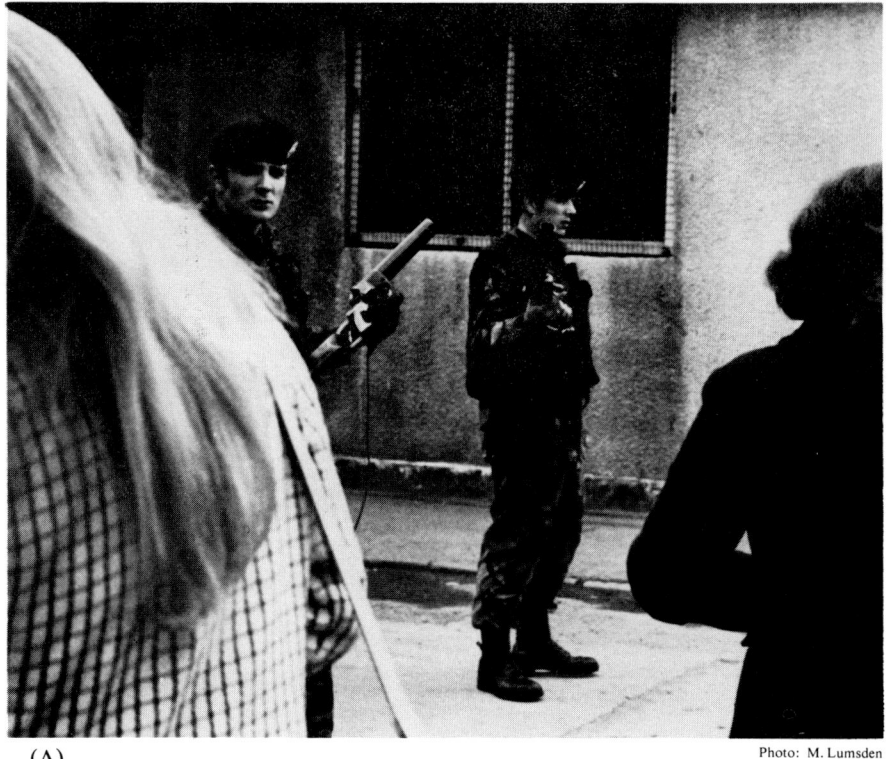

(A)

Photo: M. Lumsden

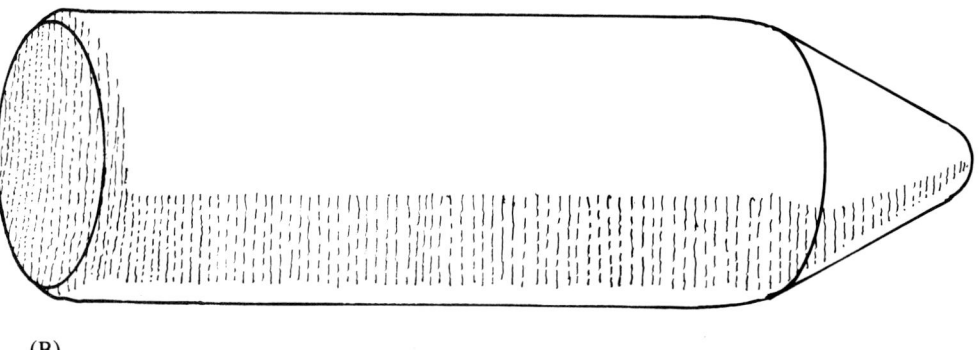

(B)

Plate 5. '... large projectiles ... can deliver a severe non-penetrating blow at some distance. ... rubber bullets are not stabilized in flight and it is difficult to hit a 2 m diameter target at a distance of 18 m .... like all other kinetic energy projectile systems, the greater the energy imparted to the projectile in order to increase the range, the greater the probability of causing severe injury or death at short range' (pp. 108, 109). Picture (A) shows British troops in Northern Ireland armed with guns for firing rubber bullets, and (B) a rubber bullet, 38 mm calibre.

(A)

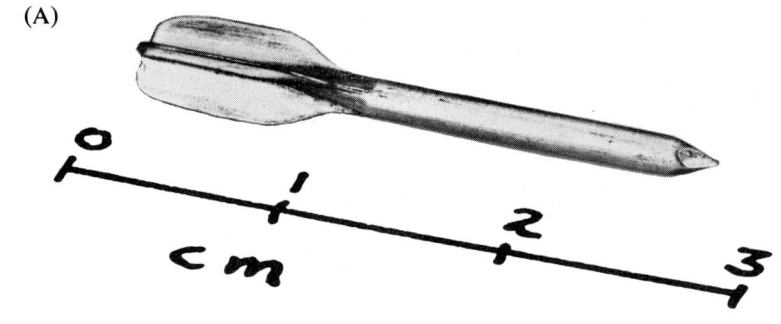

(B)

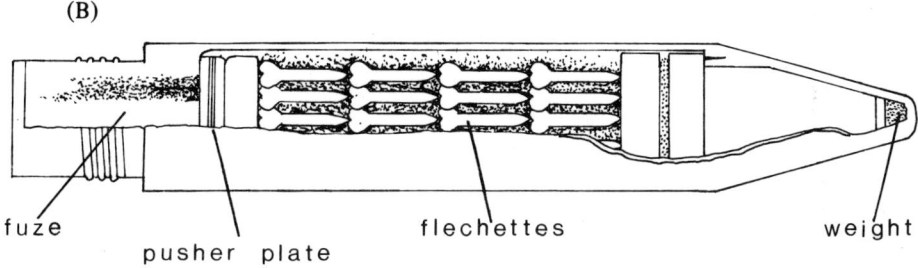

fuze

pusher plate

flechettes

weight

Source: NAVAIR 11-85-5.

(C)

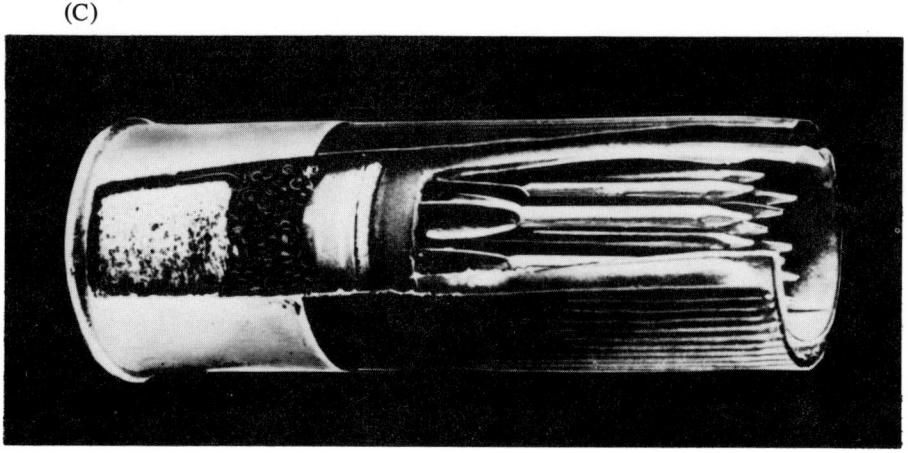

Plate 6. 'Flechettes . . . may be made of steel or . . . depleted uranium (p. 105) . . . . |they| may deform on impact, bending into a hook-like projectile . . .' (p. 67). Pictures show (A) single flechette, (B) WDU-4/4 2.75-inch rocket warhead containing 6 000 flechettes, and (C) Remington calibre 12 shot-gun shell containing 12 flechettes.

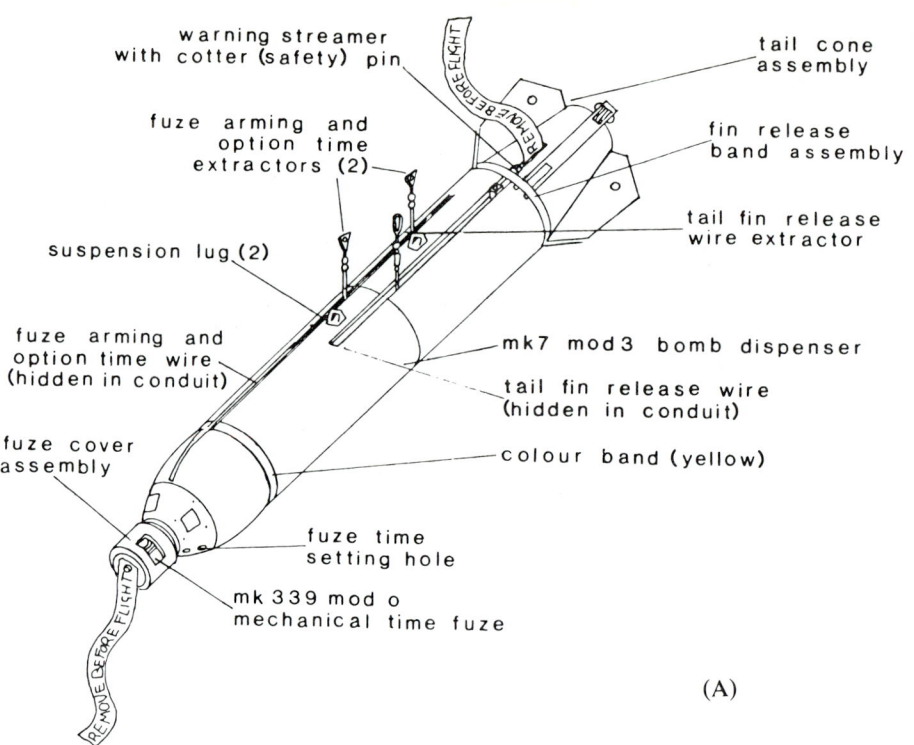

warning streamer
with cotter (safety) pin

REMOVE BEFORE FLIGHT

tail cone
assembly

fuze arming and
option time
extractors (2)

fin release
band assembly

suspension lug (2)

tail fin release
wire extractor

fuze arming and
option time wire
(hidden in conduit)

mk7 mod3 bomb dispenser

tail fin release wire
(hidden in conduit)

fuze cover
assembly

colour band (yellow)

fuze time
setting hole

REMOVE BEFORE FLIGHT

mk 339 mod o
mechanical time fuze

(A)

Source: NAVAIR 11-5A-3.

(B)

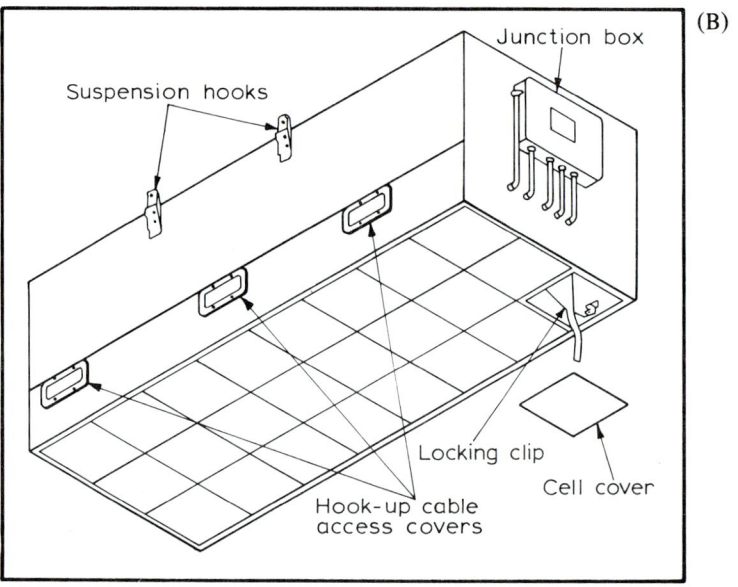

Junction box

Suspension hooks

Locking clip

Cell cover

Hook-up cable
access covers

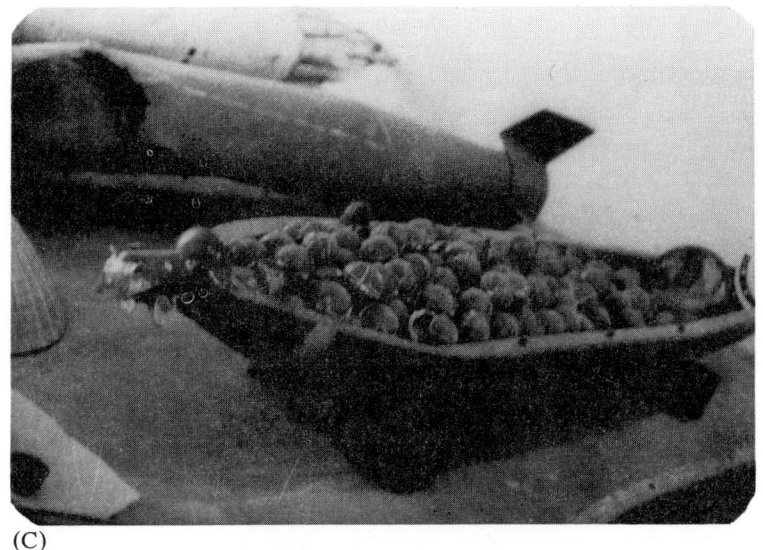

(C)

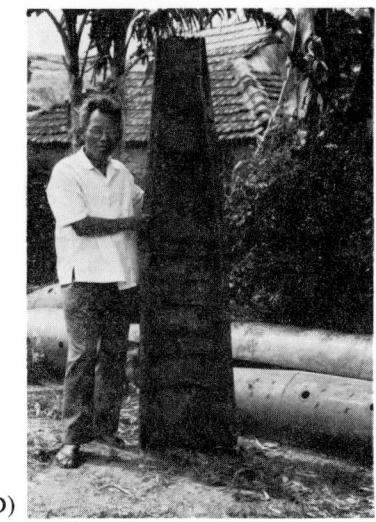

(D)

Photo: A. H. Westing

Plate 7. 'A very extensive series of cluster bombs and dispenser systems have been developed . . .' (p. 146). Pictures show (A) dispenser for free-fall delivery (Mk 20 Mod 3), and (B) fixed dispenser (SUU-24/A). The Mk 20 Mod 3/CBU-59 has a payload of 717 BLU-77 bomblets. Each of the 24 tubes of the SUU-24/A houses 3 adapters, each containing 74 BLU-3 bomblets, 535 M40 grenades or 177 BLU-26 or BLU-36 bomblets, i.e., a total of 5 328 BLU-3s, 38 520 M40s or 12 744 BLU-26s. Two SUU-24/A dispensers can be mounted in a B-52 bomber. (C) shows dud cluster bomb and bomblets, and (D) shows expended CBU-52 cluster bomb containers in North Viet Nam.

(A)

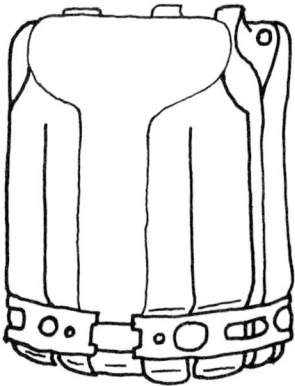

Source: TM-9-1325-207-50

(B)

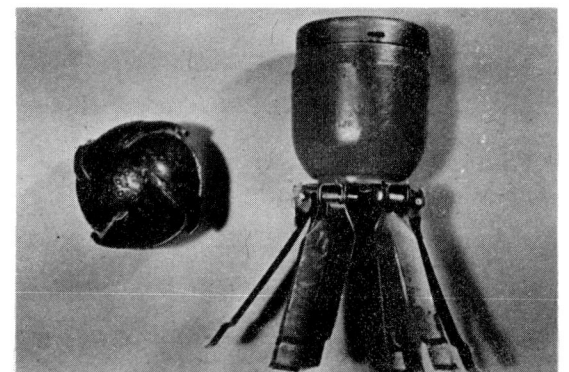

Photo: Shibata

(C)

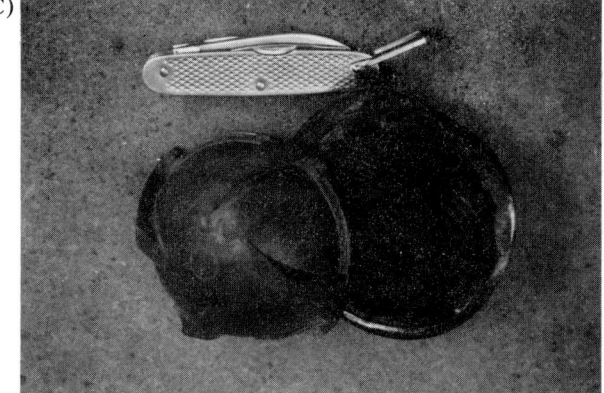

Photo: A. H. Westing

(D)

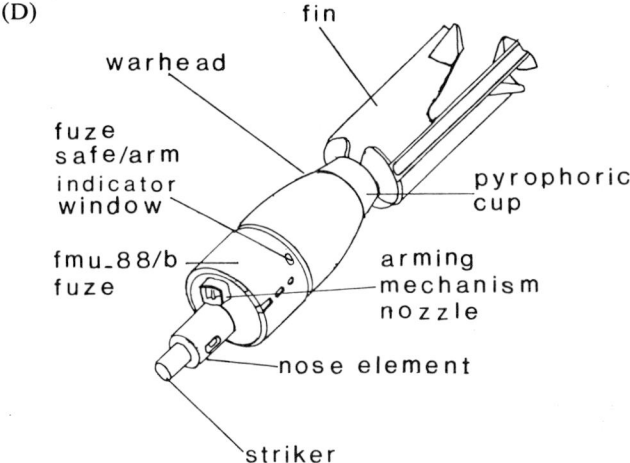

fin

warhead

fuze
safe/arm
indicator
window

pyrophoric
cup

fmu_88/b
fuze

arming
mechanism
nozzle

nose element

striker

Source: NAVAIR 11-5A-3

(E)

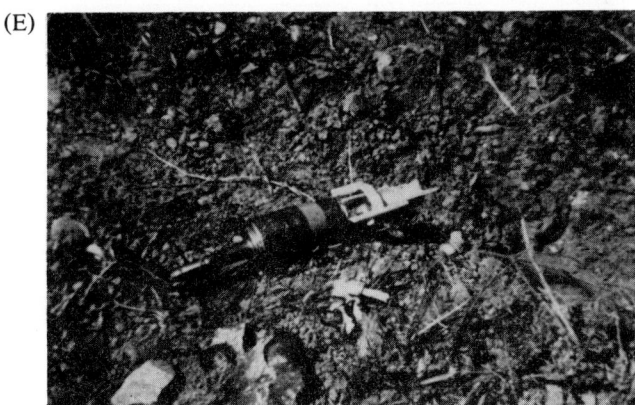

Photo: Medical Aid for Indochina

Plate 8. 'A typical bomblet is fluted, causing it to spin in the air, arming the fuze and imparting a lateral motion, thereby broadening the impact pattern. The bomblets explode in
the air or on the ground immediately or after a delay' (p. 29). Pictures show (A) BLU-3
with vanes closed; (B) BLU-3 with vanes open and BLU-26/B (impact fuze) or BLU-36/B
(random-delay fuze) steel pellet bomblets; (C) BLU-63/B bomblet with scored alloy-steel
fragmentation casing; (D) BLU-77/B soft target/hard target discriminating bomblet; and (E)
dud Mk 118 anti-tank bomblet.

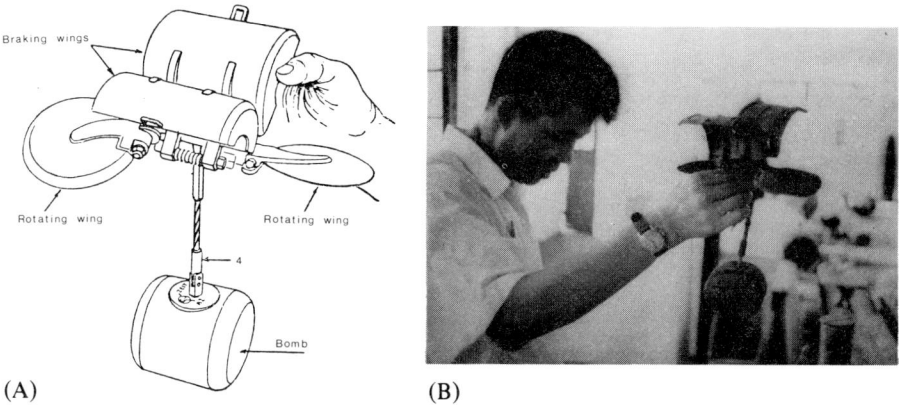

(A)   (B)

Plate 9. During World War II delayed-action bombs dropped at random added to the 'uncertainty and confusion of the defence.... Many of the anti-personnel fragmentation bombs dropped ... on Indo-China ... either remained inactive until disturbed ... or they exploded after a random delay' (pp. 179, 180). Pictures show (A) drawing of World War II German 2 kg 'butterfly' bomb with vanes open, and (B) similar bomb, presumably manufactured in the USA (see p. 146), found in Viet Nam.

(A)

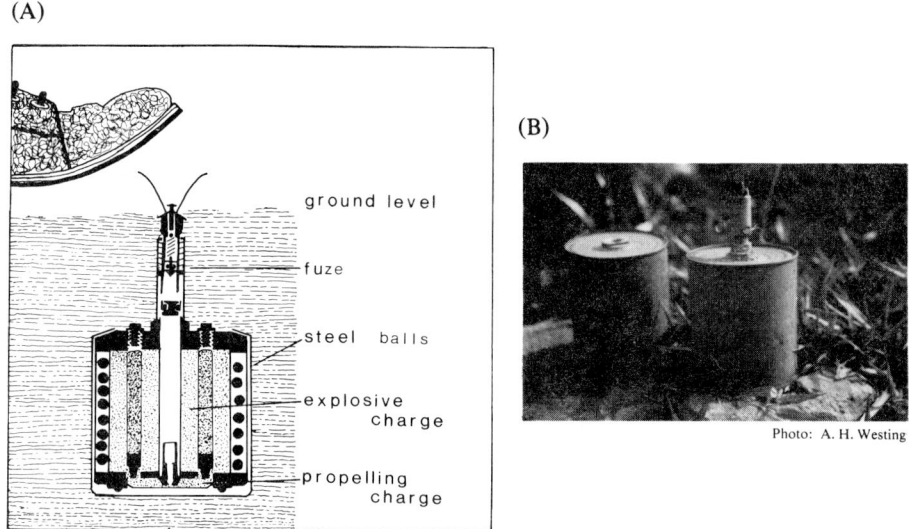

(B)

Photo: A. H. Westing

Plate 10. 'Bounding fragmentation mines are equipped with a propelling charge which throws the mine about 2 m into the air before it detonates. ... The high velocity steel fragments ejected at eye-level are particularly deadly' (p. 181). The German S mine (A) was one of the first mines of this type; during World War II most of the combatants made use of similar mines. Picture (B) shows US M16 mines in Viet Nam.

(A)

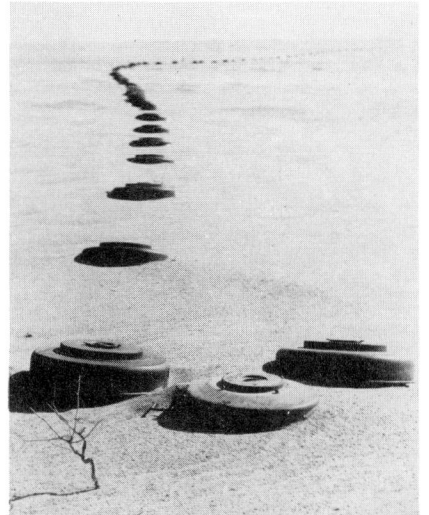

Photo: Mardell/Swedish Army

(B)

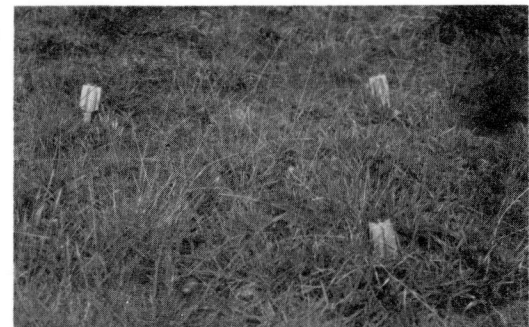

Photo: A. H. Westing

(C)

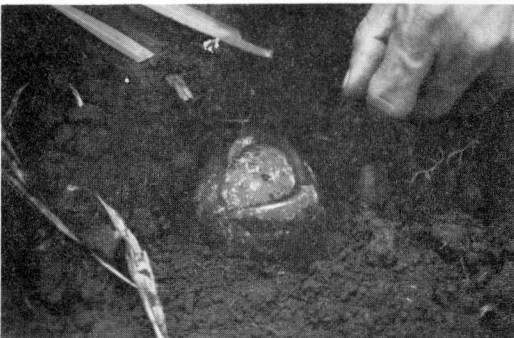

Photo: A. H. Westing

Plate 11. '... in some areas the problem of unexploded munitions – not only during the war but for many years afterwards – may be extremely great.... Reports from Viet Nam and the Middle East... indicate a large number of victims' (pp. 192, 197). Pictures show (A) anti-tank mines in desert surrounding the Suez Canal; (B) unexploded mortar shells in the Demilitarized Zone of Viet Nam; and (C) an unexploded 'guava' (BLU-26) anti-personnel bomblet in Vinh Linh, Viet Nam.

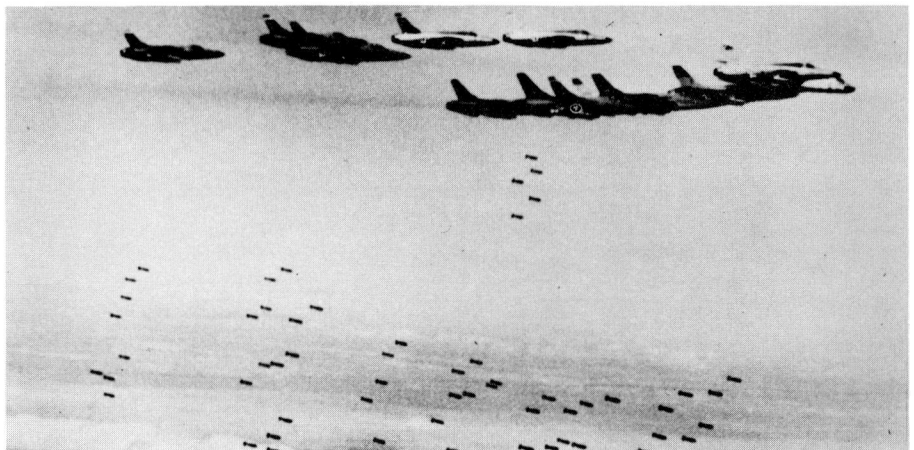

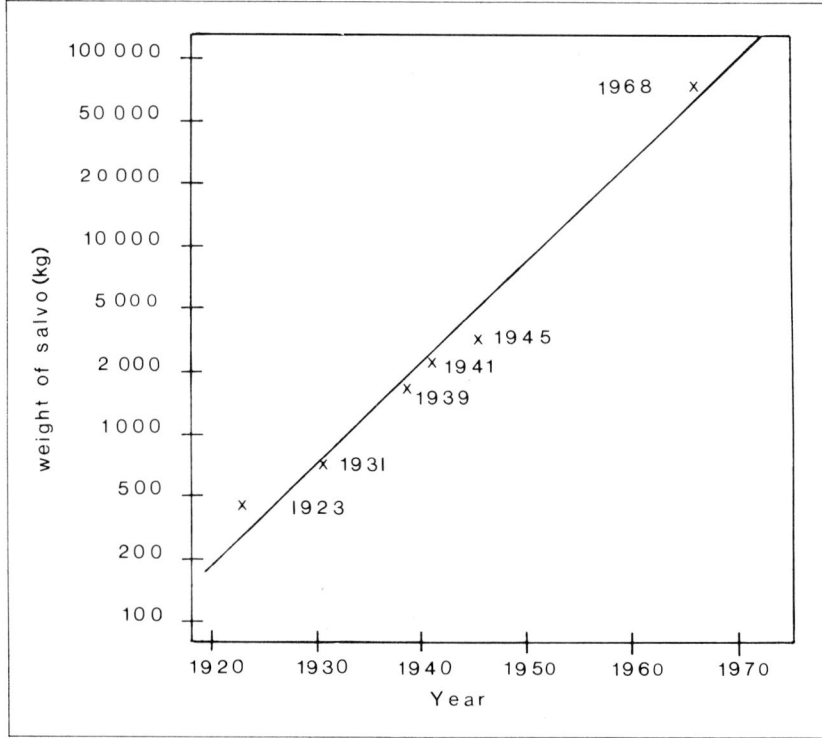

Plate 12. '... during the twentieth century... military thinking has turned from the problems of defeating groups of men whose presence on the battlefield could be observed from a commanding position to the needs of covering large areas of territory with a lethal concentration of projectiles. ... The fire-power available to front-line combat troops of the major powers has increased by as much as 26 times since World War II' (pp. 48–49). Picture shows US F-105 fighter-bombers over North Viet Nam, 1966. Diagram shows exponential increase in the weight of salvo fired by a Soviet rifle division, 1923–68 (after Sidorenko, 1970).

(A)

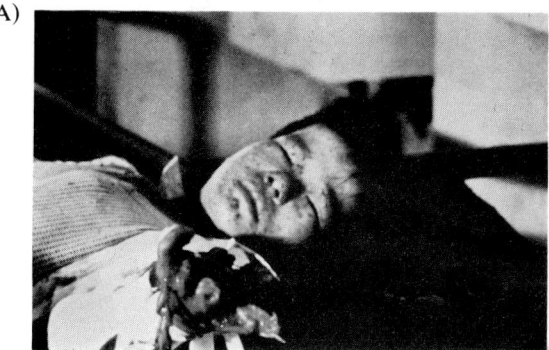

Photo: J. Champlin, MD

(B)

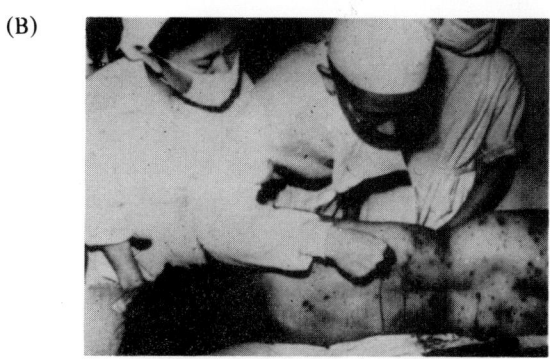

(C)

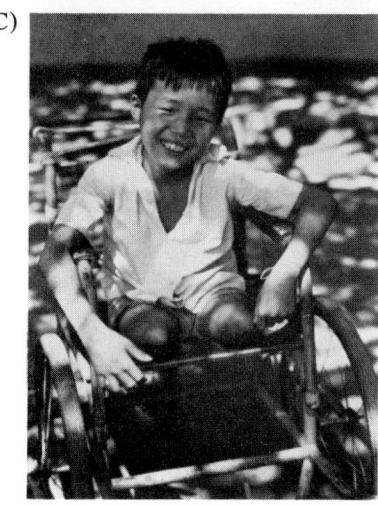

Plate 13. 'Fragmentation weapons present a difficult challenge to international law. Grenades and shells under 400 g were the first category of anti-personnel weapon to be prohibited' (p. 162). 'High velocity propellants are commonly used in mines, and the detonation usually occurs very close to the victim, so that the impact velocities attained by primary and secondary missiles are high, and wounding effects severe and multiple' (p. 192). Pictures show (A) victim of hand-grenades; (B) multiple wounds resulting from pellet bomb; and (C) one of more than 80 000 amputees in South Viet Nam, perhaps 50 per cent of them injured by land-mines (see p. 35).

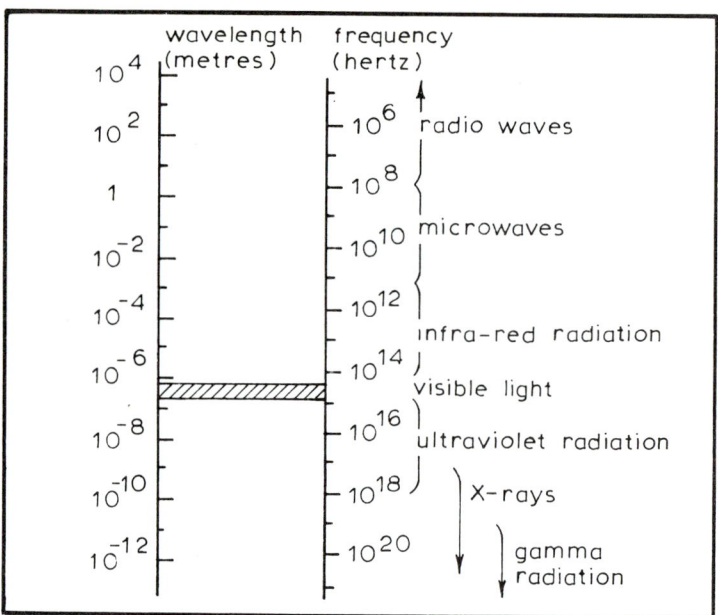

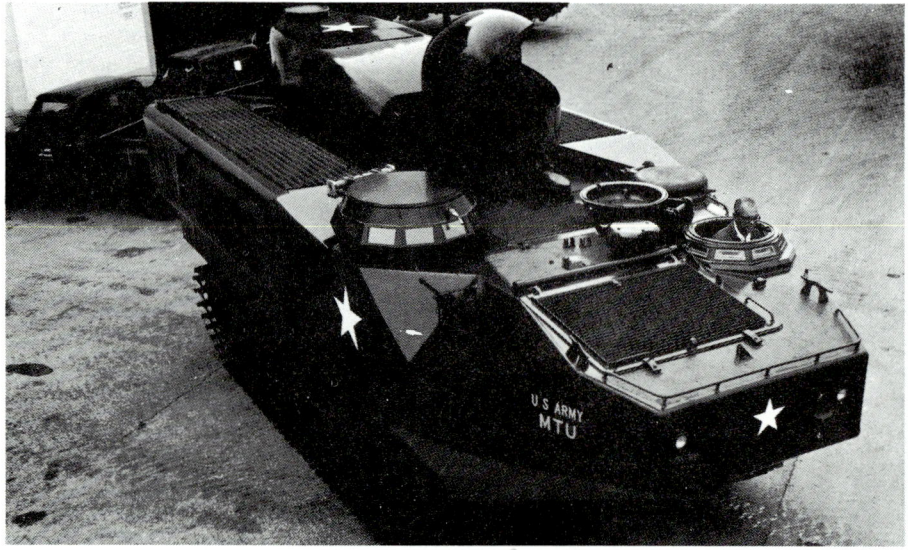

Photo: U.S. Army

Plate 14. '... electromagnetic waves have enormous military significance. ... The increase in the power of transmitting devices has led to interest in the possible biological effects of electromagnetic waves and in possible new weapons utilizing these effects. ...' (p. 205). '... the laser seems to have most potential as a battlefield weapon ...' (p. 209). Diagram shows electromagnetic spectrum. Picture shows US Army Mobile Test Unit for investigating battlefield uses of lasers, including laser weapons.

4. Small arms and ammunition

Superior numerals, thus[5], refer to notes on pages 113–114.

I. The development of ammunition

The principle issue of humanitarian concern raised by small arms ammunition has to do with the injuries caused. Rifle and machine-gun bullets have a higher relative lethality than other conventional battlefield weapons. The long range of full-power ammunition creates a danger of indiscriminate effects in inhabited areas.

Small arms are the most widely used and produced of all anti-personnel weapons. There are over 180 manufacturers of small arms in the world, of which 36 are in the USA, 32 in FR Germany, 17 in the UK and 3 in the USSR (Latour, 1974). Small arms ammunition is manufactured in about 180 factories in 50 countries (appendix 4.1). The world stock of military rifles alone numbers tens of millions.

For logistic and other reasons it is seen as desirable to reduce the size of projectiles to a minimum sufficient to disable a soldier. A smaller missile may be given the same amount of energy as a larger missile by increasing its velocity, and it is this phenomenon which has been utilized in the development of rifles and other small arms.

High velocity is mainly a function of the explosive power of the propellant, but increasing the explosive power raises the amount of recoil, which is also a function of the weight of the gun. Therefore, in practice, guns are designed to approximate a comfortable balance between the weight of the gun, the recoil, the length of the barrel, the power of the propellant and the mass and velocity of the projectile.

The function of rifling is to induce the bullet to spin as it proceeds along the barrel and out of the muzzle. This makes it more stable in flight, and therefore it has longer range and greater accuracy than an unstabilized projectile. The physics of projectile spin induced by rifling in the barrel of the gun was described by B. Robins at the Royal Society in London in 1747.

The projectile to be fired from the rifle has to have matching grooves which engage in those of the barrel, or be designed to expand in the barrel to fill the grooves. This problem occupied the attention of weapon designers for many years. Lead balls could be forced down the muzzle of a muzzle-loading rifle but the tighter the fit (and therefore the more efficient the rifle), the harder the task and the more time and energy it took. One of the most renowned early efforts to solve this problem was an invention by Captain C. E. Minié of the French Army. He made a conical bullet with an iron cup at its base which thrust itself into the lead bullet, pressing it out into the rifling grooves, when the gun was fired. This arrangement succeeded in making more efficient use of the gas pressure in the gun, giving a faster, more accurate and deadly projectile.

Other important developments led to a transition from muzzle-loading to breech-loading rifles. The first was the invention of the percussion cap by Forsyth in Scotland and Pauly in France between 1793 and 1808. The early devices placed small quantities of mercury fulminate between two layers of paper; when struck or pierced forcefully with a needle the fulminate detonated, releasing sufficient energy to initiate the oxidation of the powder in the cartridge. Forsyth invented the roll of paper 'caps' which are still used in toy pistols. In later inventions the fulminate was enclosed in a copper cap, which was subsequently incorporated into the cartridge and paved the way for modern ammunition.

This simple percussion system was used in the *Zündnadelgewehr*, or needle-gun, designed by J. N. von Dreyse about 1830 and introduced in the Prussian Army in 1841. It was a sliding bolt-action breech-loading gun in which a needle in the bolt penetrated the primer. Although the needle system is not the best it was adopted in the French *Chassepot* rifle in 1866.

A second development was a result of the increasing realization of the importance of designing a cartridge which effectively sealed the breech of the gun. Pauly experimented with metal discs in the base of the cartridge but the first successful design is attributed to Lefaucheux, working in Paris, in 1836. He used a paper cartridge with a metal disc at the base which contained the primer. When the hammer of the rifle struck the cartridge it drove a pin incorporated in the head against an 'anvil' in the base, the friction being sufficient to detonate the primer. The system, known as pinfire, was improved by another Frenchman, Houiller, in 1847, and shown at the Great Exhibition at the Crystal Palace, London, in 1851. The ammunition was demonstrated in a double-barrelled hinged gun, designed by Lefaucheux, which proved to be the first of a long line of hunting shot-guns.

At the same exhibition another Frenchman demonstrated low-powered pistol ammunition which had a rimmed percussion cap built directly into the bullet. Representatives of the US arms company, Smith & Wesson, took samples back to the United States and the company developed a low-cost method of drawing brass cartridge cases to accept a rimmed percussion cap. The Smith & Wesson .22 in (5.59 mm) rimfire cartridges produced in 1857 are almost identical with those made today.

The uneven distribution of the priming around the rim is a weakness in the rimfire cartridge and today it is only used in small calibre low-powered ammunition. A development known as the centre-fire cartridge made possible the introduction of high-powered firearms. Although a number of related patents were issued, the earliest appears to be that of Pottet in Paris in 1857.

In 1864 the British Government advertised for means of converting the existing stock of muzzle-loading Enfield rifles to breech-loaders. The conversions proposed by an American, Jacob Snider, were adopted in 1867 and were known as Snider-Enfield rifles. Snider used a centre-fire cartridge, but it was not satisfactory and was replaced by a design by Colonel Boxer of the Royal Laboratory in England. The cartridge was of coiled brass and the bullet had a hollow base containing a plug of wood or clay which caused it to expand into the grooves of the rifle.

Although the Snider-Enfield rifle was soon replaced in British service by the US-designed Martini-Henry rifle, and the coiled brass cartridge case was replaced by a drawn brass case following the campaign in Egypt in 1885, the Boxer primer system was so successful that it has remained the standard system in US ammunition until the present. A primer invented by Colonel Hiram Berdan of the US Ordnance Department in 1870 is not used in the USA but is still widely used elsewhere. While the Boxer design incorporates an 'anvil' in the primer, the Berdan design makes use of part of the primer case.

Drawn-brass percussion-fired cartridges, leading to the development of repeating breech-loading rifles, were introduced into the service of many nations in the period 1860–80. For example, in 1868, the year of the St Petersburg Declaration, Russia adopted a 10.75 mm bullet weighing 19.4 g, which was fired with a muzzle velocity of 440 m/s, giving it a muzzle energy of 2 340 J. The British adopted the .45 in (11.43 mm) Martini-Henry cartridge in 1871. At that time other powers adopted bullets between 10 and 14 mm (table 4.1).

Table 4.1. Ballistic characteristics of typical rifle ammunition

Country of origin	Calibre	Type	Year	Weight of bullet g	Muzzle velocity m/s	Muzzle energy J
First generation						
Serbia	10.15 mm	Mauser	1878	22.0	442	2 185
Switzerland	10.4 mm	Vetterli	1870	21.6	403	1 803
Russia	10.75 mm	Berdan	1868	24.0	439	2 337
Germany	11.15 mm	Mauser	1871	24.0	433	2 278
USA	12.11 mm	Remington	1867	22.4	394	1 760
UK	14.7 mm	Snider	1867	31.1	379	2 259
Second generation						
Italy	6.5 mm	Mannlicher-Carcano	1891	10.5	696	2 579
Germany	7 × 57 mm	Mauser	1892	11.2	696	2 745
Italy	7.35 mm	Carcano	1938	8.3	752	2 371
France	7.5 × 54 mm	MAS	1936	9.7	810	3 198
USA	.30–06 in	Springfield	1906	9.7	906	4 040
USSR	7.62 × 39 mm	–	1943	7.9	727	2 115
USSR	7.62 × 54 mm	–	(1891) (1903)	9.5	875	3 697
USA	7.62 × 51 mm	NATO(.308 Winchester)	1952	9.3	840	3 254
UK	.303 in	British	1888	11.3	739	3 132
Germany	7.92 × 33 mm	Mauser Kurz	1940	8.1	681	1 909
Germany	7.9 × 57 mm	Mauser	1888 (1905)	10.0	873	3 844
Third generation						
USA	5.56 mm	US M-193	1975	3.6	970	1 798
FR Germany	5.56 mm	Mauser-IWK (prototype)	–	5.0	879	1 969
USSR	5.6 mm	Sporting	–	2.76	1 090	1 671
USA	4.32 mm	–	–	1.6	1 273	1 322

Sources: Barnes (1965); Hobart, 1971a; Berlin *et al.* (1976).

Within 30 years the invention of powerful 'smokeless' powder led to the replacement of these bullets by smaller calibre, higher velocity bullets. Typical of these was the British .303 in (7.9 × 57 mm) introduced in 1888. These bullets had a muzzle velocity of some 700–900 m/s (table 4.1).

The increased velocity bullets introduced in the 1890s meant either that bullets had to be made of metal harder than lead (for example, copper–zinc alloy used by the French in World War I) or that the soft lead core had to be enclosed in a jacket of stronger metal, such as steel or copper–nickel alloy. The purpose of this jacket is to prevent deformation or break-up of the bullet in the gun but it also has the effect of reducing the likelihood of the bullet deforming when it hits the target.

It was well known that the high velocity jacketed bullets of this period could produce 'explosive-type' wounds at ranges of up to about 500 m; however, at longer ranges, and against primitive tribespeople, they were felt by some military authorities to lack 'stopping power'. A number of modifications were introduced so as to increase the severity of wounds at longer ranges. The British, having experimented with dumdum bullets having various amounts of the jacket removed from the tip, adopted for a time the Mark IV bullet, which was jacketed but hollow at the point, causing it to expand and break up on impact.

In the first decade of this century, Germany replaced the round-nosed bullet with the *Spitzer* bullet. Similar bullets were adopted by the USA in 1906 (the .30-06), and Russia in 1908, where the M-1908/1930 bullet is still in use. Around 1914 the British adopted the Mark VII, a Spitzer bullet with an aluminium- or fibre-fitted tip which made it more likely to tumble and cause a severe wound (Barnes, 1965); it remained in service until the 1950s.

Military small arms ammunition today is essentially the same as that introduced at the turn of the century. Cartridges are of the percussion type and made of drawn brass or, sometimes, steel. Bullets are jacketed, except at the base where the lead or lead alloy is filled during manufacture.

Pistol and machine-pistol bullets are usually round-nosed, about 9 mm calibre and fired with an initial velocity of about 400 m/s (table 4.2). Non-expanding pistol bullets do not cause particularly destructive wounds, though they can kill if they hit a vital part of the body.

Rifle and light machine-gun ammunition is usually pointed, of 7.62 mm calibre and with a muzzle velocity of some 800 m/s. At the long ranges (800–1 200 m) for which the older full-power ammunition was intended, wounds effectively put a man *hors de combat*, although very destructive wounds are rare. At short ranges (*c.* 100 m), where the majority of wounds actually occur in modern war, severe wounds are common, and death — especially from head wounds — is very likely.

For many military purposes the realization that the full-power 7.62 mm ammunition, with the attendant heavy rifles and severe recoil, is unnecessarily powerful has led to the introduction of either *intermediate power* or *reduced calibre* ammunition for assault rifles.

It has also been realized that in combat conditions the probability of hitting an enemy soldier is exceedingly low and various attempts have been made to design ammunition with increased *hit probabilities*.

Studies have shown that the immediate battlefield mortality due to bullet

Table 4.2. Ballistic characteristics of typical pistol ammunition

Calibre	Type	Weight of bullet g	Muzzle velocity m/s	Muzzle energy J
.22 in (5.59 mm)	Remington	2.6	515	350
6.32 mm	Automatic	3.2	245	99
7.62 mm	Tokarov	5.6	421	495
7.63 mm	Mauser	5.6	427	508
7.65 mm	Luger	6.0	378	435
7.65 mm	Browning	4.6	291	197
.32 in (8.13 mm)	Smith & Wesson	5.5	214	132
7.5 mm	Nagant	6.8	218	160
9.0 mm	Makarov	6.1	338	355
9.0 mm	Luger (Parabellum)	7.5	345	450
.38 in (9.65 mm)	Smith & Wesson	9.4	221	235
.380 in (9.65 mm)	Browning	6.2	289	260
.45 in (11.43 mm)	Browning	14.9	258	521

Source: Barnes (1965).

wounds has hardly changed in 100 years; but for those who are not immediately killed, the chance of recovery has greatly improved. This has led in some quarters to an interest in increasing the *lethality* of projectiles. Conversely, for some applications, a range of supposedly 'less-than-lethal' projectiles have appeared.

The result is that in recent years a great variety of new projectiles have appeared on the market. Many of them are being adopted by military and police forces in some parts of the world, without consideration of the legal and humanitarian implications. These new projectiles are compared with more traditional kinds in the remainder of this chapter.

II. Pistol and sub-machine-gun ammunition

Pistol ammunition is made in a range of calibres of 5–12 mm (table 4.2). For police use the .38 in (9.65 mm) is very common. Military pistols are often of .45 in (11.43 mm) calibre. For each calibre there are bullets of different weights and velocities. In general, the higher the velocity, the higher the wounding power.

Pistol bullets are of several kinds. They may be of *homogeneous* heavy metal (usually lead or a lead alloy); they may be *coated* with a thin layer of copper or other metal; and they may be wholly or partially *jacketed*. Pistol bullets are often round-nosed but may also be flat (wadcutter or semi-wadcutter) or concave (hollow-point). *Frangible* bullets are made of small pieces of iron compressed together and designed to break apart on impact. *Duplex* or tandem bullets consist

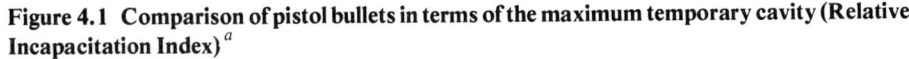

Figure 4.1 Comparison of pistol bullets in terms of the maximum temporary cavity (Relative Incapacitation Index) [a]

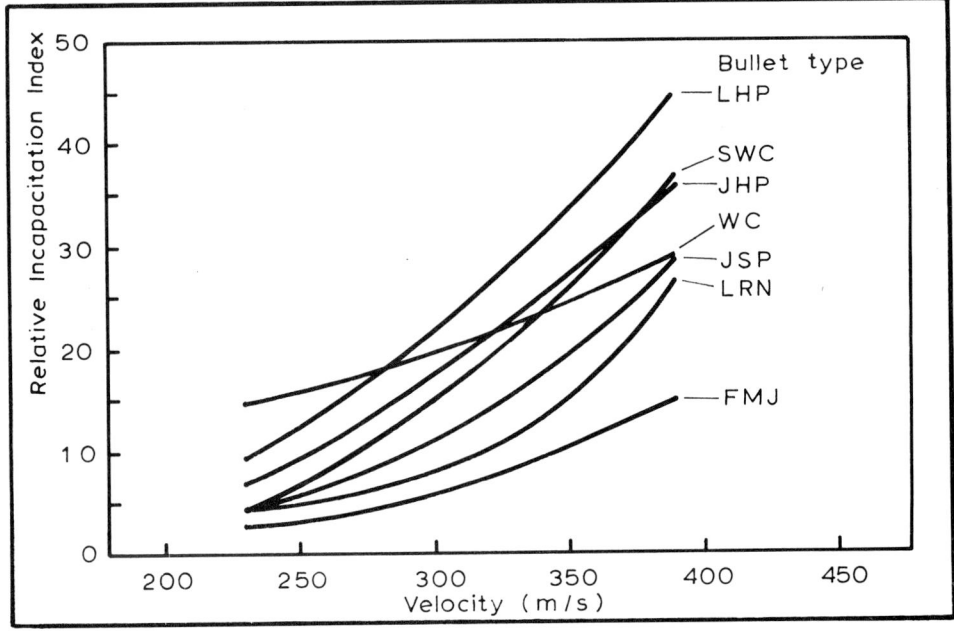

[a] All bullets are of the same calibre (.357 in = 9.07 mm) and weight (158 g). LHP = lead hollow-point; SWC = semi-wadcutter; JHP = jacketed hollow-point; WC = wadcutter; JSP = jacketed soft-point; LRN = lead round-nose; FMJ = full metal jacket.

Source: Dobbyn, Bruchey & Shubin (1975).

of two bullets, fired from the same cartridge. A bullet known as the *Super Vel.* is designed so that the soft lead core separates from the jacket on impact, and the KTW bullet is Teflon-coated and has a tungsten core, designed to penetrate cars.

In general, lead hollow-point, jacketed hollow-point and semi-wadcutter bullets have a substantially greater wounding effect (i.e., they create a larger temporary cavity) than lead round-nosed bullets. Fully jacketed bullets, as used in military service, cause the smallest temporary cavities (figure 4.1). The difference in wounding power arises from the fact that, apart from the fully jacketed bullets, all the bullets are capable of deforming on impact. Studies carried out by the Law Enforcement Standards Program of the US National Institute of Law Enforcement and Criminal Justice (NILECJ) showed that a hollow-point bullet will begin deforming at an impact velocity of 215 m/s and a lead round-nosed bullet at a velocity above 340 m/s; but lead bullets are not fired at such high velocities, whereas jacketed hollow-point bullets may be fired at 340–500 m/s and in some cases at even higher velocities (Dobbyn, Bruchey & Shubin, 1975).

The NILECJ study rated nearly 150 commercially available pistol bullets on a Relative Incapacitation Index (RII) (see p. 58). The index is derived from the maximum size of the temporary cavity on the assumption that the larger the temporary cavity, the greater the probability of affecting a vital organ. On a scale of

100 the bullets ranged from 0.4 to 54.9. The study concluded that, for police purposes, a score of 20–25 represents 'the upper limit required for reasonable reliability' (Dobbyn *et al.*, op. cit., p. 10). Some 25 bullets – most of them hollow-point or semi-wadcutter Magnum bullets – exceeded this upper limit.

Hollow-point, semi-wadcutter Magnum bullets have been issued to an increasing number of police forces in the United States and other countries. It is argued that they are required not only in order to provide the policemen with greater 'stopping power' but also because deforming bullets present less of a hazard to bystanders from ricochet. But the NILECJ study concluded that, with the exception of the Glaser Safety Slug (which also scored amongst the highest on the Incapacitation Index), 'all handgun bullets studied pose a serious hazard to bystanders' (ibid.).

Although expanding pistol bullets have been supplied to some police forces, they are prohibited for use in war by the Hague Declaration of 1899. Pistols, in fact, play a limited role in combat, although they are issued as 'personal defence' weapons to officers and certain specialists. Machine-pistols (sub-machine-guns), on the other hand, have been used extensively in combat. They are also issued to police forces. Machine-pistols are light, handy and easy to use. Their ammunition costs about one-third the price of rifle ammunition (Beer, 1975). Though they have limited accuracy, their range (c. 150 m) covers most practical combat ranges. Most military machine-pistols use 9 mm ammunition.

A typical modern sub-machine-gun is the 9 mm Israeli *Uzi*, introduced in 1954 and subsequently sold to a number of other countries, including the Federal Republic of Germany, Iran and Venezuela. It is also manufactured by the Fabrique Nationale d'Armes de Guerre (FN) in Belgium. In the Israeli armed forces about 60 per cent of infantry were equipped with sub-machine-guns (Kosar, 1974; Weller, 1972), at least until the introduction of light-weight M-16 and Galil assault rifles in 1973. Because of the low velocity it is easier to equip sub-machine-guns with an effective silencer for special operations; an example is the UK Sterling-Patchett.

A number of smaller calibre sub-machine-guns have been developed. An Austrian design, the Voere AM-180, uses .22 in (5.58 mm) long rifle ammunition with a relatively low velocity but a very high rate of fire of 1 680 rpm. The XM231 is a sub-machine-gun version of the M-16 assault rifle, designed for firing from inside an armoured personnel carrier. The *Imp* has been designed as a very light-weight weapon (1–2 kg) in several versions (Hobart, 1973*a*).

III. Full-power rifle ammunition

Modern full-power rifle (and light machine-gun) ammunition is essentially the same as that introduced at the turn of the century. It is used by armed forces the world over. Probably the most common kind is the 7.62 × 51 mm NATO

(Winchester .308 in) round, which is used by many countries outside NATO, as well as within, since 1954. It is described in more detail below, since it provides a convenient point of comparison with other kinds of ammunition. A similar round, the Russian 1908 7.62 × 54 mm, also described, is still used by the armed forces of the Warsaw Treaty Organization and in some other countries for sniping rifles and medium machine-guns; France uses a 7.5 mm round. Other varieties of basically similar ammunition are to be found elsewhere.

NATO 7.62 × 51 mm round

This type of bullet is one of the most common, being found in the armed forces of more than 70 countries. Among the more well-known of the standard rifles firing the NATO 7.62 round are the Belgian FAL (*Fusil Automatique Léger*) made by the Fabrique Nationale d'Armes de Guerre (FN) at Herstal (table 4.3). The

Table 4.3. **Distribution of the FN FAL 7.62 mm full-power rifle**

Producing countries	Importing countries	
Argentina	Brazil	Luxembourg
Australia	Burundi	Malawi
Austria	Cambodia	Morocco
Belgium	Chile	Mozambique
Canada	Cuba	Netherlands
Chile	Dominican Republic	New Zealand
India	Ecuador	Oman
Israel	FR Germany	Paraguay
South Africa	Indonesia	Peru
Norway	Ireland	Portugal
UK	Jordan	Ras al Khaimah (UAE)
	Kenya	Rhodesia
	Kuwait	Singapore
	Lebanon	Venezuela
	Liberia	Zaire
	Libya	

Source: Archer (1976).

British Army uses a version of this rifle under the designation L1A1. The Federal Republic of Germany and other countries have adopted a 7.62 mm version of a rifle developed by German engineers at the Spanish research establishment CETME (Centro de Estudios de Materiales Especiales) and manufactured by Heckler & Koch under the designation G-3 (table 4.4). The Swedish Army has introduced further modifications to this rifle and uses it under the designation AK-4. The standard US 7.62 mm rifle is the M-14. The Japanese Type 64 rifle also fires the NATO round, though normally with a reduced charge (see below, p. 89). There are many machine-guns firing the NATO round.

Table 4.4. Distribution of the Heckler & Koch G-3 7.62 mm full-power rifle

Producing countries	Importing countries	
Brazil	Abu Dhabi (UAE)	Jordan
FR Germany	Bolivia	Kenya
France	Burma	Nigeria
Iran	Chad	Philippines
Malaysia	Chile	Peru
Norway	Colombia	Qatar
Pakistan	Denmark	Sharjah (UAE)
Portugal	Dominican Republic	Sudan
Saudi Arabia	Dubai	Tanzania
Sweden	El Salvador	Turkey
Thailand	Ghana	Uganda
UK	Indonesia	Zambia

Source: Archer (1976).

In addition to their use in conventional rifles and machine-guns, these bullets are also used in a 7.62 mm version of the rapid rate-of-fire Vulcan aircraft cannon, one of a series of developments for so-called gunships and attack helicopters, intended mainly for counter-insurgency operations (chapter 2). The conventional M-60 7.62 mm machine-gun fires at 600 rpm. The General Electric M-134/GAU 2B/A 7.62 mm Minigun fires NATO 7.62 mm ammunition at 2 000–6 000 rpm.

Soviet 7.62 × 54 mm round

The Mosin-Nagant and Tokarev families of rifles, now obsolete; the SVD Sniper rifle; and light machine-guns, such as the RP-46, Goryunov SG-48 and SGM and PK light machine-guns are all designed to fire the 7.62 mm M-1908/1930 cartridge, which has a 54 mm rimmed casing. The calibre was originally adopted in 1891 and the present *Spitzer* boat-tailed shape of bullet in 1908, hence the designation. The Soviet M-1908 round is in the same class as the US Springfield .30-06, Mauser 7.92, British .303 and the current NATO 7.62 mm ammunition.

In spite of the same 7.62 mm diameter of the NATO and Warsaw Treaty Organization bullets, the rounds are not interchangeable (Stark, 1968). The Soviet bullets are slightly larger, but the differences in the sizes of the cartridges are more significant. The Soviet cartridge is 3 mm longer and 2.4 mm broader at the rimmed base than the NATO round.

Full-power 7.62 mm bullets are relatively heavy and have a high velocity, making for powerful weapons with an effective range of 800–1 200 m and a maximum range of as much as 3 500 m (Hitchman, 1952). Studies during World War II showed that the full-power rifle and machine-gun bullets then in use had a higher relative lethality rate than any other weapon on the battlefield (Beebe &

DeBakey, 1952). According to a military manual, 'the bullet sometimes sheds its jacket when passing through thick trees or large roots and the lead core continues on to deliver good destructive effect' (US Army, 1965, p. 195).

Table 4.5. Power of conventional full-power 7.62 mm NATO ammunition as shown by the penetration of inert materials

| Range
m	Material
1 200	Steel helmet
300	10 cm pine; 1/4 brick
200	16 cm pine; 8 cm oak
100	1/2 brick; 16 cm oak

Source: Gestewitz & Schwarzer (1975), p. 101.

An indication of the power of these bullets is shown by their ability to penetrate inanimate materials (table 4.5). They are quite capable of penetrating the walls of a house and killing people inside. This adds to the danger of indiscriminate effects when used in inhabited areas.

There can be little doubt that full-power ammunition is excessively powerful for use as an anti-personnel weapon at the usual combat ranges of less than 300 m. This view is shared by an increasing number of military experts, not only in the Warsaw Treaty Organization (which has relied predominantly on intermediate power ammunition for its standard infantry weapons) but also in NATO. The Editor of *Jane's Infantry Weapons 1975*, a leading Western authority on the subject, wrote:

> As a result of poor military judgement and political manoeuvring, the armies of NATO have been equipped these last 20 years with a rifle cartridge, the 7.62 mm, that is clearly too powerful for the task it is expected to fulfill and which required a rifle that is heavy to carry and uncomfortable to fire. (Hobart, 1974)

The United States has itself gone over to a smaller calibre cartridge (see below, p. 93). Arms manufacturers in many NATO countries have produced a variety of weapons to fire reduced calibre ammunition, and NATO is evaluating these weapons during 1976–78. In the meantime Japan has reduced the charge in its 7.62 mm ammunition while the USA has developed a smaller bullet for its large stock of obsolescent M-14 rifles.

It would seem likely that the days of the 7.62 mm full-power round as assault rifle ammunition are numbered. But the existence of stocks of ammunition and weapons and the cost of replacement with new ones will limit the scope for the introduction of new weapons in the short term.

IV. Intermediate-power rifle ammunition

As far back as World War II several attempts were made to fill the gap between the fully automatic sub-machine-gun, with a range of about 150 m, and the semi-automatic, full-power rifle with a range of 800 m or more. The USA introduced the .30 in (7.62 mm) carbine, the bullet for which weighed 7 g and had a muzzle velocity of 600 m/s, giving a muzzle energy of 1 285 J. The United States produced more than six million .30 carbines, more than any other single weapon (Smith, 1969). They were light and easy to use and could fire semi-automatic or, in some versions, fully automatic. But they came to be regarded as secondary weapons because of the limited power of the ammunition, and after the Korean War they went out of service.

Germany, and later the Soviet Union, developed the assault rifle, using reduced power rifle ammunition (table 4.6). The German round, the 7.92 mm Kurz, was fired from a gun originally designated as machine-pistol MP-44, and was intended for use at ranges of up to 400 m, which the Germans had concluded was the greatest range at which a rifleman could produce effective fire.

Soviet 7.62 × 39 mm round

A similar round was introduced in the Soviet Union in 1943, perhaps partly as a result of their knowledge of the German Kurz which was used against them at Cholm in late 1942 (table 4.6). Unlike the German Kurz, which fell into disuse with the defeat of Germany,[1] the Soviet M-43 round became the basis of a number of intermediate power weapons in the post-war period and is widely used today in many parts of the world. The Avtomat Kalashnikov (AK) 1947, and the later version, the AKM, has become one of the most widely used assault rifles in the world (table 4.7). It largely replaces both sub-machine-guns and rifles (except for snipers), and, with a heavier barrel, it serves as a light machine-gun (the RPD and RPK). The same round is used in the SKS carbine and in a similar Chinese weapon, the Type 68, as well as in the Chinese Type 56 (similar to the AK-47). A Finnish version of the AK-47 was introduced in 1960 (M-60) and modified later (M-62). The West German company, Heckler & Koch, chambers its HK-32 series of weapons to the 7.62 × 39 mm round, as does the Swiss SIG company for its SG 510-3 gun.

The M-43 round usually has a steel core, giving good penetration. It weighs only 85 per cent of the weight of the full-power NATO bullet and is fired at 85 per cent of the velocity. Its initial energy, therefore, is only about 65 per cent of that of the NATO round. It loses velocity more rapidly than the heavier full-power rounds, so that at 100 m its striking energy is only about 58 per cent,[2] and the energy deposit of the reduced power round in a 15 cm block of tissue simulant (gelatin) at 100 m is only 37 per cent that of the full-power round.[3] The bullet penetrates about 17 cm into soap before tumbling (Berlin et al., 1976). According to Hobart (1971a) it will incapacitate instantaneously if it hits a vital organ at

Table 4.6. Examples of intermediate-power cartridges

Ballistic characteristics	Kurz 43 (Germany)	M-43 (USSR)	M-52 (Czecho-slovakia)	— (Japan)	CETME (Spain)	XM-256E1 (USA)	.30 carbine (USA)
Calibre (*mm*)	7.92	7.62	7.62	7.62	7.62	7.62	7.62
Bullet weight (*g*)	7.96	7.96	8.54	9.70	6.14	5.8	7
Charge (*g*)	1.48	1.6	1.75	2.13	1.94	..	0.84
Muzzle velocity (*m/s*)	716	710	744	710	762	975	580
Muzzle energy (*J*)	1 958	1 993	2 018	2 372	1 095	1 599	1 285

Sources: Hobart (1973, 1975); Ludvigsen (1975); Archer (1976).

Table 4.7. Distribution of AK-47 and AKM 7.62 mm intermediate-power rifles

Producing countries	Importing countries
Bulgaria	Afghanistan
China	Albania
Czechoslovakia	Cambodia
German Democratic Republic	Chile
Finland	Cuba
Hungary	Egypt
DPR Korea	Ethiopia
Poland	Iraq
Romania	Laos
Yugoslavia	Morocco
	Pakistan
	Syria
	Tunisia
	Viet-Nam

Source: Archer (1976).

400 m, but if it hits a shoulder or a thigh it is likely to pass right through before tumbling and therefore is 'not particularly lethal'. This judgement would seem to be confirmed by smaller cavities in soap blocks (Berlin *et al.*, 1976; Switzerland, 1976).

Clinical reports suggest that the bullet occasionally breaks up so that the steel core separates from the jacket, possibly because the tip of the bullet has been filed off.

Other intermediate-power rounds

Following World War II a number of other countries, including Switzerland, France, Spain, Finland, the UK and the USA, experimented with reduced power rounds. In Spain, where German engineers worked at the CETME research and development centre, a rifle was developed which used a bullet similar to the German 7.92 mm Kurz. When NATO adopted the full-power round, the CETME rifle was modified in Germany and became the G-3. In Spain, the CETME rifle was adapted to a modified NATO round, with reduced power and a lighter-weight but longer bullet.

An advantage of intermediate power rounds is the reduction in recoil. The recoil of full-power weapons is severe and requires more training to achieve the same accuracy than less powerful weapons; this problem is particularly acute for short people. It is also easier to control the rise of the weapon during full-automatic fire, though that remains a problem even with the M-43 round.

This has been recognized in Japan where, after World War II, 7.62 mm NATO ammunition was adopted as standard. The Japanese Type 64 rifle (which is regarded as one of the best of its class), though it can fire full-power ammunition, is normally supplied with ammunition filled with only 70 per cent of the normal load of propellant. This reduces the muzzle velocity of the bullet to 807 m/s and the effective range to 400 m.

Recently the US Army Frankford Arsenal has developed a cartridge which 'could convert the Army's large stock of M-14 rifles into intermediate power automatic rifles for close-quarters fighting or special operations' (Ludvigsen, 1975, p. 118). The XM256 E1 7.62 mm cartridge fires a 5.8 g bullet at the very high muzzle velocity of 975 m/s, comparable to that of the M-16 rifle (see p. 93). The bullet has a steel core and is copper-plated and the recoil is reduced by 37 per cent. A new folding stock reduces the weight of the M-14 rifle. No information has been provided about the wounding effects of this projectile but the high velocity suggests that in 'close-quarters fighting' the effects may be more severe than those of other intermediate power bullets.

V. Reduced calibre rifle ammunition

Another approach in producing a light-weight weapon with reduced range and recoil is to reduce the calibre of the ammunition. A smaller bullet requires a less powerful propellant charge and can be fired from a lighter weapon.

Even before World War I smaller calibre bullets than 7.62 mm were in use in the armed forces of some nations, and in the UK, the USA and elsewhere experiments with smaller calibre ammunition were carried out. The experience of the Italians in Ethiopia in 1935 and of the Japanese in China in the same period led them to go in for heavier rather than lighter ammunition during World War II. But following World War II, British and Belgian designers produced an experimental light-weight rifle, the EM-2, which fired a .280 in (7 mm) bullet. These designers were convinced that the larger calibre, full-power ammunition was unnecessarily powerful. This effort to produce a light-weight rifle was given up at the time in the interests of NATO standardization on the 7.62 mm full-power round which was preferred by the USA.

The USA began a search for a new light-weight rifle in 1945. Yet 'as a consequence of unrealistic military requirements, poor management, disputes within NATO and congressional tightfistedness it took twelve years to develop a replacement for the M-1 rifle' (Ezell, 1969). The replacement, the M-14, though no doubt an improvement on the M-1, was only about 400 g lighter, since it used essentially the same full-power ammunition. The US Army, therefore, was still not satisfied with this weapon, and new design criteria were established in 1957 for an even lighter weapon.

The ORO studies

In the meantime a series of studies had been carried out by the Office of Operations Research (ORO) at Johns Hopkins University and reported by

Hitchman (1952). These studies concerned the *range, hit probability* and *lethality* of small arms weapon systems. The recommendations made by the ORO group were influential in leading to the introduction of smaller calibre, higher velocity weapons. Since these studies are not readily accessible, the findings and conclusions are summarized in some detail here.

Combat ranges

A number of studies reported by Hitchman (1952) indicated that combat ranges in modern conditions were much below what was previously supposed. Studies of the visibility of a man-sized target in various terrain conditions showed that even in open, gently rolling terrain, the probability of seeing a man approaches zero at about 1 500 m. In, for example, cultivated areas where fields are divided by hedgerows and trees and are interspersed with orchards or thickets of trees, the average probability of seeing a man approaches zero beyond 500 m. In jungle forest areas the range of visibility is even less.

In several other studies experienced soldiers were asked to estimate actual combat ranges. They estimated that 80 per cent of effective rifle and light machine-gun fire takes place at less than 200 m, and 90 per cent at less than 300 m.

At Bougainville, during World War II, nearly all US casualties caused by rifle fire were shot at ranges of less than 75 m, while a study of the Turkish Brigade in Korea showed the mean range of hits to be just over 100 m.

Studies of the ability of trained men to hit an erect man-sized target showed high hit probabilities at 100 m but a sharp decline in the hit probabilities at longer ranges, so that at 500 m even expert marksmen performed unsatisfactorily.

As a result of these studies ORO concluded that it was unnecessary to design a rifle or light machine-gun with an effective range greatly in excess of 300 m. (The same conclusion had been arrived at by German, Soviet, British and other designers many years earlier.)

Hit probability

ORO studies showed that 10 000–50 000 bullets are fired for every man hit; that amounts to between 240 and 1 200 kg of cartridges per hit (R. Robinson, 1973). Consequently there is considerable military interest in increasing the probability of a hit, $P(H)$, in order to reduce the logistic problem in supplying combat troops with such large quantities of ammunition. A further reason for increasing hit probabilities is the discrepancy in numbers of combat troops sometimes experienced by the forces of industrialized countries in combat with those of some underdeveloped countries.[4]

ORO studies concluded that more extensive training was not sufficient to increase significantly the probability of hitting a target at ranges of over 100 m. It was also discovered that it was extremely difficult to hit a target beyond 50 m by means of full-automatic fire with a full-power 7.62 mm rifle – and at 50 m an average rifleman has no great difficulty hitting a man-sized target with a single aimed shot.

ORO concluded that a weapon that dispersed a number of projectiles simultaneously with an optimal dispersion was the best means of increasing hit probability. Their reports led to a major small arms research project, Project Salvo (1952–61), in which various shotshells firing flechettes, cartridges loaded with several high velocity flechettes, a very high velocity single flechette cartridge, and various 7.62 mm multiple projectiles were tested. Some of these projectiles were tested in combat in Viet Nam (Weller, 1967). None of them met the combination of range, accuracy and dispersion recommended by ORO. In 1962 Project Salvo was superseded by the Special Purpose Infantry Weapon (SPIW) project which ended after 12 years without leading to a serviceable weapon.

In the meantime, an interim solution proposed by ORO was pursued. This was the concept of a light, rapid rate-of-fire, semi-automatic and automatic weapon designed to give low recoil and low trajectories, thereby improving the dispersion of the bullets in the area of the target. Such a weapon implied the use of a smaller calibre, higher velocity projectile. High velocity bullets of .22 in (5.6 mm) were suggested, though bullets of .14 in (3.6 mm) and .17 in (4.32 mm) were also tested.

Lethality

The ORO studies reported by Hitchman (1952) concluded that whether a bullet will incapacitate or kill immediately (or within about five seconds) is more a function of which part of the body is hit than a function of the type of bullet. ORO calculated that the 'lethality index' (the proportion of dead to wounded) due to bullets had not changed substantially in 100 years despite changes in ammunition; the proportion remained at about 35 per cent.

At about the same time studies at the US Army Ballistic Research Laboratory showed that the probability that a random hit by a given projectile would cause a fatal or severe wound was much higher than the probability of immediate incapacitation (see above, p. 60).

Faced with these conclusions, ORO recommended research in ways of increasing bullet lethality. In particular, the study of *lethal toxic* bullets was recommended. Toxic bullets were in fact produced and procured (see below, p. 107). It was pointed out that the advantage of such bullets would be that incapacitation would result *regardless of which part of the body was hit*. In this way it would be possible significantly to increase the mortality rate of bullet wounds.

It was reported that small calibre, high velocity bullets, which tumbled early and created more tissue destruction than conventional bullets, would also be a more efficient means of transmitting a dose of a toxic material.

On the basis of all these considerations – reduced combat ranges, increased hit probabilities and greater wounding power – ORO recommended, as an interim measure, the introduction of rapid-firing, very high velocity assault rifles with a calibre of about 5.6 mm. As a result of these recommendations, a new generation of small arms has emerged based on the use of a modified .223 in (5.56 mm) high velocity hunting cartridge, designated in US Army service as the M-193 round.

US 5.56 mm round

The US 5.56 mm (M-193) round, fired by the M-16 rifle and other weapons, has the highest velocity of any standard military cartridge as well as being the smallest. The round was developed from the Remington *Hornet* cartridge fitted with a 3.6 g streamlined bullet developed by the Sierra Bullet Company.

The US 5.56 mm round is said to have slightly better ballistic characteristics than the larger Soviet M-43 round. The muzzle velocity is much higher, but it loses velocity quicker. At 100 m the velocity is still 830 m/s, compared with about 600 m/s for the Soviet round.

The length–diameter ratio of the round is high, that is, the bullet is relatively long and thin, and as a result the cross-sectional density is high. The low mass and high velocity of the bullet mean that it retards rapidly, releasing a higher proportion of its energy than either full-power or intermediate-power 7.62 mm rounds.

According to a number of writers (e.g., Rathbun, 1963; Hobart, 1971a; Sie, 1972), the M-193 bullet tends to tumble earlier in the wound than 7.62 mm rounds. A military manual states that 'the bullet tends to tumble when deflected giving a good wound effect' (US Army, 1965, p. 195). Computer simulation studies also demonstrate that the M-193 bullet tumbles earlier and this is confirmed in several experimental studies which indicate that 5.56 mm rounds tumble after about 80–110 mm while the full-power NATO round tumbles after about 130–160 mm, and the reduced-power Soviet round after about 170 mm (Janzon, 1974; Berlin *et al.*, 1976; Indonesia, 1976).

This is a crucial difference, given that the average length of the wound tract in the human body is about 140 mm. It explains why the M-43 intermediate-power round will tend to pass right through, say, the shoulder or the thigh without tumbling and why it is 'not particularly lethal' (Hobart, 1971a). The M-193 reduced calibre bullet 'becomes completely unstable on impact and produces a large cavity which is the characteristic of the explosive type wound. There is ample combat evidence that a man struck in the shoulder or thigh is completely incapacitated. ... The conclusion from this is that the bullet is extremely lethal.' (Hobart, 1971a, p. 68)

Jane's Infantry Weapons 1976 writes:

> Experience in the last few years has shown that the M-193 bullet, at high impact velocities (i.e. at short range) can break up in the wound and apart from any other results, causes a very large wound. (Archer, 1976, p. 9)

All high velocity bullets have a tendency to disintegrate, but in the case of the M-193 bullet this propensity seems particularly pronounced. The following illustrative cases were published by an Australian surgical team:

> *Case 1.* A Vietnamese civilian was brought in dead after receiving a single projectile from an M-16 in the right thigh. Autopsy showed that the bullet had torn its way through the obturator foramen and disintegrated in the abdomen, only fragments of about 0.5 mm being

recovered. Within the abdomen it had wrenched the whole small bowel from its mesentery and had perforated the pancreas, stomach and spleen. Such an injury is comparable to that produced by an explosive missile.

Case 2. A Vietnamese civilian running away from an American received seven shots in the leg, the buttock, the chest and arm. The injuries outside the abdomen were minor, but several bullets must have penetrated the buttock, leaving a hole in the sacrum which accepted a fist. The rectum was transected and the small bowel perforated in eight places. Once more no trace of the projectiles could be found at laparotomy. (Dudley *et al.*, 1968)

A US surgical team reported:

> The typical minute lead splatter had not been found in other missile categories in our series of 750 missile wounds. Another factor frequently noted on X-ray is that the M-16 missile tip is intact in the wound. This is in contrast to other types of missiles where there is a breakup or marked distortion of the tip with the body of the missile remaining intact in the wound. A possible explanation of the intact tip may be the angle of impact related to the stage of tumbling. Some cases of marked M-16 missile disintegration in soft tissue only has [*sic*] been observed in this series. (Dimond & Rich, 1967)

The latter phenomenon has also been observed when firing M-16 bullets into standard gelatin blocks (Finck, personal communication, in Dimond & Rich, 1967). The break-up of these bullets has also been observed in other experiments reported above. In one experiment, 25 out of 26 reduced calibre bullets broke up in blocks of soap while none of the 14 full-power and reduced-power 7.62 mm bullets did so (Switzerland, 1976). In another experiment, 23 of 57 reduced calibre bullets broke up or deformed in the hind leg of a pig (average wound channel length, 9.5 cm); again, none of the 7.62 mm bullets broke up (Berlin *et al.*, 1976). This finding has been confirmed in a new set of experiments carried out by military experts of Austria, Sweden and Switzerland (1977).

A further feature of the weapons firing these bullets is the high rate of fire. A rate of 750 rpm means that a 20-round magazine may be emptied in 1.6 s. At 400 yards (366 m) these bullets may fall within a 150 mm diameter circle (Hobart, 1971*a*). As in one of the cases reported above by Dudley *et al.* (1968), a patient may frequently be hit by many rounds in a small area of the body. Thus these weapons may also be regarded as multiple projectile delivery systems as, indeed, they are intended to be (cf. Hitchman, 1952).

The high rate of fire of high velocity bullets places great demands on the barrel of the gun and the first weapons using the M-193 suffered from rapid barrel wear and other problems. Barrel wear may produce greater yaw in the bullet in flight which is magnified on impact with the target (see chapter 3), causing a greater wound. It has sometimes been suggested that this fact may help to explain some of the earlier reports of the excessive wounding capability of the M-193 round. In subsequent weapons the bore of the barrels was chrome-plated, the twist of the rifling increased and the rate of fire reduced to minimize wear; this in turn may have somewhat diminished the proportion of excessively severe injuries. The weapons used in experimental studies show that severe injuries may be expected even from virtually new weapons where barrel wear is not a significant factor.

To summarize, there is considerable experimental and clinical evidence to suggest that the M-193 5.56-mm round has characteristics which distinguish it from 7.62-mm rounds, particularly from intermediate-power rounds, such as the M-43 Soviet round, which is designed for a similar combat range of up to 400 m. These characteristics relate to:

(a) the high velocity at ranges where the majority of casualties occur (< 100 m);

(b) the propensity to tumble in the body within shorter distances than the average wound tract (c. 140 mm);

(c) the high probability of the bullet disintegrating; and

(d) the high probability of multiple hits.

Studies such as those of Hitchman (1952) suggest that these characteristics are not accidental but deliberately designed into the bullet.

Studies of alternative configurations of 5.56 mm bullets and of increased rifling twist suggest that bullets of this calibre can be designed that do not tumble so soon or break up so easily. Conversely, other projectile designs have produced bullets with higher velocities, greater propensity to tumble, or other characteristics, such as toxic component. Some of these designs are described below.

Other 5.56 mm bullets

In addition to the US M-193 round – the most common 5.56 mm round – a number of alternative bullet configurations have been produced (table 4.8).

Colt CMG-2 round. For its CMG-2 machine-gun the Colt Company uses a 4.4 g bullet with a muzzle velocity of 884 m/s. The barrel has a higher twist to increase the stability and range of the bullet.

Hughes plastic-cased 5.56 mm round. The Hughes Helicopter Ordnance Division has developed a plastic-cased round for its Lockless Rifle/Machine-Gun (LRMG) (see below, p. 103). Plastic-cased ammunition is lighter and more compact than conventional brass-cased ammunition. It fires a somewhat heavier bullet (4.4 g) at a muzzle velocity of 945 m/s to a range of 1 200 m.

Mauser IWK 5.56 mm round. The West German companies Mauser and IWK have produced a bullet which is somewhat heavier than the US round and is fired with a lower muzzle velocity. Its striking energy is higher than that of the M-193 round at all ranges over 50 m. In order to achieve longer ranges it requires a gun with increased twist of the rifling. The greater stability that the increased spin creates reduces the wounding effect (Hobart, 1971a).

Soviet 5.6 mm round. A Soviet 5.6 mm high velocity round is used for hunting and competition purposes. It is reported that 'there is no doubt that the Soviet Army has evaluated this cartridge for possible military use but there is no evidence so far that they intend to adopt it' (Hobart, 1975a, p. 49). The cartridge is essentially a necked-down M-43 with a smaller bullet. The muzzle velocity is higher than that of the US M-193 and tests on blocks of soap and live animals indicate that its wounding effect is greater (Jernberg, 1971; Berlin *et al.*, 1976; Switzerland, 1976).

SS-92. The SS-92 is similar to the US M-193 and is produced by the Belgian company Fabrique Nationale (FN). It is slightly heavier than the M-193 and has a slightly higher velocity at all ranges when fired from an M-16 rifle. In blocks of soap of the form and size of a human thigh, it causes larger cavities than the M-193 (Switzerland, 1976).

S-101. The S-101 is experimental ammunition also manufactured by FN in Belgium. It is somewhat longer and heavier than the SS-92, and the forward part of the core is made of steel and the rear part of lead. Soap block experiments show that it tumbles later than the SS-92. As a result, it tends to cause smaller wounds in wound tracts of up to about 150 mm. In the thighs of pigs (average depth, 95 mm), the S-101 bullet caused wounds only slightly worse than those caused by an intermediate-power 7.62 mm bullet. The wounds required less than half the amount of tissue debridement compared with the other 5.56 mm and 5.6 mm bullet wounds in the series (Berlin *et al.*, 1976).

RN-100. The RN-100 bullet is manufactured by FN in Belgium for police use and creates cavities in soap blocks similar to those caused by low velocity submachine-gun ammunition (Berlin *et al.*, 1976).

The studies of alternative bullet configurations clearly imply that it is possible to design bullets of the same calibre with greater or lesser wounding effects.

VI. The proliferation of 5.56 mm weapons

The US M-16

The first of the new generation of 5.56 mm rifles was originally known as the Armalite AR-15.[5] It was a scaled-down version of a 7.62 mm weapon known as the AR-10, which was designed by Eugene Stoner at the Armalite Division of the Fairchild Engine and Airplane Company The AR-10 had been produced in limited quantities under licence at the Netherlands Government arsenal Artillerie Inrichtingen at Hembrug. It used the gas-operated principle of semi-automatic loading used in the Swedish Ljungman (M-42) rifle and the French Model 49 and 49/56 rifles. The fixed carrying handle which incorporates the rear sight was very similar to that of the British-designed experimental .280 EM-2 rifle.

The AR-15 was derived from the AR-10 in 1957, when it was adapted to a modified 5.56 mm Remington high velocity hunting cartridge. This enabled a gun

Table 4.8. Examples of other configurations of 5.56 mm rounds

Ballistic characteristics	Mauser-IWK (FR Germany)	FN SS-101 (Belgium)	FN SS-92 (Belgium)	FN 'police' RN-100 (Belgium)	5.6 mm (USSR)	Hughes plastic-cased (USA)	M-193 (USA)	Colt CMG-2 (USA)
Bullet weight (*g*)	4.98	4.04	3.59	..	2.76	434	3.56	4.39
Muzzle velocity (*m/s*)	883	950	965	..	1 090	915	958	884
Approximate distance to tumbling (*mm*)	..	140[a]	110[a]	..	80[a]		$\left\{ \begin{array}{l} 110\,[a] \\ 98\,[b] \end{array} \right.$	

[a] Berlin *et al.*, 1976.
[b] Indonesia, 1976.

to be produced which weighed only 3.3 kg compared with the 5 kg of the US M-14 standard calibre weapon. Ten AR-15s were delivered to the US Department of Defense for evaluation in 1958 and underwent extensive testing. No further orders were placed until 1961, when the US Army bought 1 000 and sent them to Viet Nam for testing in combat, and the US Air Force police bought 8 500 (Hobart, 1971a, b).[6]

The light weight of the gun was thought to make it particularly suitable for the smaller stature of Vietnamese, Laotians and mountain peoples in Indo-China who were at that time being recruited for service against the liberation armed forces in South Viet Nam and Laos by the US Special Forces (the Green Berets) and the CIA.[7] The devastating results of the small, very high velocity bullets led to further orders. In 1963, 104 000 were purchased for $13.3 million from Colt, which had acquired the production rights. By 1967 nearly one million had been purchased, and the US Army announced that the rifle, now designated the M16A1, would be adopted as the standard infantry weapon for US forces outside NATO (*Infantry*, July—August 1967). From 1969 the weapon was supplied to US forces in NATO, though the major procurement effort at that time continued to focus on the Indo-China theatre.[8]

In addition to supplying the M-16 to its infantry, the USA has also supplied it to the Army Reserve and the National Guard (statement of Lt. Gen. Peers, Chief, Office of Reserve Components, in US Senate Committee on Appropriations, 1970). Many US police forces have also acquired it, because of its shorter range and penetration compared with larger calibre ammunition (Barnes, 1965; *Sunday Times*, 8 July 1973). More than four million have been produced to date by the Colt and General Electric companies.

The United States has supplied M-16 rifles to a considerable number of other states, either for combat use or for evaluation. In 1969, US Secretary of Defense Laird reported to the US Senate Foreign Relations Committee:

> At present we have in [the] country [South Viet Nam] 100 per cent of all the M-16 weapons that are needed to outfit the regional forces, the popular forces, and the regular forces of the South Vietnamese. Ninety-seven per cent of all those forces have this new weapon in hand at this time and have been trained to use it. (US Senate Foreign Relations Committee, 1969, p. 76)

According to *Le Monde* (3 December 1969) 750 000 M-16s had been supplied to the Saigon forces during 1969 alone as a result of the 'Vietnamization' policy. In addition, South Korean forces in South Viet Nam were issued with the new rifle (*Infantry*, July—August 1967), as were forces from Australia, New Zealand and the Philippines.

US Special Forces teams as well as local forces operating in the Philippines were supplied with M-16s (*The Guardian* (London), 11 September 1973; *Le Monde*, 14 September, 1975), and these rifles were used by some units of the British armed forces, such as the Special Air Service and the Royal Marine Commandos in Indonesia (Borneo) (Scott, 1974; *The Times*, 10 June 1972). In 1970 the USA agreed to supply M-16s to the Indonesian Government (*New York Times*, 13 July 1971).

The supply of M-16s to the Lebanese Army began in 1972 (*Le Monde*, 4 May 1973), and by 1974 it was reported that 'the United States has nearly finished re-equipping most of the 16 000-man Lebanese Army with new M-16 automatic rifles' (*International Herald Tribune*, 11 February 1974), after the supply had been stepped up sharply following fighting between the Lebanese Army and Palestinians. In 1973, Israel (which had just begun equipping its forces with its own 5.56 mm rifle – see below) was supplied with M-16s.

In Thailand, police forces as well as the Army are supplied with M-16s (*Bangkok Post*, 24 June 1974) and in 1976 it was reported that South Korea had begun licensed production of M-16s (*Far Eastern Economic Review*, 7 May 1976).

Many countries – including neutral countries, such as Austria, Sweden (*Aftonbladet*, 7 December 1968) and Switzerland – have purchased M-16s for evaluation, though companies in these countries have produced competing weapons. These rifles have also been supplied to police forces (table 4.9).

The widespread distribution of M-16s has also led to their falling into the hands of insurgent forces and criminals. Six hundred Armalite rifles were seized in the Philippines (*Far Eastern Economic Review*, 22 July 1972). In Thailand 'Southern bandits and separatists' were reported to possess M-16s (*Bangkok Post*, 24 June 1974). In Northern Ireland, Armalite rifles (sometimes AR-180s, rather than M-16s [AR-15s]; see below) have been reported in the hands of the IRA (Irish Republican Army) and the UVF (Ulster Volunteer Force) (*The Times*, 10 June 1972; *International Herald Tribune* 3 August 1972). In California, thieves stole 80 M-16s from an unguarded armoury, along with machine-guns, grenades and other ordnance (*International Herald Tribune*, 6 July 1974).

New types of 5.56 mm weapon

As a result of the great US investment in 5.56 mm weapons, an increasing number of other weapons able to use the same or similar ammunition are appearing (table 4.10). Some of these weapons are designed for special purposes, such as for firing from within armoured personnel carriers, or mounting on aircraft; others are designed to simplify manufacture, with a view to licensed production in Third World countries, either for internal use or for sale in world markets. The most important of these weapons are described briefly below.

AR-18/18S/180. The Armalite AR-18 is developed by the same company that developed the AR-15 (designated M-16 in the US Army). It is specifically designed for ease and cheapness of manufacture (Hobart, 1971*b*). As of 1971 the weapon was produced in limited numbers in the USA and Japan. Brazil, FR Germany (Mauser), Peru, Taiwan and Thailand were considering licensed production. The British Sterling Company has since produced the gun under licence. Limited supplies of the gun were sent to the Philippines, Malaysia, Brunei, and three Middle East countries. The weapon has been evaluated in the UK and Spain (Hobart, 1971*b*).

Table 4.9. Distribution of some 5.56 mm weapons

Type and producing countries	Importing countries
AR-15/M-16/M-16A1	
Philippines	Argentina
Singapore (Chartered Industries)	Australia
South Korea (Colt, Pusan)	Australia (police)
USA (Colt)	Bermuda (police)
	Brazil (police)
	Colombia (police)
	Hong Kong (police)
	Indonesia
	Israel
	Lebanon
	Malaysia
	Malaysia (police)
	Netherlands (police)
	New Zealand
	Panama
	Qatar (police)
	Saudi Arabia (police)
	South Viet Nam
	Taiwan (special forces)
	Thailand
	Thailand (police)
	UK (special forces)
	Zambia (police)
AR-18/18S/180	
Japan (Howa)	Brunei
UK (Sterling)	Malaysia
USA (Armalite)	Philippines
AR-70	
Italy (Beretta)	Italy (special units)
CAL	
Belgium (FN)	Lebanon
HK-13/33/43	
FR Germany (Heckler & Koch)	Thailand
Thailand	Malaysia
	Brazil (Air Force)
	Chile

Sources: Archer (1976); US Department of State (1976).

Beretta Model 70 series. The Italian company Beretta has produced a 5.56 mm weapon available in assault rifle (AR), special carbine (SC) and light machine-gun (LM) versions. It functions as a grenade launcher for *Mecar* 40 mm grenades. It is believed to have been purchased by Indonesia.

FN CAL and Minimi. The Belgian Fabrique Nationale, which manufactures

100

Table 4.10. Examples of current 5.56 mm weapons

Country of origin	Designation	Type[a]	Number of rounds	Muzzle velocity m/s	Muzzle energy J	Cyclic rate of fire shots/min
Austria	Steyr AUG	AR, carbine, LMG	30	970	1 668	600
Belgium	FN CAL	AR	30	970	1 668	600
	FN Minimi	LMG (belt-fed)	100, 200	895		750–1 250
France	MAS A-3	AR	25	960	1 642	900–1 000
FR Germany	HK 13	LMG (magazine)	20, 40, 100	985	1 742	800
	HK 23	LMG (prototype, belt-fed)	50	985	1 742	800
	HK 33	AR	20, 40	920	1 470	750
	HK 43	AR (semi-auto)	..	920	1 470	..
Israel	Galil	AR	12, 25, 50	970	1 668	650
Italy	Beretta AR-70	AR, carbine, LMG	30	970	1 668	630
Sweden	FFV890	AR	..	..	..	..
Switzerland	SG 530–1	AR	30	864	1 491	600
	SG 540	AR	20, 30	980	1 684	650–800
	SG 543	Carbine	20, 30	875	1 373	650–800
UK	Parker-Hale	(semi-auto)	..	970	1 668	..
	Sterling AR-18 BP	AR	20, 30	990	1 745	650
USA	AR15 (M-16)	AR	20, 30	970	1 668	850
	AR18/AR180	AR	20, 30	970	1 668	800
	AR18S	SMG	20, 30	780	1 085	800
	Stoner 63 system	AR, SMG, LMG, MMG, FVG	30	990	1 749	650
	Colt CAR 13	HAR	30	985	1 742	750
	Colt CMG-2	LMG	150	..	..	650
	XM214 Minigun	AC	2 × 500	990	1 749	400–4 000

[a] AR = assault rifle; SMG = sub-machine-gun; LMG = light machine-gun; MMG = medium machine-gun; FVG = fixed vehicle gun; HAR = heavy assault rifle; AC = aircraft cannon.

Sources: Hobart (1971a, 1971b); Weller (1973); Archer (1976).

the very widely used 7.62 mm FAL rifle and MAG machine-gun, has produced a 5.56 mm assault rifle, the CAL (*Carabine Automatique Légère*), and a light machine-gun, the *Minimi*. They are designed to fire the US M-193, the FN SS-92 or the S-101 round with a supplementary propellant charge, giving a muzzle velocity of 895 m/s; this makes the *Minimi* capable of penetrating a steel helmet at 800 m. It can also be fitted with a special long barrel allowing the launching of anti-personnel and armour-piercing grenades, as well as increasing the muzzle velocity. The *Minimi* has been entered in the SAWS (Squad Automatic Weapons System) competition for the US Army. The CAL, which was one of the first European 5.56 mm weapons (1966), has been supplied to Lebanon. For the NATO small arms competition, FN is believed to have entered a new version with an increased twist in the rifling and a more stable bullet, giving increased range.

Galil. The Israeli armed forces have adopted a 5.56 mm weapon, the *Galil* (named after the chief design engineer, Israel Galili), produced in Israel by IMI (Israel Military Industries). It was adopted after extensive tests of effectiveness and suitability for Israeli conditions had placed it ahead of the *New Uzi* (a competing Israeli design by Major Uziel Gal, inventor of the *Uzi* sub-machine-gun), the AK-47 and the M-16 (in that order), as well as other foreign designs, including the HK-33, Stoner 63, AR-18, AR-70 and the Austrian AUG.

The *Galil* is heavier than its competitors and fires more slowly. It serves as a grenade launcher for a 225g anti-personnel grenade, using a blank cartridge, with a range of about 250 m. The weapon is manufactured for the US 5.56 mm round, apparently mainly because of its availability rather than because it was necessarily regarded as the most suitable round. According to Weller (1973), some Israeli generals would have preferred a somewhat heavier round, more suited to the light machine-gun role.

The *Galil* is manufactured in two versions, the standard assault rifle (ARM) which also serves as a light machine-gun, and a short assault rifle (SAR), with slightly shortened barrel, reduced weight and less muzzle velocity. The action of the *Galil* is similar to the Finnish Valmet M-62, modified from the Soviet AKM. Vents in the piston guide-ring allow some of the gas to blow back to remove dirt particles from the moving parts, thereby increasing reliability in adverse climatic conditions. After its adoption, which was announced in May 1973, it was only used on a small scale in the war of October 1973, during which Israel purchased US M-16s as an emergency measure. These M-16s have since been used in operations in the South Lebanon border area. The Netherlands MD 1 and the Swedish FFV 890 are derived from the *Galil* under licence.

GEC 5.56 mm Minigun. The General Electric Company has produced a scaled-down version of the M-61A1 20-mm Vulcan aircraft cannon. It is designed to be fitted to helicopters or light attack aircraft. Operating on the Gatling multi-barrel principle, it has a rate of fire of 400 to 4 000 rpm. A 7.62 mm version of this gun was employed in Indo-China.

HK-13/23/33/43/53. In association with the US company Harrington & Richardson the West German company Heckler & Koch has developed a scaled-down version of the standard 7.62 mm German rifle, the G-3. The 5.56 mm version is known as the HK-33 in Europe and as the H & R G-3 (modified) in the

United States. Weller (1967) reports that Australian forces tested it in combat in Viet Nam. It has been manufactured under licence by MAS in France and is also believed to have been purchased by Malaysia. The HK-43 is described as the non-military version of the HK-33 (company brochure, undated); it is identical but lacks full-automatic capability. The HK-43 is produced in Thailand, and it is reported that the Thai Government authorized the sale of 4 400 to Chile (*Wehrtechnik*, no. 10, 1975, p. 535). The HK-53 is a sub-machine-gun version of the same weapon. A derivative, the HK-53 KL, has been designed for firing from a combat vehicle. The HK-13 and HK-23 are light machine-gun versions.

Hughes 5.56 mm lockless rifle/machine-gun (LRMG). Based on research originally sponsored by the US Advanced Research Projects Agency (ARPA) and the US Army Armament Command, the Hughes Helicopter Ordnance Division has developed a lockless automatic rifle/light machine-gun which permits the use of special plastic-cased ammunition (see p. 111). It has a rate of fire of 420 rpm.

MAS Type A-3. The French company Manufacture d'Armes de Saint Etienne (MAS) has produced a 5.56 mm weapon of less conventional design. It is reported that the French Army decided in 1970 to adopt the 5.56 mm calibre for infantry weapons in the future; but in 1976 no final decision on a specific weapon had been made. Trade unions in France urged the adoption of the MAS weapon, which was to undergo further tests (*Le Monde,* 12 February 1976).

MKS 5.56 mm assault rifle and carbine. A small Swedish company, Inter-dynamic, Stockholm, has developed a 5.56 mm weapon as a private venture.

Parker-Hale .223 in (5.56 mm). The British company Parker-Hale of Birmingham, England, markets a 5.56 mm rifle which has been sold to some British police forces.

SIG SG-530-1/540/543. The Swiss company SIG has produced prototypes of 5.56 mm rifles to be manufactured in Switzerland. The company was reported to be experimenting with several kinds of 5.56 mm ammunition. The guns are designed to launch a STRIM (Société Technique de Recherches Industrielles et Mécaniques) anti-personnel grenade without the need for an additional attachment. A competing Swiss weapon has been designed at the Eidgenössischen Waffenfabrik, Bern (*Neue Zürcher Zeitung*, 3 June 1977).

Steyr AUG 5.56 mm assault rifle. The Austrian company Steyr, in association with the Austrian Army, is developing a modern assault rifle, the AUG (*Armée-Universal-Gewehr*). Several kinds of ammunition are being tried, including a 6 mm round as well as 5.56 mm rounds (Widhofner, 1974*a, b*). Austria has now placed an order believed to be for some 80 000 AUGs, with the twist of the rifling increased so as to improve the stability of the bullet.

Stoner 63 system. The designer of the M-16, Eugene Stoner, designed a system of weapons in 1963 using many common components. The rifle and the light machine-gun version are the most used. The rifle is somewhat heavier than the M-16 since some of the internal components were designed to take the stresses of a medium machine-gun; the additional weight is compensated for by reduced recoil, which makes for greater accuracy.

XM177E1/XM177E2 (Colt Shorty). The Colt Shorty is a short version of the

M-16, intended for a sub-machine-gun role.

XM231. The XM231 is a new adaptation of the M-16 to a sub-machine-gun role.

VII. Other small calibre, high velocity bullets

In spite of the great investment in weapons designed for the US 5.56 mm M-193 round, a number of other bullet configurations have been developed. There appear to be two main reasons for this. Firstly, there is a notion that even greater logistic savings can be achieved by using still smaller calibre bullets with increased velocity. Secondly, the range and penetration of the M-193 round is not regarded as sufficient by some military experts, particularly for the machine-gun role. Smaller calibre bullets have reduced range and penetration and therefore these two considerations tend to contradict each other. The result has been the development of a range of 'compromise' rounds with varying calibres and ballistic characteristics, in addition to those of the same calibre but different mass and other characteristics (see below).

US 4.32 mm (.17 in) round. The US 4.32 mm bullet has a weight of only 1.6 g. It is fired at a muzzle velocity of 1 272 m/s and retains a velocity of 1 000 m/s at 100 m, but has less range than an M-193 round. It was used in one of the SPIW (Special Purpose Individual Weapon) variations. The manufacturer, Remington, already markets a hunting rifle using the ammunition and has produced two military assault rifles for it, a standard version and a sniper's rifle (Beer, 1975).

West German 4.6 mm round. Heckler & Koch have designed two 4.6 mm bullets for firing from a new assault rifle, the HK-36. The tip of the *Löffelspitz* (spoon-point) anti-personnel bullet is bevelled to cause maximum tumbling which, as Hobart (1975c) implies, is one way of circumventing the intentions of the Hague Declaration on expanding bullets. The hard-target bullet has a tungsten carbide core.

British 4.85 mm round. The Royal Small Arms Factory at Enfield, England, has developed a 4.85 mm round for a new assault rifle, the British entry in the competition for a new standard NATO assault rifle and light machine-gun. The gun is derived from the British EM-2, which was developed after World War II to fire a short 7 mm (.280 in) cartridge. The new assault rifle is complemented with a light support weapon (light machine-gun) firing the same ammunition. The bullet has a muzzle velocity of 900 m/s from the rifle and 930 m/s from the machine-gun. It is reported that it can penetrate a steel helmet at 550 m, whereas the US M-193 5.56 mm cannot. This suggests that the ballistic characteristics are dependent upon a configuration with a high-sectional density but which will tumble readily on impact, causing a large temporary cavity.

US .221 in (5.613 mm) round. The Remington *Fireball* cartridge has been utilized for a prototype weapon, the GUU-4/B *Imp*, which may be developed as a survival rifle, using 4.32 mm ammunition or a standard rifle using 5.56 mm ammunition (Hobart, 1973c). The *Fireball* bullet weighs 3.24 g, slightly lighter than the standard M-193 bullet, and it has a lower muzzle velocity.

US 6 mm round. For some years the USA has had a programme to develop a Squad Automatic Weapon (SAW), firing a bullet with tracer and target penetrating capability at 1 000 m range. Several rounds have been produced, with brass, steel or aluminium cartridge cases. The most prominent, the XM732, fires a high-sectional density bullet weighing 6.86 g at a muzzle velocity of 762 m/s (Archer, 1976).

VIII. *Unconventional small arms projectiles*

Flechettes

Flechettes are small needle-like metal darts or arrows which may be made of steel or other metal such as depleted uranium. They are fin-stabilized and usually designed to be fired at very high velocities of about 1 450 m/s. A wide variety of flechette rounds were tested in the USA and in some other countries. The most common US types of flechette round (XM110, XM144, XM215, XM645) consisted of 5.56 mm cartridges loaded with flechettes of various lengths and weights (0.05–1.3 g). Other flechette cartridge calibres included 7.62 mm, 10.4 mm, 0.45 inch (11.43 mm). The Amron Corporation developed an 8.35 mm cartridge firing four flechettes, and several multi-flechette shot-gun cartridges have been produced (see p. 108). Some flechettes are composed of two metals, to give greater weight at the front; others have a split tip, to increase wounding power; and others with a coating of a lethal toxic agent have been evaluated.

Since the expanding gas produced by the detonation of the propellant rushes past the projectile as it emerges from the muzzle, the accuracy of the flechette is very sensitive to the launching conditions. Firing a flechette from a rifle therefore requires that it be enclosed in a cartridge case in a sabot which drops away as the flechette emerges from the barrel. Flechette cartridges of this kind were designed for the US XM19 SPIW which was tested for about 12 years with only limited success. Its successor, the XM70, was converted from a flechette-firing to a 4.32 mm bullet-firing weapon in 1974–75. Flechette cartridges were also produced for the M-14 7.62-mm rifle and the M-16 5.56-mm gun.

Descriptions of the wounding effects of rifle-fired flechettes suggest that they are capable of causing severe wounds. A leading small arms authority writes:

> Due to its long, thin shape, there is a lack of rigidity, and the flechette turns into a hook on impact with the target. It becomes totally unstable and imparts its full kinetic energy to the target, producing an explosive-type wound. (Hobart, 1973a, p. 314)

> Flechettes tend to buckle into a hook upon impact with flesh, and since this is a very poor ballistic shape, and since flesh is about 800 times denser than air, the buckled flechette gyrates and gives up its energy very rapidly, thus earning high marks as an effective projectile. (Archer, 1976, p. 13)

A US military writer suggests that the US Army was concerned about possible public reactions to the use of flechettes:

> The attitude of the American public is of real concern to the Army for a very practical reason. By influencing their Congressmen, citizens can thwart even what the military chiefs believe are their best ideas. The horror with which the public regards chemical and biological warfare is reflected in the Army's relatively low budget for research and development in this area. The service wanted to avoid a similar fate for SPIW. The reason for the Army's anxiety is that the wound from a SPIW arrow is usually big, nasty and fatal. The effect is similar to that of the soft-nosed dum dum bullet, which was condemned by most of the major powers during the Hague Peace Conference of 1899 ... [The] tumbling action of flechettes which is induced by their hitting an object, is what accounts for the gravely torn wounds they can inflict on human targets. (Beller, 1968, pp. 81–82)

A French manufacturer has designed flechette-like ammunition for pistols. Each projectile is 30 mm long, tapering to a point from a maximum diameter of 3 mm, and weighs 0.53 g. The projectiles are launched in salvos at a velocity of 150 m/s.

The USA has also experimented with Scimitar projectiles which rely on a cutting mechanism, rather than kinetic energy, to attain lethal effects.

Salvo and Salvo Squeezebore ammunition

Experiments were carried out early in this century with Duplex and Triplex ammunition, designed to fire two or three bullets from a single cartridge. During the 1950s this concept was taken up again in the course of Project Salvo in the USA, and elsewhere. Duplex and Triplex loadings were made for 7.62 mm NATO ammunition and 6.35 mm ammunition, and a French 7.5 mm Triplex round was also developed. It proved difficult to design these projectiles in such a way that they could achieve an adequate dispersion on the target at 400 m.

The Salvo Squeezebore (SSB) technique was developed as a means of improving the dispersion of multiple projectiles. Conical bullets are nested into each other as in salvo ammunition, but the cones are squeezed into more conventional shape by a tapering construction in the bore of the gun. The system was first publicly demonstrated in the USA in 1962 using two calibres: .50 in (12.7 mm) swaged down to .30 in (7.62 mm) in the barrel; and a .30 in (7.62 mm) swaged down to .15 in (3.8 mm). The larger calibre was employed by the US Navy in riverine operations in Viet Nam in 1967. Salvo Squeezebore bullets have since been made in a number of other calibres, including 9 mm (jointly developed by the USA and Israel) (R. Robinson, 1973; Archer, 1976), and have been evaluated in a number of countries. The USA has also experimented with a projectile on to which fins are moulded as it proceeds down the barrel.

'Gyrojet' or self-propelled ammuniton

A range of self-propelled ('Gyrojet') recoilless ammunition for rifles and pistols has been developed by US and French manufacturers. The series includes a 13 mm round incorporating a solid propellant booster charge which is 50 mm long and weighs 13 g. It has a maximum velocity of 430 m/s and is said to penetrate 25 cm of wood at 17 m. There is also an 11 mm percussion-fired round.

Toxic projectiles

A number of small arms projectiles designed to infect the body of the victim with a toxic agent of the nerve gas type have been studied in military laboratories. In 1964 the US Army procured 85 000 E-2 separable bullets (US Department of Defense procurement data (unpublished); see also *New York Times*, 31 October 1969).

In a study of new infantry weapons, Hitchman (1952) explains the advantages of toxic projectiles:

> [The effects of toxic missiles] constitute an order of lethality not achieved by any missile ground weapon yet devised . . . The progress of the physiological symptoms is demoralizing to watch; thus real psychological effects not normally characteristics of weapons design are added . . . It has been found that small missiles (such as .22 cal [5.6 mm]) are more efficient vehicles for such toxic agents than are the larger calibres . . . Thus would be achieved a genuine innovation in a weapons system which has exhibited through history a constancy in lethal effects. (Hitchman, 1952, pp. 29–30)

As pointed out by Hitchman, the lethality of conventional bullets depends not so much on the bullet as on the part of the body hit. But any area of the body would be able to absorb a toxic agent, so that even relatively minor wounds could prove lethal. Smaller calibre bullets are presumably more effective in this respect because they retard more in the body and may dispense more of their toxic agent.

IX. Shot-guns

Smooth-bore shot-guns firing a multiplicity of hardened lead balls lack the range and accuracy of rifles. But by dispersing a number of projectiles simultaneously in the vicinity of the target they may increase the probability of a hit, particularly when fired at small moving targets. They are commonly used for hunting birds.

Shot-guns are often issued to police forces but are not very common in military service. They were made available to US troops in Indo-China, some of whom apparently preferred them to rifles for certain purposes. The use in Viet Nam of an experimental .50 in (12.7 mm) machine-gun fitted with a special shot-gun barrel and firing 00 Buck pellets, 36 per charge, has been reported (Weller, 1967).

Flechette shot-gun ammunition has also been produced. The AAI company produced a 12-gauge [18.5 mm] shell in 1957, known as the A-LI. It fired 32 flechettes of 0.84 g weight at a muzzle velocity of 426 m/s. Another design fired 26 flechettes at a muzzle velocity of 548 m/s. Flechettes of the 'mass (weight) stabilized' type are used in some other shot-gun ammunition; these flechettes are thicker at the front, which is made of a heavier metal, and have no fins. In one shot-gun shell, 18 flechettes of this kind are fired at a muzzle velocity of 518 m/s. According to a US patent application, flechette shot-gun shells have 2–3 times the effective range of conventional shot-gun ammunition (Shellnut & Jenkins, 1971).

A 12-gauge flechette cartridge appears in the US Department of Defense ammunition code list (US Defense Supply Agency, 1971, p. 21). According to Weller (1967), 12-gauge flechette shot-gun shells were used by US troops in Viet Nam, 'particularly in river boat operations by the US Navy.' They were also fired from the specially adapted machine-gun referred to above.

More recently the USA has been experimenting with the XM261 cartridge which fires 9–16 tungsten alloy pellets. Metal-piercing loads and cartridges for launching gas grenades are also available for shot-guns. A US designer, Atchisson, has developed an automatic assault shot-gun which fires from a 20-round magazine at a rate of 360 rpm. Semi-automatic shot-guns are also available and have been supplied to some police forces.

X. Non-penetrating kinetic energy projectiles

Non-penetrating kinetic energy weapons are perhaps the oldest of all, ranging from sticks and stones to a variety of modern devices. Although the club is hardly used in modern warfare, truncheons and batons are still widely used by police forces. Improperly used they can cause severe injury, particularly to the head.

The use of batons is limited by the need to be very close to the target. This limitation has led to the development of 'baton rounds', large projectiles which can deliver a severe non-penetrating blow at some distance. The original baton rounds, sometimes called 'broomstick' rounds, were made of wood and it is believed that they were first used by police in Hong Kong. They were cylindrical in form and produced a whistling sound which can have added to their effectiveness in their main use of dispersing crowds. They are normally aimed at the legs or at the ground so that they ricochet. Field tests showed that they could cause serious internal injury or death and they sometimes splintered. A wooden multiple block, 37 mm round, was used by police in Berkeley, California (Applegate, 1971).

Early in its engagement in Northern Ireland, the British Army made use of CS munitions. Although often referred to as 'tear-gas', CS is in fact a smoke of fine particles with a highly irritant effect. It was fired in cartridges from 1.5-in (38-mm) Very signal guns or the specially adapted US Federal Riot Gun, which has a longer barrel. The indiscriminate effects of CS, which was extensively used in Viet Nam, and is now supplied to many police forces, led to its withdrawal in 1970. At that time the British Army was issued with L2A2 rubber baton rounds, fired from the same 1.5 inch guns; CS and CN gas projectiles are now also often made of rubber. The L2A2 rubber projectile weighs 149 g and is fired at about 70 m/s.

Since the weapons firing these rounds were originally designed only to fire signal rounds into the air they are smooth-bore and not very accurate. The rubber bullets are not stabilized in flight and it is difficult to hit a 2 m diameter target at a distance of 18 m. Later a PVC round, the LR L3A1, with longer range and accuracy was introduced, but it proved more dangerous at short ranges. More recently it has been announced that a rifled version of the British L48 riot gun is being developed in order to improve accuracy (*Daily Telegraph,* 4 August 1976).

Other kinetic energy rounds have been developed for similar purposes. These include golf-ball-like projectiles, and rubber balls filled with water, other liquid or gas. The Belgian Fabrique Nationale has developed a rubber projectile to be launched from the 40 mm grenade launcher or rifle attachment.

Another development is the Stun Gun, developed by MB Associates of California, which fires a 'bean bag' consisting of a canvas bag filled with lead shot. The bag is rolled up in the cartridge and unfolds as it is fired, giving it very limited range and penetrating ability. One version weighs 227 g and is fired at a velocity of 45 m/s. It is able to administer a severe, and possibly fatal, 'punch' at short range (Security Planning Corporation, 1972).

The Ring Aerofoil Grenade (RAG) developed at the US Army Edgewood Arsenal led to the idea of a lower velocity, soft-rubber projectile, the XM743 Sting Rag, for use in civil disturbances. This ring-like device is launched at a velocity of 60 m/s by a blank cartridge fired from an M-16 rifle. The projectile has aerodynamic, rather than ballistic, characteristics, which enable it to deliver accurately a powerful blow at ranges beyond which it is possible to throw stones (*US Army Research & Development News Magazine,* November–December 1974).

All of these munitions are intended to be non-lethal. But, like all other kinetic energy projectile systems, the greater the energy imparted to the projectile in order to increase the range, the greater the probability of causing severe injury or death at short range. Experimental studies on the effects of blunt projectiles impacting

Table 4.11. Effects of non-penetrating missiles impacted against the lateral thoracic wall of dogs[a]

Biological effects observed	Threshold velocities (m/s) for missiles of indicated weights	
	360 g	180 g
Lung haemorrhage		
Unilateral only	13.7	24.3
Bilateral	33.4	38.0
Rib fracture	18.2	36.5
Internal lacerations from rib fracture	27.4	36.5
Fatality within 1 hour	47.1	51.7

a The missiles were 7 cm in diameter and fired from an airgun.

Source: White & Richmond (1959).

on the chests of dogs showed that serious and even fatal injury could occur at relatively low velocities (table 4.11). The figures in this table are fully comparable with the weights and velocities of the 'non-lethal' kinetic energy rounds described above. This is confirmed by studies of British rubber bullets, bean-bag type projectiles and other kinetic energy projectiles carried out by the US Army Human Engineering Laboratory on behalf of the US Law Enforcement Assistance Administration (Egner *et al.*, 1973; Thein *et al.*, 1974; Wargovitch *et al.*, 1975; see also Rosenhead, 1976).

In a survey of casualties caused by rubber bullets in Northern Ireland, over a two-year period during which some 33 000 rounds were fired, Belfast surgeons counted two fatalities, 17 persons permanently disabled or disfigured and 73 others injured (*Sunday Times*, 27 May 1973; Millar *et al.*, 1975); a third person died shortly after (Rosenhead, 1976). The rubber bullets are supposed to be used at ranges of 6–25 m, and the plastic ones at longer ranges. Most of the severe injuries arise because the troops fire them at short ranges – more than half of the persons treated in hospital had been hit at ranges of less than 15 m (Rosenhead, 1976; Wade, 1972).

Obviously, the basic laws of physics apply as much to non-penetrating as to penetrating kinetic energy projectiles: additional energy applied to propel the missile further results in unnecessarily severe injuries at close range.

XI. Trends in ammunition technology

The trend in projectile development has been successively to increase the velocity of projectiles as well as the rate of fire of the delivery system. These trends are restrained by a number of natural limitations. Higher velocities and higher rates of fire can be produced with existing technology, but the exceedingly high temperatures produced cause rapid corrosion or failure of the gun. A 7.62 mm aircraft 'Minigun', for example, may fire 2 000 rounds in 20 seconds; but the barrels become red-hot, are prone to fail and the rifling is eroded (Heiney, 1973). Therefore only shorter bursts of 2–3 seconds are fired. With current propellants it is not possible to increase muzzle velocity significantly without reducing gun-barrel life below acceptable levels.

A high rate-of-fire gun also consumes huge amounts of ammunition and this creates a logistic problem. To reduce this problem, as well as to save copper used in cartridge cases, aluminium and plastic cartridge cases are being developed and even caseless ammunition. But with the high temperatures produced there is a danger that aluminium cartridge cases will ignite.

Research is going on into alternative propellants (by-products of rocket technology) to make possible higher muzzle velocities and rates of fire. A series of compounds containing cyclic or linear nitramines as oxidizers have been tested as potential new propellants and show significantly reduced temperatures (Heiney, 1973).

The development of caseless ammunition began during World War II and has now reached an advanced stage in the USA and FR Germany. It reduces the weight and the cost of the round by 40–50 per cent and eliminates the need for brass – which may be a critical material in wartime. The 'cartridge' consists of a sleeve of compressed, heat-resistant particles of propellant, containing a core of standard propellant. (Sie, 1972; *US Army Research & Development News Magazine,* July–August, 1973)

Cartridge cases, however, serve many purposes, including sealing the chamber, protecting the propellant from contamination, and serving as a flame barrier, as a heat remover, and as packaging during handling and loading (Davis, 1973). Caseless systems must provide for these other functions in some other way. For high rate-of-fire weapons this may require more complex mechanisms which are not justified except where weight savings are especially critical (as in air superiority aircraft) (Davis, 1973). For more general use, aluminium, plastic and aluminium–plastic composite ammunition cases are being investigated.

None of these developments in itself has legal or humanitarian implications, but a further development may have such implications. Most bullets are made by first drawing out the copper-alloy or steel jacket and then filling it with lead from the rear. The lead core does not usually separate from the jacket unless the bullet tumbles significantly. In some modern bullets, the core is injected from the tip instead of the base. This enables the tail of the bullet to be manufactured with greater precision, increasing the accuracy of the bullet. These bullets have proved very successful in shooting competitions. In a soft target, however, the open tip means that these bullets will function as dumdum bullets. The fear has been expressed that the step from military shooting competitions to sniping is a small one and that in this way such bullets may enter into military service.

XII. Summary and conclusions

By the end of the past century, high explosive propellants, percussion-fired cartridges, and automatic weapons were coming into use. The effects of high velocity rifle bullets were the subject of intensive study at that time. The powerful propellants, which gave a bullet a range of several kilometres, made a small bullet a deadly projectile at close range, but jacketed bullets would frequently pass right through the victim, causing in many instances milder wounds than the older lead bullets.

The principal reason for developing high velocity ammunition was to attain increased range, but there is a widespread view that the full-power 7.62 mm ammunition in use by most countries since the turn of the century is unnecessarily powerful for modern combat conditions. For short range, low velocity pistols and machine-pistols (sub-machine-guns) have been used until the present. Since World War II there has been a strong trend towards replacing both long range rifles and light machine-guns and machine-pistols with intermediate range automatic rifles.

There have been two approaches to designing intermediate range weapons. One is to reduce the *power* of the cartridge, thereby reducing its size and recoil and therefore the weight of the gun. Reduced-power bullets, in general, have less wounding power than full-power cartridges. The second approach is to reduce the *calibre* but to increase the velocity. Small calibre, high velocity bullets have about the same range as reduced-power bullets but some types – including that most widely used – are more inclined to tumble early in the wound, and to deform or disintegrate, depositing more of their energy.

From the military point of view, the principal advantage of the reduced-power approach is that the projectile maintains its velocity better than the reduced-calibre projectile and, particularly with a steel core, may penetrate a target better at longer ranges. It is thus relatively suitable for use in the light or even medium machine-gun role. The principal advantage of the reduced calibre, higher velocity projectile, apart from a greater weight saving, is its flat trajectory, which increases accuracy of shooting and decreases dispersion at longer ranges.

Most armed forces of the NATO alliance, as well as many others, have adopted the full-power 7.62 mm NATO round as standard. They are now searching for a less powerful alternative, such as the US 5.56 mm round. But opinion remains divided as to whether this round is suitable for the machine-gun role. Some alternatives have a smaller calibre; others have the same calibre but a heavier bullet; while yet other possible machine-gun rounds have larger calibres, for example, 6 mm. Clearly, it is difficult to find a single weapon which adequately performs all the tasks expected of a pistol, sub-machine-gun, rifle and machine-gun.

It is equally difficult to conceive of a single bullet/weapon combination which is fully acceptable from a humanitarian point of view, since more powerful ammunition intended for long range will always tend to cause unnecessarily severe wounds if used at short range.[9] Therefore, from the humanitarian point of view, the combination of low-powered ammunition for short range and high-powered ammunition for long range is preferable to the present trend towards intermediate-power weapons for both short and longer ranges.

Any attempt to find a compromise solution to the conflicting military considerations should not be at the expense of humanitarian concerns. If a single type of ammunition is adopted for the several military roles, it should be designed to keep the probability of excessive injury at close range to a minimum. This requires that the bullet should be designed according to the following criteria: (*a*) the bullet should not deform or disintegrate on impact; and (*b*) the bullet should not yaw significantly within 140 mm of a medium having the density of human tissue.

These criteria apply equally to pistol ammunition. In addition, it might be argued that a limitation on the maximum velocity of about 400 m/s for pistol ammunition and 800 m/s for rifle ammunition should be determined.

Table 4.12. Safety zones for small arms with regard to military personnel in training and combat conditions [a]

Weapon	Dispersion around target *m*	Safety zone beyond target *m*
Training		
Assault rifle	10	2 000–3 500
Light or medium machine-gun		
With risk of ricochet	150–200	2 000–3 500
Combat		
Assault rifle	> 3	1 400
Machine-gun	> 3	1 500

[a] Assumes target fired upon at average combat range of 200 m.

Source: Swedish military regulations.

The power of long-range rifles and machine-guns also makes them unsuitable for use, whether by military or police forces, in inhabited areas, due to the danger of indiscriminate effects. From table 4.12 it can be seen that there is a risk zone of several thousand metres associated with the use of small arms ammunition.

Notes to Chapter 4

1. German designers working at the Centro de Estudios Tecnicos de Materiales Especiales (CETME) in Spain after World War II utilized a 7.92 × 41 mm cartridge and the Belgian Fabrique Nationale made a version of its FAL rifle for it.
2. These figures are calculated from data obtained from a Swiss Army study carried out in association with Austrian and Swedish experts and presented at the Lugano Conference of Government Experts in Switzerland, 1976.
3. This figure is calculated from data obtained from a US Department of Defense study presented at the Lugano Conference of Government Experts (ICRC, 1976).
4. The ORO study, written at the time of the Korean War, put it as follows: 'It appears almost certain that future large-scale ground operations will involve a numerically superior enemy . . . to increase each infantryman's capability with respect to defensive rifle fire becomes highly desirable' (Hitchman, 1952, p. 6).

113

5. In 1954 Armalite produced the AR-5, a bolt action 'survival rifle' using the .22 in (5.6 mm) *Hornet* ammunition which was later modified for use in the AR-15 (Hobart, 1971*b*).

6. The apparently greater enthusiasm of the US Air Force for an infantry weapon was later explained by a retired US Air Force officer who was responsible for liaison with the US Central Intelligence Agency (CIA). A US Army officer who was an advocate of the gun had trouble getting his service to adopt it; a fellow officer engaged in a secret project was also interested. Together they arranged for the manufacturer to demonstrate the weapon to a mixed group of officers from the Army and Air Force. Afterwards there were meetings at a special section of the office of the Secretary of Defense with an official having long experience of special operations. 'The meeting ended with a consensus that the gun should be purchased in trial numbers by the Air Force for security reasons for use by the Air Force Air Police Units. Later, the Air Force did purchase tens of thousands of the new weapons, and they disappeared into the security-covered inventory of the CIA' (Prouty, 1972).

7. 'In the late 1950s we began to arm, resupply and advise the Meo, and their hill-tribe peers, the Lao Teung, and the Yao ... Initially this program was master-minded under the auspices of the US Special Forces "white star" teams that were attached directly to the field units and co-ordinated guerrilla activities. Then after the restrictions placed on overt U.S. military involvement in Laos by the Geneva Accords of 1962, the role of advising the guerrilla forces fell under the operational wing of the CIA' (Ronald J. Rickenbach, former refugee officer with the US Agency for International Development in Laos; in US Senate Committee on the Judiciary, 1970).

8. In July 1968, US Secretary of Defense Clifford announced: 'We will be turning out M-16s at a substantially more rapid rate and giving them to all ARVN (South Vietnamese Army), even at the expense of our own forces, just as soon as we can' (*Keesing's Contemporary Archives*, 1968, p. 23139).

9. This problem was already appreciated by military experts at the end of the past century when bullets of the 7.62 mm class were first adopted. A British official report of a trial of various dumdum bullets stated: 'Inspector General of Ordnance remarked that a bullet was required which ... should be capable of stopping, at a moderate range, a horse in a charge of cavalry or a man on foot, while retaining, as far as might be, accuracy at all ranges and power of penetration, and at the same time not infringing the spirit of St. Petersburg. It was doubtful whether any bullet would meet the conditions required, which would not inflict a severe wound at short ranges' (UK War Office, 1898).

Appendix 4A

Principal manufacturers of military small arms ammunition

Country	Factory	Identifying code
Australia	Footscray	MF
Austria	Hirtenberger	H
	Österreichische Jagdpatronenfabrik	OJP
Argentina	..	FAMAP
	..	FMC
	..	FMCSF
	..	FMMAP
	..	FMSF
	..	FMSL
	..	IMPA
	Cartucheria Orbea	ORBEA
Belgium	Fabrique Nationale	FN
	Poudrières Réunies de Belgique	PRB
Brazil	..	CBC
	..	FNCM
	..	FR
	..	R
Bulgaria	..	10
Canada	Dominion Arsenal	DA, DAC
	Defence Industries	DI
	Dominion Cartridge Company	DC
	Industrie Valcartier	IVI
Chile	..	FAMAE
	..	FME
	..	FMEP
	..	FMG
China	..	11
	..	31
	..	41
	..	61
	..	71
	..	81
	..	121
	..	321
	..	451
	..	(661)
	..	671
	..	791
	..	21215

Country	Factory	Identifying code
Colombia	. .	IM
Czechoslovakia	. .	AYM
	. .	BXN
	. .	Z
	. .	ZV
	. .	0
Denmark	Ammunitionsarsenalet	AA, AMA
	Haerens Ammunitionsarsenalet	HA
Dominican Republic	San Cristobel	AC
	. .	RD
Finland	Lapua	Lapua, VPT
	Sako	S, SAKO, SO
France	Atelier de Construction de Tarbes	TS
	Le Mans	LM
	Manhurin	MR
	Etablissement Rey à Nimes	RY
	Gevelot (formerly SFM)	SF
	Toulouse Arsenal	TE
	Valence	VE
Germany, Federal Republic of	Dynamit AG	DAG
	Deutsche Waffen und Munitionsfabrik	DWM
	Genschow	G, GECO
	Heckler & Koch	HK
	Industrie Werke Karlsruhe	IWK
	Maschinenfabrik Elisenhütte, Hessen	MEN
	Manusear, Budingen	MS
	RWS, Nuremberg	RWS
German Democratic Republic	. .	04
	. .	05
	. .	22
Greece	Greek Powder and Cartridge Company	EK, EMK, HXP
Hungary	. .	23
India	Kirkee	KF
	. .	OFV
Indonesia	. .	AD
	. .	PSM
Israel	. .	AE
	. .	E
	Israel Military Industries	IMI
	. .	TA

116

Country	Factory	Identifying code
Italy	Bombrini Parodi Delfini	AOC, BPD
	Fiocchi	GFL
	Leon Beaux	LBC
	Societa Metallurgica Italiana	SMI, SYI
Japan	..	JAO
	..	JTE
	..	TE
Korea, North	..	93
Korea, South	Pusan	KA
Malaysia	..	MAL
Mexico	Fabrica Nacional de Municiones	FNM
	..	CDM
Morocco	Fabrique Nationale	FNAM
	..	MNAM
Netherlands	Artillerie Inrichtingen	AI
	Eurometaal, Zandam	EMZ
	Nederland Wapen & Munitiefabriek	NWM
New Zealand	Colonial Ammunition Company	CAC
Nigeria	Ordnance Factory, Nigeria	OFN
Norway	Raufoss Arsenal	RA, AYR
Pakistan	Pakistan Ordnance Factory	POK
Peru	..	FAME
Philippines	..	RPA
Poland	..	21
	..	343
Portugal	..	ASC
	Fabrica Nacional de Municiones de Armas	FNM
Romania		CMC
	..	RPR
	..	21
	..	22
	..	23
Singapore	Chartered Industries	CIS, GB
	Singapore Arsenal	SGA
South Africa	..	A.74
	Pretoria Metal Pressings	PMP
	South African Mint	SAM
Spain	Palencia Arsenal	FNP, P
	Toledo	FNT, T
	..	MMM
	Seville Arsenal	PS, S
	..	SBLT
	Sociedad Santa Barbara	SB

Country	Factory	Identifying code
Sweden	..	AMF
	Karlsborg	K
	Förenade Fabriksverken	FFV
	..	SM
Switzerland	Altdorf	A
	Thun	T
	Oerlikon	OE
Thailand	Royal Thai Arsenal	RTA
Turkey	..	MKE
UK	British Manufacturing & Research Co.	B.MARCO
	Greenwood & Batley	GB
	Imperial Chemical Industries (Kynoch)	ICI,K
	Radway Green Royal Ordnance Factory	RG
	Royal Laboratory, Woolwich	RL
	Spennymore Royal Ordnance Factory	SR
USA	Frankford Arsenal	FA
	Federal Cartridge Company	FC
	Lake City Arsenal	LC
	Military Armament Corporation	MAC
	Remington Arms Company	RA
	Remington UMC	Rem-UMC
	Twin Cities Ordnance Plant	TW
	Winchester Repeating Arms Co.	WRA
	Winchester-Western Company	W-W
USSR	..	3
	..	10
	..	17
	..	30
	..	38
	..	46
	..	50
	..	58
	..	60
	..	179
	..	(184)
	..	188
	..	270
	..	304
	..	513
	..	529
	..	539
	..	540
	..	541
	..	543
	..	545
	..	547
	..	611

Country	Factory	Identifying code
USSR (*continued*)	..	710
	..	711
Yugoslavia	..	IK
	..	NK
	..	NNY
	..	NR
	..	PP
	..	PPU
	..	PPL
	..	PPYU
	..	11
	..	12
	..	14

Source: Archer (1976).

5. Fragmentation weapons

Superior numerals, thus [5], refer to notes on pages 162–163.

I. Wounding effects of fragmentation weapons

Anti-personnel fragmentation munitions produce a large number of fast-moving fragments of material intended to incapacitate several people simultaneously. They give rise to the questions: How much incapacitation is 'enough'? And, how many people is it 'enough' to incapacitate, both from the military and humanitarian points of view?

The commonest type of fragmentation munition is one which derives its 'splinters' from the break-up of a metal case ('body') by detonation of an explosive charge contained within it. Other fragmentation munitions include canisters containing round lead shot, steel balls or other small projectiles, which rupture at the muzzle of a gun, dispersing the contents as from a shot-gun shell; shrapnel projectiles, similar to canisters, but which open in the air; and shaped-charge/fragmentation munitions combining a shaped charge (or 'hollow charge') for armour penetration and a metal case whose fragments can incapacitate people nearby.

Fragmentation weapons have been known for centuries. Since World War II, two trends have been outstanding: (*a*) an increase in the number of fragments produced by a munition, with a concomitant decrease in their size; and (*b*) the emergence of delivery systems for dispersing large numbers of small fragmentation munitions (essentially grenades) over wide areas. Both trends contribute to the increased effectiveness of modern fragmentation munitions as compared with those of World War II. An increase in the number of fragments means an increase in the probability of hitting people nearby, and the improvement in delivery systems means that people will be hit over a greater area (Wulff *et al.*, 1973; ICRC, 1973, 1974).

Increases in the numbers of fragments in high explosive munitions are brought about principally by changes in the explosive charge and in the material and construction of the case. Increases in area coverage are brought about by the use of bomblets (small bombs) dispersed from bomb dispensers, shells or rocket warheads.

Effectiveness calculations for fragmentation munitions use the same basic formula as for small arms ammunition (chapter 3, pp. 57–59) but they consider hits on several people spread out over an area rather than hits on single persons.

For many years it was commonly accepted that a missile with approximately 80 J of kinetic energy was capable of producing a casualty upon hitting the body. A modern refinement of this criterion, accepted in France, states that an effective fragment is one that has a penetration energy of 1.5 J per square millimetre. Such a criterion has the virtue of simplicity and can readily be stated in terms of the wooden board penetration tests, widely used in Europe. For example, an effective fragment, as defined in the French criterion, will penetrate 41 mm of poplar wood or 37 mm of pine (French & Callender, 1962; Le Gall, 1974; Crevecoeur, 1973; Hobart, 1974).

In the USA, the 78 J criterion and the pine board penetration test have been superseded by elaborate instrumented panel tests and by casualty criteria which take into account the time within which a person is to be incapacitated. There is, for example, a 30-second incapacitation criterion which can be used in connection with small arms ammunition (US Military Academy, 1968–9; Hobart, 1974).

Once a casualty criterion is decided upon, the effectiveness of a weapon can be calculated from the expected numbers, masses and velocities of fragments at various distances from the point of explosion. Effectiveness can be stated in terms of a 'lethal area', which is obtained by integrating the probability of incapacitation over the area within which there are effective fragments.[1]

Once the lethal area of a munition is known, it can be used to determine how many casualties the munition will inflict. If people are distributed uniformly over the target area with a density of u people per unit area, the expected number of casualties due to a single warhead, N, will be equal to the product of the lethal area, A_L and the density of people:

$$N = A_L.u$$

The US Army defines the 'effective casualty radius' of a fragmentation munition as 'the radius of a circle about the point of detonation in which it may normally be expected that 50 per cent of the exposed personnel will become casualties' (US Department of the Army, 1966).

These measures of effectiveness, however, give little idea of the wounding effects of fragmentation munitions on individuals. As in the case of the development of small arms, there appears to be only a limited consideration of medical data in the design of weapons. In the case of the multiple wounds caused by fragmentation weapons these data are extremely difficult to interpret in the relatively simple mathematical formula required by the weapon designer. Therefore the weapon designer generally ignores this problem and adopts a simple criterion of the wounding power of a single fragment. He then seeks to design a munition capable of approaching an optimum distribution of such fragments in a given space.

Medical studies have shown that while fragmentation munitions are responsible for the greatest proportion of combat casualties, the mortality of these casualties is less than the mortality due to bullet wounds. This is not surprising since fragmentation munitions are designed to maximize hit probability rather than incapacitation.

It should also be recalled that the bullets currently in use tend to be used at ranges substantially less than the range for which they are designed to incapacitate.

II. Further design considerations

A munition design incorporates 'trade-offs' between such factors as effectiveness, cost, ease of manufacture, safety and reliability. For example, tungsten fragments will penetrate metal targets better than steel fragments, so the higher cost of the tungsten will be justified if fewer rounds are needed. A shell whose body is a steel coil may fragment better than an ordinary steel shell, but the coiled body may weaken the shell to the point where it ruptures when fired from a gun.

The effect of the trend towards more and smaller fragments is to increase the probability that persons within the area of effect will be hit by one or more fragments, since the hit probability, $P(H)$, is mainly a function of the number (or density) of fragments in space. The smaller fragments have higher initial velocities than the larger fragments of older munitions, but the smaller fragments have a shorter effective range. Therefore these smaller modern fragments have a lower conditional incapacitation probability $P(I|H)$, that is, the probability that a given hit, H, will actually incapacitate, I. The greater likelihood of multiple wounding helps to offset the reduced wounding effect of single fragments.[2]

Fragmentation munitions are often divided into two classes: *natural fragmentation* munitions, which have a simple metal case, and *controlled fragmentation* munitions, where the case is designed to produce uniform fragments of a predetermined size and shape. In natural fragmentation, fragment sizes can be decreased by the proper selection of casing materials, and fragment shapes can to some extent be influenced as well. In controlled fragmentation, fragment shapes and sizes are determined by scoring or moulding grooves in the case, by the use of spirals of notched wire, or by the use of pre-formed fragments. All of these techniques add to the cost of a munition.

Since World War II, naturally fragmenting munitions with improved fragmentation characteristics have been developed using two casing materials, cast irons and high fragmentation steels. Grey cast iron had been used in British shells in World War II, but it pulverized if used with TNT or a higher-brisance explosive. In the United States interest in cast irons revived in 1950 when US forces in Korea were bombarded with Chinese grey iron mortar shells that were more effective than their own mortar shells. With this stimulus, US ordnance engineers examined a number of types of cast iron and selected pearlitic malleable iron and, later, ductile iron (also known as nodular graphitic iron) and ferritic malleable iron for use in mortar shells and certain other munitions (tables 5.3 and 5.4). Some experimental work was also done on cast-iron artillery shells.

In the United States and elsewhere there has also been interest in high fragmentation steel for natural fragmentation munitions. Sweden has a 155 mm high fragmentation steel artillery shell (table 5.4), and Australia has cooperated with the United States in a joint research project on fragmentation.

Modern controlled fragmentation munitions derived largely from developments that took place in the 1950s, a time when there was interest in fragmentation warheads in both anti-aircraft and anti-personnel munitions. Grooved casings, notched wire and pre-formed steel balls are among the techniques used.

In one important study (patent submitted in 1958), three US Navy scientists devised a multi-walled shell with helical grooves in a cross-hatched pattern cut in the inside surface of each wall. An experimental grooved two-walled shell yielded 7 per cent more fragments than a comparable shell with no grooves; the fragments were smaller, and there was less dust (pulverized casing material) (US patent no. 3,566,794, 2 March 1971).

Another means of making a fragmentation munition more effective is to increase the velocity of the fragments. The initial velocity of fragments can, in principle, be changed by using an explosive of higher brisance, or by increasing the charge-to-mass ratio (using a thinner-walled case and packing it with more explosive).

In practice, since World War II such changes have been much less important than changes in the construction and materials of casings. The shape of a munition is usually dictated by factors other than effectiveness. Explosives have remained essentially the same since World War II (TNT and cyclotol, a mixture of RDX and TNT, are among the commonest). A thinner wall, although making for faster – and smaller – fragments, also means that there is less total mass of metal available for target destruction.

The striking velocities of fragments can be enhanced by improvements in aerodynamic shape; here the trade-off is a decline in the wounding effect at low velocity, associated with the shape. A polished steel ball slows down less rapidly in air than a jagged fragment of the same mass, and it therefore has a greater striking velocity, but a jagged fragment may be more readily retarded in flesh.

Flechettes pose a similar problem: they travel readily through the air, but below a certain velocity they can also pass straight through the body without causing much harm, unless they are adapted to inflict worse wounds. At high velocities, flechettes may buckle on impact and cause severe injury (see p. 106).

Square wire, wound around an explosive charge and notched on the inside surface, was used in grenades developed in the 1950s (tables 5.1 and 5.2). This technique may be compared with the spirals of steel bar stock that were used in the casings of World War II fragmentation bombs and with the grooved ring shell developed for test purposes in the late 1940s.

Pre-formed rectangular and spherical pellets have been used in grenades, bomblets and other munitions. They are comparable with similar shapes used earlier in canister and shrapnel ammunition. In the 1930s the Swedish Army introduced an artillery shell containing steel balls and in the USA an experimental hand-grenade with steel balls was developed in 1951 (Dunn & Sterne, 1952).

Since shrapnel-type munitions using small spheres had tended to fall into disfavour during the first half of the twentieth century, it is interesting to consider the reasons for their apparent re-emergence in the second half. As with any attempt to force many objects through a bottle-neck, the earlier shrapnel designs tended to dissipate much of the propelling energy in the competition of the projectiles to emerge from the canister. The lead balls originally used were frequently deformed in the process, which further increased the rate at which their velocity retarded in flight, although they caused serious wounds at short ranges. By the time the individual projectiles hit the target they had a relatively low energy. Newer designs try to avoid bottle-necks and to use steel balls which are less likely to deform and can stand up to the forces exerted by more powerful explosives. The result is that the steel balls projected by modern munitions have a high velocity, whereas those projected by older munitions had a low velocity. High velocity spheres and fragments are capable of causing large soft-tissue wounds, shattered bones and other severe injuries (Mendelson & Glover, 1967; Charters & Charters, 1976).

Another means of making a fragmentation munition more effective, especially against people who are prone or in foxholes or trenches, is to make the munition explode above the ground. This is done by making the munition bound in the air before exploding, or by detonating it by means of a time fuze or a proximity fuze before it hits the ground. Proximity fuzes are coming into increasing use as their cost is reduced through innovations in microcircuitry and production techniques.

III. Modern types of fragmentation munition

The commonest fragmentation munition is still the conventional 'HE', or high explosive, munition, consisting of an explosive charge enclosed in a metal case. When the explosive is detonated, the case breaks into fragments which are hurled outwards at high velocity. The design features of a high explosive munition can be varied to increase either the blast effect or the fragmentation effect; but for most high explosive munitions, the fragmentation effect is more important in damaging targets. Ordinary high explosive munitions occur as hand-grenades, mortar and artillery shell, rocket and guided missile warheads, bombs and mines.

Other designs, of varying importance, for fragmentation munitions are:

1. a fragmentation face in front of a layer of explosive, as in the US Claymore mine (chapter 8);

2. 'mass-focus' designs consisting of a layer of high explosive with a fragmentation face on either side, something like a pancake; the fragments are projected outward from each face in a slightly conical pattern. Mass-focus warheads have been in development since the 1960s;

3. end-projection warheads in which fragments are propelled forward from the nose of the munition by means of a high explosive or a propellant charge; end-projection warheads were in development in the mid-1960s as air-to-surface munitions for close support of ground troops;

4. canister or shot-gun-type ammunition in which pre-formed fragments are ejected from a shell, their velocity being essentially that imparted to the shell by the gun or other projecting device. Among such munitions are ordinary shot-gun ammunition and canisters and shrapnel shell. A similar munition is the US Mk-44 missile cluster adapter, or Lazy Dog, in which 10 000 small, solid, bomb-shaped iron missiles are dropped from an aircraft; their downward velocity is imparted by gravity;

5. shaped charge or 'hollow charge' munitions consisting of a block of high

124

explosive, of which the nose is hollow and lined with metal, the cavity of which is typically in the shape of a cone. Detonation from the base converts part of the metal liner into a forward-moving jet of metal particles that will bore through armour plate or concrete and kill or injure people on the other side as well as ignite fuel and explosives. Shaped-charge munitions are meant primarily for use against tanks, armoured vehicles, and concrete fortifications; if they are enclosed in a fragmentation case, people outside the tank or other hard target under attack will also be hit. Further, they may also be used together with fragmentation warheads in mixed munitions of the cluster-bomb type.

IV. Grenades

Hand-grenades were used as early as the fifteenth century. They went out of use for a time but were revived with the Russo–Japanese War of 1904 and World War I (Hobart, 1974). They are primarily intended for close-range infantry combat, providing the infantry with a weapon with limited area coverage.

The British Mills grenade of World War I and the similar US Mk-2 and Soviet F-1 grenades were still widely used in World War II and for many years after. All three grenades were barrel-shaped and had a heavy cast-iron body with deep exterior grooves in a grid pattern. *Jane's Infantry Weapons 1975* states with reference to one grenade of this type, the British no. 36M hand-grenade, that

> the original idea was that the body would break up into pieces corresponding to the notched segments but it was found that the fragment size is in no way related to the notches and in fact the grenade produces a relatively limited number of very large fragments and also a lot of cast iron dust. (Hobart, 1974, p. 588)

At the same time, as the re-examination of the Mills-type grenade showed, the fuze and the base plug remained relatively intact and could be projected as far as 200 m on explosion. If the grenade landed on its side, as usually happened, many of the casing fragments would shoot up into the air or down into the ground, while the fuze and base plug were projected so far as to endanger the thrower (Hobart, 1974; Crevecoeur, 1973).

The inadequacies of the Mills grenade led to the re-examination of design and performance characteristics. Effectiveness close to the point of explosion, it was recognized, should be combined with an absence of dangerous fragments further away. Probably the first country to re-examine its hand-grenade was the USA when, as a result of experience gained during the Korean War, the US Army formulated a demand for a grenade that would be as dangerous as possible within 5 m of the point of explosion and as safe as possible to the thrower (Dunn & Sterne, 1952). A contrast of this sort is achieved in modern grenade designs by producing a large number of small fragments with sufficient velocity to be incapacitating close to the point of explosion but which are so small that they will be stopped by air resistance before they travel as far as the throwing range of the grenade.

It is usual to assume that a fragment weighing between 0.2 and 0.65 g and with a kinetic energy of approximately 80 J is sufficient to incapacitate a man. Modern grenade designs attempt to produce fragments of that calibre at a density of one per square metre some 5–10 m from the point of explosion.

In order to test these characteristics of grenades it is usual to surround a grenade with pine boards at varying distances. In one such study, using the Belgian PRB-423 grenade, one perforation per square metre was reported at 9.5 m range whereas at 20 m there was less than a 10 per cent chance of causing a perforation. At 4 m range there was an average of over six perforations (Crevecoeur, 1973).

The US M-26 series grenade, developed in the 1950s and incorporating a coil of notched steel wire around a high explosive charge, was probably the first of the new grenade designs. In other countries, the redesign of hand-grenades has resulted in grenades in a variety of shapes, and sizes as small as 120 g (in the Dutch V-40 'mini' grenade). Several fragmentation techniques are used, including notched wire, as in the US M-26 series grenade and the Belgian PRB-423 grenade; nodular cast iron, as in the Argentinian FMK-2 grenade; notches on the interior surface of the case, as in the Dutch 'mini' grenade; and small metal balls cast in a plastic matrix surrounding an explosive charge, as in the German Diehl DM-51 grenade, which contains 5 900 2-mm balls (table 5.1).

Several factors are taken into account in hand-grenade designs. The shape of a grenade affects the throwing characteristics, directional pattern and initial velocity of the projected fragments. Some modern grenades are so designed that fragments are projected from the bottom as well as the sides, thus improving the performance if the grenade lands on its side. The Belgian PRB-423 grenade, for example, has notched wire around the side and steel balls in the base and near the top. Hand-grenades normally have fuzes that function after a fixed time delay of several seconds. Some modern grenades have fuzes that also function on impact, so that an enemy soldier cannot pick up the grenade and toss it back (Crevecoeur, 1973; Hobart, 1974; Le Gall, 1974; Crossman, 1966).

Older grenades usually weighed 400–700 g but there is a tendency to reduce the weight. A standing soldier can throw a 400 g grenade about 30 m, and a 250 g grenade about 40 m (Crevecoeur, 1973). More of the smaller grenades can be carried and each one has only a slightly smaller lethal area. Hobart (1974) says 'it can be argued that the lighter grenades ... will, over several engagements, produce more casualties than the same weight of heavier grenades' (p. 522).[3]

Fragmentation grenades are often known as 'defensive' grenades in contrast to 'offensive' grenades, which produce blast without fragmentation and are therefore effective over a narrower area and can safely be thrown by troops as they advance. Several modern grenades consist of a cylindrical-shaped 'offensive' grenade over which a fragmentation coil or cylinder can be slipped, converting it into a 'defensive' grenade. Some hand-grenades are designed so as to be readily convertible into rifle grenades.

126

Table 5.1. Examples of hand and rifle grenades

Producing country and designation	Weight g	Manufacturer	Casualty agent	Remarks
Argentina				
FMK2	165	Fabricaciones Militares	Nodular iron case	Can be rifle-projected
Austria				
HdGr 69	485	Arges	3 500 steel balls (in plastic matrix)	
HdGr0 69	220	Arges	Blast	
Belgium				
PRB-8	440	Poudrières Réunies de Belgique (PRB)	Notched 4 mm square wire	Produces c. 500 0.55-g fragments; impact fuze
PRB-7	116	PRB	Blast	Wire produces c. 900 0.1-g fragments; casualty radius, 9 m
PRB-423	235	PRB	Notched wire; 520 1-g steel balls in base and upper part	
PRB-446	115	PRB	Blast	
PRB-404	..	PRB	Notched steel coil	Casualty radius, over 14 m; convertible into offensive or rifle grenade
PRB-434	555	PRB	Notched steel coil	Rifle grenade
PRB-103	665	PRB	Notched wire	c. 500 fragments; casualty radius, 40 m; polyvalent: hand/rifle, offensive/defensive
MECAR 50 mm	220	Mecar SA	900 steel balls	Casualty radius, 50 m
HE-RFL-60N	470	Mecar SA	500-plus fragments	Casualty radius, 30 m
FRG-RFL-40N	220	Mecar SA	300 fragments	
FRG-RFL-40BT (5.56 mm)	255	Mecar SA	300 fragments	Fired by 5.56 mm rifle; casualty radius, 30 m
FRG-RFL-40BT (7.62 mm)	325	Mecar SA	300 fragments	Casualty radius, 30 m; fired by 7.62 mm rifle

Table 5.1 (*continued*)

Producing country and designation	Weight g	Manufacturer	Casualty agent	Remarks
Belgium (*continued*)				
AP 32 Z	515	Fabrique Nationale, Herstal	Steel fragments	Casualty radius, 20 m; combined anti-vehicle/anti-personnel; rifle grenade
AP 32 ZA	495	FN	1 000 spheres, 3.2 mm diam.	Casualty radius, 20 m
AP 32 ZB	495	FN	1 250 fragments	Casualty radius, 20 m
China				
Type 42	385	State factories	Plain steel case	Copy of Soviet RG-42
Type 1	581	State factories	Cast iron	Copy of Soviet F-1 (World War II)
Type 59	308	State factories	Serrated steel	Similar to Soviet RGD-5
M-32	310	State factories	Steel case	Similar to Soviet RGD-5
Czechoslovakia				
RG-4	300	State factories	Steel case/cast-iron jacket	Has upper and lower bursting charges; convertible into defensive grenade by addition of cast-iron jacket; casualty range, 15–25 m
RG-34	300	State factories	Steel case/cast-iron jacket	Cast-iron jacket converts into defensive grenade; casualty radius, 15–25 m
France				
MDF	414	Losfeld	Controlled fragmentation; 1 000 fragments	Impact/delay fuze; convertible into offensive or rifle grenade
M-1948	485	..	Metal fragments	Rifle grenade
M-1952	500	..	Metal fragments	Rifle grenade
M-1937	140	Luchaire	Blast	Aluminium body

DM-46	540	Luchaire	Cast-iron fragments	Similar configuration to M-1937
STRIM F1 40 mm	510	Luchaire	Steel fragments	Anti-personnel/anti-vehicle rifle grenade; casualty radius, 100 m
A-45	556	Luchaire	Steel fragments (plus shaped charge)	Anti-personnel/anti-vehicle rifle grenade; under development (1976)
Alsetex No. 1	140	Société Alsacienne d'Etudes et d'Exploitation (Alsetex)	Blast, thin metal case	
Alsetex No. 2	540	Alsetex	Thick metal case	Plastic case (small size)
Alsetex No. 3	220	Alsetex	Blast	Plastic case (large size)
Alsetex No. 4	310	Alsetex	Blast	
FR Germany				
M-DN11	470	Diehl	3 800 2.5–3 mm steel balls	Delay fuze
M-DN21	225	Diehl	2 200 2.0–2.3 mm balls	Delay fuze
M-DN31	248	Diehl	3 000 2.0–2.3 mm balls	Delay fuze
DM-51	480	Diehl	5 900 2-mm metal balls	Convertible into offensive grenade; adopted by German Army
DT-11B1	330	..	Blast	
Hungary				
M-42	310	State factories	Steel fragments	World War II model, still in service; several grenades can be screwed together to form demolition device
Israel				
No. 14	325	..	Blast	Paper case
M-26	426	..	Notched steel coil, 1 000 fragments	US model, licensed production
Netherlands				
No. 1	..	..	Cast iron	
No. 1C1	670	..	Cast iron	Similar to above but with different fuze assembly

Table 5.1 (*continued*)

Producing country and designation	Weight g	Manufacturer	Casualty agent	Remarks
Netherlands (*continued*)				
Mk 2	630	..	Cast iron, notched	Copy of US Mk 2
No. 13	475	..	Blast	Tin-plate body
No. 17	475	..	Blast	Plastic body
EMZ	330	Eurometaal	c. 2 100 steel balls and fragments	Plastic body
V40 Mini-grenade	120	NWM de Kruithoorn	Notched steel body, c. 380 incapacitating fragments	
Poland				
Model 31	..	State factories	Cast iron	Similar to Soviet F1
F 1/N60	630	State factories	Notched cast iron	Adaptation of Soviet F1 for use as rifle grenade
Spain				
PO I	285	Plasticas Oramile (PO)	Blast	Plastic case
PO II	255	PO	Light metal body	Offensive/defensive
PO III	325	PO	Metal coil	
POM-I	326	PO	Metal coil	Development of PO III
POM-II-R		PO	Blast; optional steel collar	
Posare VI	170	..	Blast	'Mini' grenade
Posare VII	210	..	Blast; optional metal coil sleeve	
E.A. M5	290 (500)	Explosives Alaveses SA	Blast; optional metal sleeve	Delayed action or impact fuze; can be rifle-launched
G.L. Type II, model 63B	510	Instalaza	Steel fragments and shaped charge	Combined anti-vehicle/anti-personnel rifle grenade; casualty radius, 6 m
Sweden				
FFV 542	460	Försvarets fabriksverk	Controlled fragmentation, 500 × 0.02–0.05 g fragments	Impact/delay fuze

UK				
L2 A1	510	Royal Ordnance Factory	Notched steel wire	Produces c. 1 200 0.1–0.2 g fragments; similar to US M26 grenade
M-36	700	Royal Ordnance Factory	Cast iron	Obsolescent
USA				
M-26, M-61	454	US Army	Notched steel wire	Produces more than 1 000 fragments; effective casualty radius, 15 m
M-33, M-67	398	US Army	Steel body	Delay fuze; effective radius, 15 m
M-59, M-68	398	US Army	Steel body	Impact fuze
MK 3A2	227	..	Blast	
USSR				
RGD-5	310	State factories	Serrated liner	Effective radius, 15–20 m
RG-42	420	State factories	Sheet steel	Delay fuze; World War II model, still in service
Viet Nam				
..		State factories	Balls in aluminium matrix	
Yugoslavia				
M-69	600	State factories	Serrated steel	
M-60	520	State factories	Steel fragments	Rifle grenade

Sources: Archer (1976); Crevecoeur (1973); *Guide to Viet Cong Ammunition* (1971); Hobart (1974); *International Defense Review* **7**(2), April 1974, p. 233; US Departments of the Army and the Navy (1971).

Rifle grenades are adapted for projection from rifles. Their principal advantage is the greater distance (several hundred metres) they can be projected. A variety of rifle grenades are in service in many Western countries. Poland is the only Warsaw Treaty Organization country to equip its forces with a rifle grenade.

In the USA, the Army undertook in the 1950s to develop a weapon that would be 'capable of projecting the lethality of the 60 mm mortar cartridge to ranges between those of hand grenades and light mortars' (Chase, 1973, p. 1). The development led to the introduction around 1960 of the M-79 40-mm grenade launcher, a shoulder-fired, low-recoil weapon that launched projectiles at low velocity up to a range of 400 m. About four rounds per minute can be fired, each having an effective radius of about 5 m.

The ammunition originally used with the M-79 was the M-406 cartridge containing a spherical 'grenade' with a body of notched steel wire that broke into fragments weighing on average only 0.13 g and projected at over 1 000 m/s, giving the grenade a lethal radius of 5 m. With the widespread use of the M-79 in Viet Nam, many other cartridges were developed (table 5.2), and European manufacturers, such as FN in Belgium and Heckler & Koch in FR Germany, have produced launchers to fire them, as well as an increasing number of other 40 mm grenades. A 40 mm grenade launcher attachment was developed for the M-16A1 rifle, with 'the potential of making every rifleman a grenadier' (Chase, 1973, p. 2). An automatic low velocity launcher with a range of about 375 m was developed and tested in Viet Nam. High velocity launchers with a range of about 2 000 m were also developed for helicopter use (Chase, 1973; Hobart, 1974).

A Swiss company, Sarmac, has developed a light launcher, the *Falconet*, for a 24 mm grenade which contains 12 'bomb-shaped' darts with a range of about 700 m. A blast-effect grenade is also available. The US Army has been developing a 30 mm grenade.

A Belgian company, PRB, has produced a small disposable grenade launcher or mortar for its 404 anti-personnel fragmentation grenade and 422 blast grenade; the range claimed exceeds 400 m.

V. Mortar and recoilless rifle ammunition

Mortars were also used as early as the fifteenth century. They fell into disuse but were revived in the early twentieth century and are now a standard infantry weapon. Since World War II, the light-weight mortar, easily portable, has become a favourite weapon in guerrilla warfare.

The mortar has been defined as 'a high trajectory fire weapon in which the recoil force is passed directly to the ground through a baseplate' (Hobart, 1974). Although mortars may be rifled, they usually have a smooth bore and are loaded at the muzzle with a fin-stabilized shell and a propelling charge. Mortars are 'indirect fire' weapons, that is, they are fired in a high trajectory at a target which often cannot be seen by the user. Thus, in order to hit a particular target,

Table 5.2. Examples of 40 mm grenade ammunition for US M-79 launchers

Designation	Description	Remarks
M-381	High explosive	Contains spherical grenade
M-386	High explosive	Airburst cartridge, contains spherical grenade
M-397	High explosive	Contains spherical grenade, notched steel wire yielding 0.13 g fragments; effective casualty radius, 5 m
M-406	High explosive	
M-433	High explosive dual purpose (HEDP)	Shaped-charge fragmentation round; anti-personnel effectiveness equal to M-406; development began in early 1960s; standardized 1970; supersedes 40 mm light explosive cartridges
M-441	High explosive	Smokeless, flashless cartridge
M-463	High explosive	Shot-filled, effective to 40 m
XM576E1	Canister	Product improvement, contains more balls than XM576E1; never produced
XM576E2	Canister	
..	High explosive, rocket booster	Anti-personnel/anti-matériel cartridge; range, 1 000 m; in development (1973)
..	High explosive	Belgium/FN bouncing grenade; 450 × 0.135 g, 3.2-mm steel balls embedded in plastic in case; development cancelled in 1973

Sources: Chase (1973); Harvey (1972); Hobart (1974); US Army Munitions Command (1970); US Department of the Army (1972).

calculations have to be made with the aid of tables enabling the user to adjust the amount of propellant (and hence the range of the projectile) and the angle of elevation of the mortar tube.

Typical light mortars have a calibre up to 60 mm and weigh less than 20 kg. They fire a shell weighing between 450 and 1 350 g from 500 to 2 000 m. Medium mortars, of 60–100 mm calibre, fire a 3–7 kg bomb 2 000–6 000 m, and heavy mortars, exceeding 100 mm calibre, fire bombs of about 7 kg and more to a range of up to 13 km.

Because of their simplicity of construction and relative lightness, mortars can be transported to and used in areas inaccessible to vehicles. The high trajectory means that they can be fired from behind barriers, such as hills or forests, but this also means that they are liable to be affected by cross-winds and that they are very susceptible to radar tracking and subsequent counter-fire. Due to the system of projection, mortars are not as accurate as guns. In general they are not suitable for use against targets such as tanks, their main use being against troops in the open or in open trenches.

Several steps have been taken in the design of modern mortars to reduce the dispersion caused by the propulsion system. The increasing field use of electronic calculators and computers may improve the precision of aiming corrections necessary to compensate for weather conditions.

In addition to mortars of Soviet, Chinese, Czech, British and US manufacture, much of the world market is dominated by the French firm Hotchkiss-Brandt and the Finnish Tampella Company (table 5.3). Perhaps because of a more restrictive arms export policy in the home country, Tampella has a working arrangement with Israel to produce mortars under the 'Soltam' mark, which are sold to a very large number of countries (Hobart, 1974). Brandt, Tampella and the Israeli Government company IMI have introduced rocket-assisted mortar projectiles in the larger calibres. The incorporation of multiple sub-projectiles, perhaps including shaped-charge anti-tank grenades, in a single large-calibre mortar projectile has been suggested (Hobart, 1975a). Soltam has produced a self-propelled heavy mortar by mounting the Tampella 160 mm model on a Sherman tank chassis. The West German Army mounts an Israeli-made Tampella 120 mm mortar in an M-113 armoured personnel carrier and other vehicles, and the 120 mm Brandt mortar in an HS-30 armoured personnel carrier.

Mortar ammunition is designed to be of maximum effectiveness against personnel and light matériel, and mortar bombs are made of forged steel or cast iron of various kinds. According to Hirshman (1973), a new type of steel increases the lethality of the US 4.2 inch mortar by a factor of 1.58.

Proximity fuzes, such as those produced for the US Army by the Norwegian Raufoss Company, are said to improve the anti-personnel effectiveness of mortar ammunition by 100 per cent (Hobart, 1974).

Recoilless rifles are breech-loading, portable weapons mainly intended for attacking armoured vehicles. They may be fired from the ground or from light vehicles, and a number of anti-personnel rounds have been produced.

For its 57 mm recoilless rifles, the USA developed the T25E5 canister round, as well as the M306 and M306A1 high explosive rounds. For the 75 mm recoilless

Table 5.3. Examples of mortar ammunition

Producing country and ammunition calibre	Designation	Manufacturer	Body material	Remarks
Belgium				
60 mm	..	PRB	..	Controlled fragmentation
81 mm	..	PRB	..	Controlled fragmentation
Czechoslovakia				
82 mm	M48	State factories	..	
France				
60 mm	M61	Hotchkiss-Brandt	Pearlitic, malleable iron	..
60 mm	M72	Hotchkiss-Brandt	Pearlitic, malleable iron	..
60 mm	..	..	..	Canister round for Panhard mortar for armoured vehicles
81 mm	M57D	Hotchkiss-Brandt	Steel or pearlitic, malleable iron	..
81 mm	M61	Hotchkiss-Brandt	Steel or pearlitic, malleable iron	..
USSR				
82 mm	VO-832D	..	Cast iron	..
107 mm	..	..	..	Scaled-down model of 120 mm
120 mm	VOF-843A	..	Cast iron	..
United Kingdom				
51 mm	L1A1	..	..	Controlled fragmentation; in development
81 mm	L15	..	Ductile cast iron	..
USA				
60 mm	M49A3/A4	..	Pearlitic, malleable iron	Entered production c. 1966

Table 5.3 (*continued*)

Producing country and ammunition calibre	Designation	Manufacturer	Body material	Remarks
60 mm	M49A4E1	..	High fragmentation, A151 1340 steel	Thin-walled shell; in development (1973); 1.3 times effectiveness of the M49A4
60 mm	XM720	..	High fragmentation, A151 1340 steel	Same body as M49A4E1; in development for new 60 mm Light-weight Company Mortar System (1973)
81 mm	M374	..	Pearlitic, malleable iron	Approved for mass production in 1964; superseded by steel projectile
81 mm	M374A2	..	High fragmentation, A151 1340 steel	Entered production c. 1968
4.2 in	M329A2	..	High fragmentation, A151 1340 steel	In development (1973); 1.58 times effectiveness of standard 4.2 inch steel shell
4.2 in	M453	..	..	Anti-personnel shell containing 'submissiles' (probably bomblets)
107 mm	XM572	..	High fragmentation steel	In development 1965–67
Yugoslavia				
50 mm	M8	..	..	Modified British 2 inch Mk8
60 mm	M57	..	..	Copied from US M2 (World War II)
81 mm	M31	..	..	Based on French designs
81 mm	M68	..	..	
82 mm	BB1	..	..	
120 mm	..	..	..	

Sources: Archer (1976); *International Defense Review* (November 1967; August 1973; June 1975); UK Ministry of Defence (1974); *Guide to Viet Cong Ammunition* (1971).

Table 5.4. Examples of 'improved' fragmentation artillery ammunition

Producing country and ammunition calibre	Designation	Weapon	Body material	Remarks
Sweden				
84 mm	FFV41	Recoilless rifle	..	High explosive warhead with metal balls
155 mm	..	Howitzer	High fragmentation steel	
UK				
105 mm	..	Gun	Spheroidal graphite cast iron	In development
USA				
90 mm	XM591	Recoilless rifle	Pearlitic, malleable iron	Developed for Viet-Nam; not widely used
105 mm	M1	Howitzer	High fragmentation HF-1 steel	Accepted but not yet in production (1972)
105 mm	M548	..	High fragmentation A151 52100 steel	Rocket-assisted projectile
	XM710	Howitzer	High fragmentation steel	In development (1974)
5 in	..	..	High fragmentation, steel	Composition similar to A151 06 steel; specified in 1966
152 mm	XM657	Gun	High fragmentation A151 52100 steel	
155 mm	M549	Howitzer	High fragmentation A151 52100 steel	Rocket-assisted projectile
155 mm	XM708	Howitzer	High fragmentation HF-1 steel	In development (1973)

Sources: Jane's Infantry Weapons 1975; Jane's Weapon Systems 1974–75; International Defense Review (February 1972); US Department of the Army (1967); Magis (1967); US Army Munitions Command (1973).

rifle there are the M309 and M309A1 high explosive rounds. For the 90 mm recoilless rifle there are the XM590 and XM590E1 canister (flechette) rounds as well as high explosive rounds. For the 105 mm rifle there is a high explosive round, and for the 106 mm rifle there is the XM581 anti-personnel-tracer (flechette) round.

The Swedish 84 mm FFV 41 recoilless rifle has an anti-personnel munition which combines a high fragmentation steel case with metal balls.

VI. *Artillery ammunition*

Artillery weapons continue to account for a very high proportion of battlefield casualties. Though small calibre guns in the 20–60 mm range are widely used against aircraft and vehicles, and though larger calibre guns and howitzers can be fired with some precision at point targets, both smaller and larger calibre weapons continue to have important anti-personnel applications.

Smaller calibre artillery projectiles of the HEI (high-explosive–incendiary) type typically have a lethal radius due to blast, fragments, fire and toxic gases of about 5 m. They can be fired at high rates and have been used against guerrilla and conventional forces.

Even against highly mechanized forces, such as those typical of NATO and the Warsaw Treaty Organization, it has been estimated that 54 per cent of the potential targets for a modern 25–30 mm gun are made up of personnel, compared with 29 per cent light armoured vehicles, 13 per cent aircraft (including helicopters) and 4 per cent other vehicles. This conclusion, arrived at in a design study for the Bushmaster gun carried out by the US Army Infantry School (US Senate Committee on Armed Services, 1974, part 6, p. 2803), indicated that the anti-personnel applications of such weapons are far from negligible.

Larger guns are usually deployed in batteries of four or six and used as area weapons against troops in the open or in field fortifications. They are not used in an indirect fire role except in self-defence when the position is about to be or is actually being overrun. For this eventuality, special canister and flechette rounds are available.

The most common type of artillery ammunition consists of a 'shell' of iron or steel containing a quantity of high explosive which is detonated by a fuze. The fuze may be of impact type (instantaneous or delayed to ensure penetration of the target) or proximity type. Sometimes time fuzes have been used to permit the detonation of the shell over the target. Although the blast overpressure resulting from explosion of the shell may cause casualties and damage near to the point of impact, fragments of the casing are the more significant anti-personnel agent. Artillery shells typically break up into more than 1 000 effective fragments, each propelled at over 1 000 m/s. But the high fragmentation steels and more powerful explosives used in some modern shells (table 5.4) may produce more than six times as many effective fragments as do older types of shell.

Table 5.5. Canister and Beehive (flechette or shrapnel type) artillery ammunition

Producing country and ammunition calibre	Designation	Type	Weapon	Wounding agent	Remarks
Belgium					
90 mm	..	Canister	Gun	1120 × 3.6-g spheres	Operational range 300 m
UK					
76 mm	..	Canister	Gun	..	
105 mm	..	Canister	..	..	500 m range; in development (1972)
USA					
76 mm	..	Beehive	Gun	Flechettes	In development (c. 1972)
90 mm	M377	Canister	Gun	c. 5 600 × 0.5-g flechettes	Maximum effective range 400 m; standardized in 1958; never produced
90 mm	XM580E1	Beehive	Gun	4 100 × 0.5-g flechettes	
90 mm	XM590E1	Canister	Recoilless rifle	2 400 flechettes	Maximum effective range 300 m; rapid response development for Viet Nam
105 mm	XM494E3	Beehive	Gun	5 000 × 0.84-g flechettes	
105 mm	XM546	Beehive	Howitzer	8 000 × 0.5 g flechettes	
115 mm	..	Beehive	Gun	Flechettes	Feasibility study (1959)
117 mm	..	Beehive	Gun	Flechettes	In development (c. 1972)
152 mm	XM617	Beehive	Gun	Flechettes	
152 mm	M625	Canister	Gun	10 000 × 0.84 g flechettes	
155 mm	XM396	Beehive	Howitzer	Flechettes	Design study reported in 1963
175 mm	..	Beehive	..	Flechettes	Design analysis reported in 1965
8 in	..	Beehive	..	Flechettes	

Sources: Jane's Weapon Systems 1974–75; International Defense Review (February, 1972, February, 1973); US Department of the Army (1967); US Army Material Command (1969); Painter (1974); US Army Munitions Command (1972).

Table 5.6. US anti-personnel bomblet-filled artillery ammunition

Calibre	Designation	Remarks
105 mm	M444	Contains spherical bomblets with folding wings
155 mm	M449A1	Payload of M43A1 anti-personnel grenades
8 in	M404	Payload of M43A1 anti-personnel grenades
8 in	M509	
16 in	MK19	Developed (in *c.* 6 months) in 1968 for Viet Nam

Sources: US Army Project Manager for Selected Ammunition (1972), *Commerce Business Daily* (5 March, 1974, p. 15), *International Defense Review* (February 1977).

Canister and shrapnel rounds were widely used until World War I but were much less prevalent in World War II. After the Korean War, the USA developed a number of flechette-filled canister and shrapnel-type shells (Beehive rounds) (table 5.5). These rounds release thousands of 0.5 g (or larger) steel flechettes, either directly from the muzzle of the gun or at some distance down range. They are primarily intended for use where an artillery battery is in danger of being overrun, and during the Viet Nam War cases were reported where hundreds of enemy soldiers were killed in a single engagement against a battery firing flechette rounds.

In the USA artillery ammunition has been developed to eject a number of anti-personnel bomblets (table 5.6).

Artillery batteries are frequently targeted on an 'area of effect' of 1 ha (100 × 100 m) at a range of some 10 or 20 km. Often all the batteries in a battalion or larger unit will be firing simultaneously, covering a wide area. When artillery is used as an area weapon in this way, calculations are made as to the number of shells to be fired per hectare, depending upon the degree of protection of the enemy troops within the area and other tactical factors.[4]

Table 5.7. Safety zone for conventional high explosive artillery shells with regard to military personnel in training and combat conditions

Calibre *mm*	Risk distance for fragments, f *m*	Longitudinal dispersion, l *m*	Horizontal dispersion, h *m*	Safety zone, $(f + l) \times (f + h)$ *m*
Training				
75– 80	300	500	100	800 × 400
105–122	500	550	120	1 050 × 620
155	600	600	150	1 200 × 750
Combat				
75– 80	50	150	75	200 × 125
105–122	100	200	75	300 × 175
155	200	225	75	425 × 275

Source: Swedish military regulations.

It can be readily understood that the employment of artillery in this manner leads to the delivery of very large numbers of shells, often leading to great destruction over wide areas. In the Viet Nam War, for example, it has been calculated that over 200 million 105 mm artillery shells were fired by USA and allied forces alone (SIPRI, 1976*b*).

In order to avoid casualties to his own troops, the artillery commander must take certain considerations into account, namely, the average dispersion of the shells (longitudinally and horizontally) and the distance travelled by the fragments when the shell explodes. These factors may be combined to give a 'safety zone' for each calibre of artillery (table 5.7).

It will be seen that the safety range is always more than 100 m and may exceed 1 000 m, depending upon the conditions. (These figures, provided by the Swedish Army, apply to soldiers in peace-time and wartime conditions and assume that civilians are evacuated from the area.)

VII. Rocket and missile warheads

High explosive surface-to-surface rockets have been extensively used since World War II. The USA phased out the 2.36 in (60 mm) and 3.5 in (89 mm) infantry rocket launchers after the Korean War but 76 mm and 106 mm rockets continue in service in Soviet-supplied forces. Soviet 122 mm rockets are fired in salvos from a mobile launcher, as are a number of other rockets (table 5.8).

A Swiss company, Sarmac, produces a novel infantry weapon called the Rattlebox. It consists of a series of small rocket launchers mounted on a tripod and firing 50 mm rockets to a range of 800 m. The anti-personnel warheads have preformed fragmenting steel bands.

Rockets may also be fired from fixed-wing and rotary aircraft. Most notable is the US 2.75 in (70 mm) rocket, for which a number of fragmentation and flechette warheads are available (table 5.9). They were widely used in Viet Nam (chapter 2). Air-to-surface rockets are usually fired in salvos from pods slung under the wings of the aircraft.

Unguided rockets are not very accurate and often have indiscriminate effects. The safety zone required is large (table 5.10). This problem is likely to be compounded in the case of the few bomblet-filled rocket warheads which have been developed (table 5.8).

A number of guided missiles have been adapted for use as anti-personnel as well as anti-matériel munitions. The French Rafale and the US Little John and Honest John have been adapted to carry a quantity of grenades. The US Lance, originally a tactical nuclear missile, has been adapted to carry a payload of bomblets (table 5.9). The cost of these munitions makes their use unlikely except against high-value targets.

Table 5.8. Examples of surface-to-surface anti-personnel rockets and missiles

Producing country and weapon	Remarks
Belgium	
RL-83	83 mm anti-personnel and combined anti-personnel/anti-tank warheads
RL-100	101 mm
Brazil	
114 mm	Spin-stabilized, fired from 5-tube launcher; range 25 km
108R	Spin-stabilized, fired from 16-tube launcher; range believed to be about 12 km
Czechoslovakia	
RM-130	130 mm, fired from 32-tube launcher; range 8 km
M-1972	122 mm BM-21-pattern rocket, fired from 40-tube launcher; range (short and long versions) 11 km and 21 km
France	
ACRA (Anti-Char RApide)	142 mm anti-tank gun-launched guided missile with optional cast-iron anti-personnel warhead
Harpon	Battlefield missile with optional anti-personnel warheads
SARPAC	68 mm, 1.8 kg HE and fragmentation warhead producing 800 g of splinters
SS11	High fragmentation anti-personnel warhead (optional)
ACL/APX 80	80 mm
Rafale	145 mm, fin-stabilized rocket; range 9–30 km; anti-personnel warhead contains 35 ball-grenades, each releasing 360 steel spheres
RAP-14	140 mm; range 16 km (20 km version in development); fragmentation and multiple-grenade warheads; CEP 90 m
FR Germany	
BO 810 *Cobra 2000*	Shaped-charge/fragmentation warhead, with 10 m casualty radius
Mamba	As above
LARS	110 mm multiple rocket launcher system with choice of warheads
Israel	
Ze'ev (Wolf)	2 versions used in 1973 War: (*a*) 170 kg warhead with 1 000 m range; (*b*) 70 kg warhead with 4 500 m range; area weapon for use against concentrations of troops and vehicles
Italy	
Bora	Artillery rocket family with 20 kg warhead and 10 km range
BR 51	158 mm artillery rocket, with optional warheads including preformed fragmentation and canister; under development (1976)
Mira	108 mm artillery rocket carrying 10 kg warhead 5 km
Attila Mk II	82.5 mm artillery fired from man-pack or multiple launcher; 3 kg anti-personnel fragmentation warhead with 4.5 km range
Samurai	76 mm artillery or air-to-ground rocket; under development (1976); 3 kg warhead

142

Table 5.8 (*continued*)

Producing country and weapon	Remarks
Japan	
Type 30	300 mm rocket, largest of series; range 25 km
Poland	
WP-8	8-tube launcher for 140 mm rockets; range 10 km
Spain	
D-3	300 mm artillery rocket; range 17.0 km
E-3	216 mm artillery rocket; range 14.5 km
R-2B	108 mm artillery rocket; range 7.5 km
Sweden	
M-2 *Carl Gustaf*	84 mm anti-tank rocket, with optional anti-personnel warhead; in service with Canadian, Danish, Norwegian, Swedish and British forces
Switzerland	
DIRA	81 mm rocket, various versions with 3 kg and 7 kg warheads
USA	
MGR-1B *Honest John*	Tactical nuclear missile with optional high explosive and M-38/M-40 grenade warheads
Little John	Version with M-38/M-40 anti-personnel grenades
Lance	M-251 warhead contains 860 BLU-63 bomblets
M-21	114 mm artillery rocket launcher, primarily chemical
M-91	115 mm artillery rocket launcher, primarily chemical
Slammer VI	6 × 19-tube 2.75 inch rocket launcher system
GSRS	General Support Rocket System; in development
USSR	
. .	107 mm infantry rocket
BM-14	140 mm artillery rocket launched from 8-, 16- or 17-tube launcher; range 9 km
BM-21	122 mm artillery rocket launched from 40-tube launcher; range 11 km (46 kg rocket) or 21 km (64 kg rocket)
BM-24	240 mm rocket launched from 12-tube launcher; range 7 km
BM-28	280 mm rocket launched from 6-tube launcher; range 30 km
BMD-20	200 mm rocket launched from 4-tube launcher; range 18 km
BMD-25	250 mm rocket launched from 6-tube launcher; range 20 km
Yugoslavia	
M-63	128 mm artillery rocket launcher, similar to Czech RM-130; range 9.6 km

Sources: International Defense Review (August 1971; February 1977); Pretty & Archer (1974); Pretty (1976); US House Committee on Armed Services (1972).

Table 5.9. Examples of anti-personnel aircraft rockets and missiles

Producing country and weapon	Warhead designation	Warhead type	Remarks
France			
68 mm SNEB rocket	253	Shaped-charge/fragmentation	In service
68 mm SNEB rocket	265P	Fragmentation	In service
AS11 missile	..	Fragmentation	Airborne version of SS11
USA			
40 mm 'grenade' launcher	XM683	..	Rocket booster cartridge
2.75 in (70 mm) rocket	M151	High explosive	Pearlitic, malleable iron or other cast-iron case
2.75 inch rocket	M229	High explosive	Pearlitic, malleable iron case
2.75 inch rocket	WDU-4/A	Flechette	Contains 6 000 flechettes; Model 113A acceleration-deceleration fuze; superseded by WDU-4A/A
2.75 inch rocket	WDU-4A/A	Flechette	Contains 2 200 flechettes; Model 113A fuze
5 in (127 mm) *Zuni* rocket	MK-32	Shaped-charge/fragmentation	Impact, proximity fuzes
5 in (127 mm) *Zuni* rocket	MK-63	High explosive	Thin-walled aluminium alloy case; proximity fuze, lethal area much greater than with MD-32 warhead against personnel in open
Wasp	—	—	0.5 kg spin-stabilized rocket for helicopter use; under development in mid-1960s
Bullpup missile	—	—	Anti-personnel warhead under development (1966)
Shrike missile	—	High explosive	Rectangular fragments

Sources: Hobart (1974); US Department of the Navy (1972); *Ordnance* (September–October 1966); *Missiles and Rockets* (25 October 1965, p. 15).

Table 5.10. Safety zones for air-delivered rockets and bombs with regard to military personnel in training conditions[a]

Munition	Longitudinal dispersal of munition[b] m	Horizontal dispersal of munition m	Dispersion of fragments m	Required safety zone m
Rockets (135–150 mm)	− 1 500 + 3 000	150	600–1 000	4 000 × 1 000
Bombs (50–500 kg)	− 500 + 2 000	300	800–1 000	3 000 × 1 100

[a] Assumes target area of 100 × 100 m.
[b] 'Minus' figure is risk zone in front of target, 'plus' figure risk zone behind target.

Source: Swedish military regulations.

VIII. Bombs

General purpose (GP) bombs. Made up of about 50 per cent high explosive filler and 50 per cent fragmenting steel case, these bombs are still widely used against troops (chapter 2) though they are not very cost-effective except against well-protected troops. A typical 250 kg bomb has an effective casualty radius of about 30 m against troops in the open (i.e., it is expected to incapacitate 50 per cent of persons within 30 m of the explosion), but individual fragments may travel much further. To cope with the dispersion of fragments and aiming errors, a safety zone of about 1 000–3 000 m is required, depending on bombing tactics (high or low level), type of aircraft, and other factors (table 5.10).

Fragmentation bombs. These bombs may be similar to GP bombs but have a higher proportion of fragmenting steel, sometimes in the form of an additional layer of steel wire wrapped around the body. (Conversely, demolition or concussion bombs have a thinner case and a higher proportion of explosive.) Large fragmentation bombs may be effective against some matériel targets, but studies have shown that against personnel it is more effective to disperse a larger number of smaller bombs (Green, Thomson & Roots, 1955).

The 20 lb (9 kg) Hales bomb was used by the British during World War I and in 'pacification' operations between the two World Wars (chapter 2). The US M-41 20-lb fragmentation bomb was used in World War II and usually dropped in clusters of six (M1A1 cluster). About 30–50 bombs could be dropped by a single World War II bomber aircraft. The explosive charge made up about 15 per cent of the weight. A steel wire, wrapped around the body, broke up into pieces about 20 mm long. With a TNT charge it produced about 1 000 fragments, and with ednatol or RDX Compound B, about 1 400–1 600 fragments. The effective casualty radius when the bomb exploded in a vertical position was estimated at 15 m (using a criterion of two hits) (Beyer, 1962, appendix G). During World War II a fairly detailed study of the effects of one of these bombs was made following an accident involving 24 men, of whom 17 were injured and 6 died. Thirteen of the wounded suffered multiple injuries, including 10 who suffered multiple fractures. Four casualties suffered a total of 10 traumatic amputations of limbs or parts of limbs (Beyer, op. cit.).

Similar bombs used during World War II included the German S.C.10 12-kg bomb, usually carried in clusters of five; Italian 12 kg bombs; and Japanese 15 kg bombs.

During World War II much smaller anti-personnel fragmentation bombs were also widely used. Italy made a 2 kg *bombetta spezzone* as well as a 3 kg anti-personnel bomb. The German S.D.1 1-kg bomb was made from a modified 50 mm mortar shell and was carried in containers holding as many as 700. The German 2 kg 'butterfly' bomb – so nicknamed because of the vanes which opened out from the body – was carried in containers holding up to 80. This bomb was copied and manufactured in the United States (Green, Thomson & Roots, 1955) and some were dropped in Viet Nam (plate 9).

During World War II it was standard practice to add a number of exploding or combined-effect bombs to clusters of incendiary bombs, with the object of harassing or deterring salvage and rescue personnel. Examples include the Japanese 1 kg incendiary/anti-personnel bomb; the German 1 kg incendiary bomb with explosive pellet, or, as a 2.2 kg bomb, with anti-personnel attachment; and the US M-50X 1.7 kg incendiary bomb with explosive charge.

Several larger anti-personnel bombs were also introduced during World War II. Examples are the German S.Be.C. 50 and S.Be.C. 250 bombs, which consisted of a steel tube filled with a high explosive bursting charge surrounded by a concrete matrix embedded with small pieces of steel (US War Department, 1943). The Swedish 120 kg *Virgo* bomb is an example of a modern, large fragmentation bomb designed for use against light matériel and troops in the open.

Cluster bombs and bomblet dispenser systems. A cluster bomb may be similar in external appearance to a conventional 250 or 350 kg bomb, but it is designed to burst open in mid-air and release a large number of grenades or bomblets. Cluster bombs have developed into significant weapons during the last two decades, though an early form, a bundle of grenades projected from a mortar, was in use over a century ago (plate 1). Many varieties of bomblet have been developed and several varieties may be mixed in the same cluster. Bomblet dispenser systems constitute an alternative means of dispersing a large number of bomblets but they are fixed to the aircraft and may be reloaded (plate 7).

A very extensive series of cluster bombs and dispenser systems have been developed by the USA. The typical US cluster bomb consists of a dispenser (SUU) containing a large number of bomblets or grenades (BLUs) (table 5.11). Each combination of SUU and BLU receives a different ADU, CDU or CBU number, and since the SUUs and BLUs have been modified at various stages there is a bewildering variety of designations. One common type of dispenser for example, the pea-pod-like SUU-30, is found as SUU-30/B, SUU-30A/B, SUU-30/B (mod) and SUU-30C/B, each of which is slightly different.

Table 5.11. Index of US munitions and submunitions in the BLU series

Designation	Weight kg	Dispenser	Type
BLU-1	325	..	Fire-bomb (750 lb rating) dispensing 280 kg M2 napalm
BLU-2	..	..	..
BLU-3	0.79	SUU-7, SUU-14, SUU-24[b], B-57MBD[b], NC-123X[b], PWU-1[b], PWU-4[b]	Anti-matériel fragmentation bomblet ('Pineapple'); cylindrical, with pop-out drag-vanes; 0.16 kg cyclotol projecting about 250 steel pellets
BLU-4	0.54	SUU-7	Anti-personnel fragmentation bomblet; cylindrical, with pop-out drag-vanes; on impact, throws up an explosive hemisphere to 3 m
BLU-5	..	..	..
BLU-6	..	TMU-10	Smoke sphere; payload for TMU-10 smoke tank
BLU-7	0.64	SUU-10	Anti-armour shaped-charge bomblet; parachute-armed and -stabilized
BLU-8	..	..	..
BLU-9	..	..	..
BLU-10	c. 115	..	Fire-bomb (250 lb rating) dispensing 100 kg napalm
BLU-11	c. 230	..	Fire-bomb (500 lb rating) dispensing 200 kg napalm; modified M116A1
BLU-12	..	..	..
BLU-13	..	..	..
BLU-14	c. 345	..	Skip bomb (750 lb rating) for low-level penetration; modified MLU-10
BLU-15	..	..	Anti-matériel
BLU-16	0.73	SUU-7	Smoke (HC) bomblet; cylindrical; modified M8 grenade
BLU-17	0.5	SUU-7, SUU-14	White phosphorus bomblet; cylindrical; modified M15 grenade
BLU-18	0.19	SUU-13[c]	Anti-personnel fragmentation bomblet; triangular shape, delay fuze
BLU-19	..	SUU-13[c], TFD[c]	Chemical warfare bomblet: GB nerve gas, explosive burst
BLU-20	..	SUU-13	Chemical warfare bomblet: BZ incapacitant, thermal generator, parachute-retarded
BLU-21	..	..	Biological warfare bomblet: dry agent, such as UL2
BLU-22	..	SUU-13	Biological warfare bomblet: wet agent, such as UL1
BLU-23	c. 230	..	Fire-bomb (500 lb rating) dispensing 200 kg napalm
BLU-24	0.73	SUU-14, SUU-50	Anti-personnel fragmentation bomblet; spherical, plastic fins, cyclotol filler; spin-delay fuze allowing jungle penetration; ('Orange')

Table 5.11 (*continued*)

Designation	Weight kg	Dispenser	Type
BLU-25	..	SUU-13	Anti-personnel bomblet (flechette?); cylindrical
BLU-26	0.43	SUU-24[b], SUU-30, SUU-31, B-57MBD[b], NC-123X[b], PWU-1, PWU-4[b], *Bullpup*	Anti-personnel/anti-matériel fragmentation bomblet ('Guava'); spherical, 6 cm diameter, vaned surface, impact detonating; cyclotol A3, projecting about 300 steel pellets
BLU-27	400	..	Fire-bomb (750 lb rating) dispensing 360 kg napalm B
BLU-28	..	..	Biological warfare bomblet, self-dispersing
BLU-29	73	SUU-24(?)	Flame-agent (napalm B?) canister
BLU-30	..	SUU-13	Chemical/biological warfare bomblet; dry incapacitant filler
BLU-31	350	..	Bluff-shape anti-ricochet demolition bomb (750 lb rating), Destex filler; functions as a land-mine, set off by oncoming heavy vehicles
BLU-32	270	..	Fire-bomb (500 lb rating) dispensing 240 kg napalm B
BLU-33	c. 690	..	Demolition bomb (1 500 lb rating), bluff shape, tritonal filler
BLU-34	c. 1 380	..	Hard-surface demolition bomb (3 000 lb rating), bluff shape
BLU-35	150	..	Modular fire-bomb (250 lb rating) dispensing 140 kg napalm
BLU-36	0.43	SUU-24[b], SUU-30, B-57MBD[b], NC-123X[b], PWU-1[b], PWU-4[b]	BLU-26 anti-personnel/anti-matériel fragmentation (pellet) bomblet fitted with random-delay fuze
BLU-37	..	..	..
BLU-38	..	..	..
BLU-39(XM16)	..	SUU-13[b], strongback[b] used in the CBU-19 munition	Chemical warfare bomblet: CS irritant; burning type, skittering along ground; flashlight-cell size and shape; less than 80 g
BLU-40	0.78	..	Fragmentation bomblet, random-delay fuze
BLU-41	..	SUU-24[b], B-57MBD[b], NC-123X[b], PWU-1[b], PWU-4[b]	Fragmentation bomblet; spherical; spin-armed, spin-delay fuze
BLU-42	..	SUU-38[b]	Anti-personnel minelet; spherical, vaned surface; trip-wire sensors, anti-disturbance features, self-destruct timer; 0.12 kg comp B
BLU-43	0.02	SUU-13[b]	Anti-personnel minelet ('Short Dragontooth'); triangular; blast
BLU-44	0.02	SUU-13[b]	Anti-personnel minelet ('Long Dragontooth'); triangular; blast
BLU-45	9.1	SUU-36	Anti-vehicle mine, anti-tank optimized; shaped charge; timed self-destruct

BLU	Weight (kg)	Carriers	Description
BLU-46	::	::	Anti-personnel bomb; in Honeywell R&D in 1968
BLU-47	::	::	General-purpose bomb; in Honeywell R&D in 1968
BLU-48	::	SUU-30, SUU-37[b]	Fragmentation bomblet, jungle penetration; presumably spherical
BLU-49	6.1	SUU-13	Fragmentation bomb; ringtail; cyclotol 70/30 filler
BLU-50	::	SUU-13[b]	Chemical warfare bomblet: BZ incapacitant; bursting type
BLU-51	::	::	Fire-bomb
BLU-52	160	::	Chemical warfare bomb; BLU-1 fire-bomb adapted to dispense 123 kg micronized CS irritant
BLU-53	c. 9	SUU-51	Napalm B canister
BLU-54	::	SUU-38[b]	Anti-personnel minelet, long life; bounding; identical with BLU-42 apart from timer
BLU-55	::	SUU-13	Bomblet
BLU-56	::	::	Anti-personnel mine
BLU-57	c. 230	::	Fragmentation bomb (500 lb rating), bluff shape
BLU-58	c. 230	::	General purpose bomb (500 lb rating), bluff shape
BLU-59	0.43	SUU-30	BLU-26 anti-personnel/anti-matériel fragmentation (pellet) bomblet fitted with random-delay fuze; shorter delay than BLU-36
BLU-60	5.9	SUU-13	Fragmentation bomb; cyclotol filler
BLU-61	1.0	SUU-24[b], SUU-30, B-57MBD[b], NC-123X[b], PWU-1[b], PWU-4[b]	Anti-matériel fragmentation/incendiary bomblet; spherical; zirconium and composition B filler
BLU-62	0.43	::	Anti-personnel/anti-matériel fragmentation bomblet; pop-up; cyclotol filler
BLU-63	0.43	SUU-24[b], SUU-30, SUU-54, B-57MBD[b], NC-123X[b], PWU-1[b], PWU-4, Lance	Anti-personnel/anti-matériel fragmentation bomblet; spherical; scored steel case, cyclotol filler; 1971 replacement for BLU-26
BLU-64	c. 350	::	Fuel-Air Explosive (FAE) bomb; 200 kg hydrocarbon fuel
BLU-65	372	::	Fire-bomb
BLU-66	0.73	SUU-7	Anti-personnel fragmentation bomblet; spherical; plastic tailfins
BLU-67	c. 5	SUU-13	Cratering bomb
BLU-68	0.42	SUU-24[b], SUU-30, B-57MBD[b], NC-123X[b], PWU-1[b], PWU-4[b]	Anti-personnel/anti-matériel incendiary bomblet; zirconium-sponge filler; presumably spherical
BLU-69	0.73	SUU-14	Anti-personnel/anti-matériel incendiary bomblet
BLU-70	0.4	SUU-24[b], SUU-30, B-57MBD[b], NC-123X[b], PWU-1[b], PWU-4[b]	Anti-personnel incendiary bomblet, presumably spherical
BLU-71	::	::	Mine
BLU-72	1 100	::	FAE bomb, low-speed carriage ('Pave Pat I'); drogue-chute retarded; 450 kg propane fuel

Table 5.11 (*continued*)

Designation	Weight kg	Dispenser	Type
BLU-73	60	SUU-49	FAE canister; drogue-chute retarded; long probe; 33 kg ethylene oxide fuel
BLU-74	107	SUU-48	Modular fire-bomb (250 lb rating), napalm B filler
BLU-75	..	..	Chemical warfare bomb
BLU-76	1 200	..	FAE bomb, high-speed carriage, low-speed delivery ('Pave Pat II'); streamlined version of BLU-72
BLU-77	..	Mk7 Mod3 *Rockeye*	Anti-armour/anti-personnel shaped-charge/fragmentation bomblet; cylindrical; pop-up, hard-target/soft-target discriminating
BLU-78	..	..	..
BLU-79	..	..	..
BLU-80	..	..	..
BLU-81	..	..	..
BLU-82	6 800	..	Blast bomb, 3.35 m long; 5 700 kg DBA-22M filler
BLU-83	..	..	..
BLU-84	..	..	..
BLU-85	..	..	..
BLU-86	..	..	..
BLU-87	..	..	Photograph published in December 1972

a Several types of dispenser have been developed for air delivery of small munitions: (1) *Free-fall dispensers.* These streamlined tailfinned containers are dropped from aircraft like general-purpose bombs but open in mid-air to release or eject their payloads of submunitions which impact on the target in a circular or elliptical pattern. The Mk5 Universal Weapons Dispenser ('Sadeye'), the SUU-30 dispenser and the SUU-31 dispenser are of 750 lb rating and open like clamshells. The Mk7 'Rockeye' dispenser is of 500 lb rating, and the SUU-54 dispenser of 2 000 lb rating. The SUU-51 is a cartridge-ejection dispenser, apparently of the free-fall type, used to dispense flame-agent submunitions. (2) *Fixed dispensers.* These remain attached to the aircraft during use, thus dispensing lines of submunitions along the aircraft flight path. They may dispense submunitions singly or pre-clustered in opening free-fall canisters. There are three main varieties: (2.1) *Rearward-ejection (RE) dispensers.* These are used by ground-support aircraft from low altitudes. For dispensing bomblets, the principal ones comprise a sheaf of tubes of about 70 mm calibre, the tubes each being loaded with several submunitions and being dischargable successively (in some cases) or simultaneously. The SUU-14 is a light (22 kg unladen weight) unstreamlined 6-tube cartridge-ejection dispenser, about 200 cm long, for helicopters and other low-performance aircraft, for use at speeds of up to 300 knots; the bomblet impact pattern for a 90 knot delivery is typically about 280 m long. The SUU-7 and SUU-10 are streamlined 19-tube dispensers for high or low performance aircraft, looking rather like aircraft multiple rocket launchers pointing backwards; their tubes, which are about 300 cm long, are discharged by a combination of ram-air and spring-loaded piston. The SUU-50 is a 12-tube cartridge-ejection dispenser, apparently of the RE type with tubes similar to those of the SUU-14. (2.2) *External-carriage downward-ejection (DE) dispensers.* These are used from ground-support aircraft, those that can function at supersonic delivery speeds being known as *Tactical Fighter Dispensers* (TFDs). Some versions – though not TFDs – comprise a strongback fastened to the aircraft to which several releasable canisters of submunitions are attached, a streamlined cowling being provided for those that are for high-speed carriage: the Mk4 Universal Weapons Dispenser ('Gladeye') is a 7-module dispenser of this type. Other versions for high-speed carriage comprise a streamlined elongated box, the interior of which is divided into cylindrical or other shaped bays having openable floors. One or more submunitions or clusters of submunitions are loaded into each bay. The SUU-13 is a 40-bay dispenser (the bays – tubes about 12 cm in diameter and 28 cm long – being opened explosively) that can be used only at subsonic speeds, though it can be carried by high-performance aircraft; the bomblet impact pattern at 450 knot delivery is typically 1 110 m long and 60 m wide (with a cluster canister loading); loaded, its weight seems usually to lie in the 250–400 kg range; its dimensions have been quoted as 250 cm in length and 36 cm square in section. The SUU-36, SUU-37,

SUU-38 and SUU-41 dispensers are 10-bay TFDs; the SUU-45 is a TFD using SUU-13 tubes. (2.3) *Internal-carriage DE dispensers.* These are fastened inside the bomb-bays of bomber aircraft and comprise large box-like containers divided into rectangular cells with openable floors. Each cell is loaded with one or more boxes of submunitions, the boxes acting as free-fall dispensers. For B-52 bomb-bays there is the 24-cell SUU-24 Hayes Dispenser (which also fits the B-47 bomb-bay) and the PWU-1/A Big Belly Hayes Dispenser; for B-57 bomb-bays there is the 22-cell Modular Bomb Dispenser (MBD). each cell having one-third the capacity of SUU-24 cells, and the 22-cell PWU-4/A; and for the C-123 cargo plane modified for bombing operations there is the Black Spot NC-123X dispenser, which has 12 SUU-24-sized cells, designed to be used in pairs, one on top of the other. Fully loaded, these dispensers may weigh about three tonnes.

b The BLUs are clustered into ADU or CDU modules (see table 5.12) for discharge from these dispensers.

c The BLUs are presumably discharged in clusters from these dispensers.

Source: This index was compiled by Julian Perry Robinson, using data collected by himself and by Eric Prokosch from US Defense Department publications, Defense Department Congressional testimony and aerospace trade journals. Not all the items listed are standard munitions; some are now obsolete, some are still in development, and some were abandoned in development. There are no doubt others that are not listed.

Table 5.12. Index of US cluster bombs and dispenser munitions

Designation and type		Weight kg	Dispenser[a] or adapter	Submunitions		Remarks
				Number	Designation	
M1	Bomb cluster	58	M1 cluster adapter	6	M41 bomb fragmentation	Anti-personnel/anti-matériel; the M41 is a 9 kg wound steel bar fragmentation bomb
M4	Bomb cluster	40	M3 cluster adapter	3	M40 bomb fragmentation	Anti-personnel/anti-matériel; the M40 is an 11 kg heavy-case parachute-retarded bomb
Mk 12	Bomblet dispenser munition	270	Padeye	..	..	Smoke; Padeye is also used for chemical-warfare bomblets: BZ incapacitant filler
Mk 15	Cluster bomb	c. 370	Mk 5 Sadeye	..	..	..
Mk 17	Bomblet dispenser (DE) munition	230 500	Mk 4 Gladeye	7	Bomblet canister	..
Mk 21	Cluster bomb	c. 370	Mk 5 Sadeye	..	..	
Mk 20	Cluster bomb	220	Mk 7 Rockeye	247	Mk 118 bomblet shaped-charge/fragmentation	Anti-armour/anti-personnel
Mk 22	Cluster bomb	c. 370	Mk 5 Sadeye	..	..	..
Mk 44	Cluster bomb (?)	280	M16 cluster adapter	10 000	'Lazy Dog' shaped iron fragment	Anti-personnel
ADU-253	Bomblet cluster[b]	62	CBU-27 cluster adapter	74	BLU-3 bomblet fragmentation (pellet)	Anti-matériel
ADU-256	Bomblet cluster[b]	78	CBU-27	535	M40 grenade fragmentation	Anti-personnel; M40 grenade is a spherical 0.14 kg vaned-surface bomblet, 4.7 cm diam.
ADU-272	Bomblet cluster[b]	80	CBU-27	177	BLU-26 bomblet fragmentation (pellet)	Anti-personnel/anti-matériel
ADU-285	Bomblet cluster[b]	80	CBU-27	177	BLU-36 bomblet fragmentation (pellet)	Anti-personnel/anti-matériel

Designation	Type				Payload	Description
ADU-313	Bomblet cluster[b]	..	CBU-27	..	BLU-61 bomblet fragmentation/incendiary	Anti-matériel
CDU-2	Minelet cluster[c]	c. 5	..	120	BLU-43 minelet 'Short Dragontooth'	Anti-personnel; for SUU-13 dispenser (see CBU-28)
CDU-3	Minelet cluster[c]	c. 5	..	120	BLU-44 minelet 'Long Dragontooth'	Anti-personnel; for SUU-13 dispenser (see CBU-37)
CDU-4	Minelet cluster[c]	20	..	147	XM41 minelet 'Gravel'	Anti-personnel; for SUU-41 dispenser; the XM-41 weighs 65 g; 7.1 g RDX + 3.2 g lead azide filler
CDU-5	Minelet cluster[c]	21	..	750	XM40 'Sandwich Button Bomb' minelet	Anti-intrusion; for SUU-41; the XM40 weighs 6 g and consists of a match composition between plastic friction plates
CDU-9	Bomblet cluster[c]	..	..	..	BLU-50 bomblet BZ incapacitant	Chemical warfare; for SUU-13 dispenser (see CBU-16)
CDU-10	Minelet cluster[c]	21	..	680 + 48	XM40 SBB, and XM44 'Microgravel'	Anti-intrusion; for SUU41; the XM44 is very similar to the XM40 (see above)
CDU-11	Minelet cluster[c]	..	..	..	XM40 or XM48 'Button Bomb' minelets	Anti-intrusion; for SUU-41 dispenser
CDU-12	Bomblet cluster[c]	c. 5	..	32	BLU-39 bomblet CS irritant	Chemical warfare; for SUU-13 dispenser (see CBU-30)
CDU-13	Bomblet cluster[c]	..	..	..	BLU-48 bomblet fragmentation	For SUU-37 dispenser (see CBU-43)
CDU-14	Minelet cluster[c]	20	..	147	XM65 minelet 'Gravel'	Anti-personnel; for SUU-41; the XM65 is very similar to the XM41 (see above)
CDU-15	Bomblet cluster[b]	..	CBU-27	177	BLU-68 bomblet incendiary	Anti-personnel/anti-matériel
CDU-16	Minelet cluster[c]	..	..	238	XM43 minelet	Anti-personnel (?); for SUU-41 dispenser; the XM43 contains RDX explosive
CDU-17	Bomblet cluster[b]	..	CBU-27	177	BLU-70 bomblet incendiary	Anti-personnel
CDU-18 CDU-19	Minelet cluster[c]	..	..	54	BLU-42 minelet	Anti-personnel; for SUU-38 dispenser (see CBU-34)
CDU-20 CDU-21	Minelet cluster[c]	..	..	54	BLU-54 minelet	Anti-personnel; for SUU-38 dispenser (see CBU-42)

Table 5.12 (continued)

Designation and type	Weight kg	Dispenser[a] or adapter	Submunitions		Remarks
			Number	Designation	
CDU-22	Bomblet cluster[b]	80	CBU-27	163	BLU-63 bomblet fragmentation	Anti-personnel/anti-matériel
CBU-1	Bomblet dispenser (RE) munition	340	SUU-7	509	BLU-4 bomblet fragmentation	Anti-personnel
CBU-2	Bomblet dispenser (RE) munition	370	SUU-7	360 409	BLU-3 bomblet fragmentation (pellet)	Anti-matériel
CBU-3	Bomblet dispenser (RE) munition	300	SUU-10	352 371	BLU-7 bomblet shaped charge	Anti-armour
CBU-4	..	..				
CBU-5 (M43)	Cluster bomb	360	M30 cluster adapter	57	M138 bomblet BZ incapacitant	Chemical warfare; subsonic carriage; M138 10 lb bomb comprises four thermal generator canisters nested in a tube Redesignated CBU-13 (q.v.)
CBU-6	..	..	..	..	..	Anti-personnel
CBU-7	Bomblet dispenser (DE) munition	..	SUU-13	1 200	BLU-18 bomblet[d] fragmentation	
CBU-8	Bomblet dispenser (RE) munition	390	SUU-7	409	BDU-40 practice bomblet	Training version of CBU-2
CBU-9	Bomblet dispenser (RE) munition	390	SUU-7	406	BDU-28 dummy bomblet	Training version of CBU-2
CBU-10	Dispenser (RE) munition	..	SUU-7	..	..	..
CBU-11	Bomblet dispenser (RE) munition	..	SUU-7	261	BLU-16 bomblet smoke (HC)	Smoke
CBU-12	Bomblet dispenser (RE) munition	290	SUU-7	261	BLU-17 bomblet white phosphorus	Smoke
CBU-13	Bomblet dispenser (RE) munition	..	SUU-7	261	BLU-16, BLU-17 HC and WP bomblets	Smoke
CBU-14	Bomblet dispenser (RE) munition	..	SUU-14	..	BLU-3 bomblet fragmentation (pellet)	Anti-matériel

CBU	Type			Bomblet		Role
CBU-15	Bomblet dispenser (DE) munition	..	SUU-13	BLU-19 bomblet[d] GB nerve gas	..	Chemical warfare
CBU-16	Bomblet dispenser (DE) munition	..	SUU-13	CDU-9 cluster BZ incapacitant	..	Chemical warfare
CBU-17	Bomblet dispenser (DE) munition	..	SUU-13	BDU-34 practice bomblet[d]	1 200	Training version of CBU-7
CBU-18	Bomblet dispenser (DE) munition	..	SUU-13	BLU-25 bomblet flechette (?)	..	Anti-personnel
CBU-19 (E159)	Bomblet dispenser (DE) munition	59	Twin strongback	Module of BLU-39s CS irritant	16	Chemical warfare; the module holds 33 BLU-39 (XM16) bomblets
CBU-20	..	..	..	..	..	..
CBU-21	..	..	..	..	..	..
CBU-22	Bomblet dispenser (RE) munition	60	SUU-14	BLU-17 bomblet white phosphorus	72	Smoke
CBU-23	Cluster bomb	..	SUU-31	BLU-26 bomblet fragmentation (pellet)	..	Anti-personnel/anti-matériel
CBU-24	Cluster bomb	380	SUU-30	BLU-26 bomblet fragmentation (pellet)	670	Anti-personnel/anti-matériel; primarily for use against trucks
CBU-25	Bomblet dispenser (RE) munition	..	SUU-14	BLU-24 bomblet fragmentation	..	Anti-personnel, jungle penetration
CBU-26	Bomblet dispenser (RE) munition	296	SUU-10	BDU-37 practice bomblet	352	Training version of CBU-3
CBU-27	Unfilled canister for DE dispensers	..	..	..	..	Becomes an ADU or CDU when filled with submunitions
CBU-28	Minelet dispenser (DE) munition	..	SUU-13	CDU-2 cluster of Dragonteeth	40	Anti-personnel
CBU-29	Cluster bomb	380	SUU-30	BLU-36 bomblet fragmentation (pellet)	670	Anti-personnel/anti-matériel
CBU-30	Bomblet dispenser (DE) munition	..	SUU-13	CDU-12 cluster CS irritant	40	Chemical warfare
CBU-31	..	..	..	..	..	..
CBU-32	..	..	..	..	..	..
CBU-33	Mine dispenser (DE) munition	c. 350	SUU-36	BLU-45 mine shaped-charge	30	Anti-vehicle (particularly tanks)

Table 5.12 (*continued*)

Designation and type	Weight kg	Dispenser[a] or adapter	Submunitions		Remarks
			Number	Designation	
CBU-34	Minelet dispenser (DE) munition	..	SUU-38	10	CDU-18, CDU-19 minelet clusters	Anti-personnel; 'Wide Area Anti-personnel Mine' (WAAPM)
CBU-35	..	..	..	..	..	..
CBU-36	..	..	..	..	..	..
CBU-37	Minelet dispenser (DE) munition	..	SUU-13	40	CDU-3 cluster of Dragonteeth	Anti-personnel
CBU-38	Bomb dispenser (DE) munition	..	SUU-13	40	BLU-49 bomb fragmentation	..
CBU-39	..	..	..	..	..	..
CBU-40	..	..	..	..	..	..
CBU-41	Cluster bomb	c. 220	SUU-51	18	BLU-53 canister napalm B	Anti-personnel/anti-matériel
CBU-42	Minelet dispenser (DE) munition	..	SUU-38	10	CDU-20, CDU-21 minelet clusters	Anti-personnel; long-life WAAPM
CBU-43	Bomblet dispenser (DE) munition	380	SUU-37	..	CDU-13 cluster fragmentation bomblets	Jungle penetration
CBU-44	Bomblet dispenser (DE) munition	..	TFD	..	..	Anti-personnel
CBU-45	Minelet dispenser (DE) munition	..	TFD	..	..	Multi-purpose
CBU-46	Bomblet dispenser (RE) munition	400	SUU-7	444	BLU-66 bomblet fragmentation	Anti-personnel; jungle penetration
CBU-47	Bomblet dispenser (DE) munition	..	SUU-13	..	BLU-55 bomblet	..
CBU-48	..	..	..	..	..	..
CBU-49	Cluster bomb	380	SUU-30	670	BLU-59 bomblet fragmentation (pellet)	Anti-personnel/anti-matériel

CBU-50	Bomb dispenser (DE) munition	..	SUU-13	40	BLU-60 bomb fragmentation	..
CBU-51	Bomb dispenser (DE) munition	..	SUU-13	40	BLU-67 bomb	For cratering
CBU-52	Cluster bomb	c. 350	SUU-30	254	BLU-61 bomblet fragmentation/incendiary	Anti-personnel/anti-matériel
CBU-53	Cluster bomb	c. 370	SUU-30	670	BLU-70 bomblet incendiary	Anti-personnel
CBU-54	Cluster bomb	c. 370	SUU-30	670	BLU-68 bomblet incendiary	Anti-personnel/anti-matériel
CBU-55	Cluster bomb	c. 230	SUU-49	3	BLU-73 bomblet fuel–air explosive	Anti-personnel/anti-mine; low-speed carriage
CBU-56	..	..	..	..	..	Chemical/biological warfare munition (?)
CBU-57	Bomblet dispenser (RE) munition	118	SUU-14	132	BLU-69 bomblet incendiary	Anti-personnel/anti-matériel
CBU-58	Cluster bomb	c. 380	SUU-30	670	BLU-63 bomblet fragmentation	Anti-personnel/anti-matériel; replaced CBU-24
CBU-59	Cluster bomb	c. 230	Mk 7 Mod 3 *Rockeye*	717	BLU-77 bomblet shaped-charge/fragmentation	Anti-armour/anti-personnel, discriminating
CBU-60	Bomblet dispenser (RE) munition	230	SUU-50	264	BLU-24 bomblet fragmentation	Anti-personnel; jungle penetration
CBU-61	..	..	..	..	CS irritant	Chemical warfare
CBU-62	Cluster bomb	c. 380	SUU-30	2 025	M38 grenade fragmentation	Anti-personnel/anti-matériel; the M38 weighs 0.14 kg and is random-delay fuzed
CBU-63	Cluster bomb	c. 380	SUU-30	2 025	M40 grenade fragmentation	Anti-personnel; the M40 grenade is described above (see ADU-256)
CBU-64	..	..	..	..	..	..
CBU-65	..	..	..	..	..	..
CBU-66	..	..	..	..	..	..
CBU-67	..	..	..	..	..	..
CBU-68	Cluster bomb	..	SUU-30	..	BLU-48 bomblet fragmentation	..

Table 5.12 (*continued*)

| Designation and type | Weight kg | Dispenser[a] or adapter | Submunitions | | Remarks |
			Number	Designation	
CBU-69	—	—	—	—	—
CBU-70 Cluster bomb	—	SUU-30	—	—	Anti-personnel/anti-matériel; submunitions are random delay fuzed; replacing CBU-49
CBU-71 Cluster bomb	—	SUU-30	650	fragmentation	
CBU-72 Cluster bomb	c. 230	—	3	BLU-73 bomblet fuel–air explosive	Anti-personnel/anti-mine; streamlined CBU-55; high-speed carriage, low-speed delivery
GBU-2 Guided cluster bomb	1 050	SUU-54	1 800	BLU-63 bomblet fragmentation	Anti-personnel/anti-matériel ('Pave Storm'); target homing by KMU-421 laser bomb guidance kit

[a] For details of some of the dispensers, see note *a* to table 5.11.

[b] These clusters are for loading into the cells of DE dispensers mounted inside bomber or cargo aircraft: they are boxes that open to release their payloads during descent. Seventy-two may be dropped from an SUU-24 dispenser, of which two may be accommodated in a B-52 bomb-bay; 22 from a Modular Bomb Dispenser for B-57 bombers (one per B-57); and 36 from a Black Spot NC-123X dispenser for C-123 cargo-bays (two per C-123).

[c] These clusters are for loading into the cells of DE dispensers mounted on tactical ground-support aircraft.

[d] The bomblets are presumably clustered as a CDU or other module.

Source: This index was compiled by Julian Perry Robinson, using data collected by himself and by Eric Prokosch from US Defense Department publications, Defense Department Congressional testimony and aerospace trade journals. Not all the items listed are standard munitions; some are now obsolete, some are still in development, and some were abandoned in development. There are no doubt others that are not listed.

When filled with 670 BLU-26/B anti-personnel bombs with an instantaneous detonation fuze, the SUU-30/B is known as the CBU-24/B; when filled with 670 BLU-36/B anti-personnel bombs with a random delay fuze, it is known as CBU-29/B; with 670 BLU-59/B random delay anti-personnel bombs it is known as the CBU-49/B; with 2 025 M38 grenades with a random delay fuze as the CBU-62/B; and with 2 025 M40 instantaneous detonation grenades as the CBU-63/B (US Department of the Navy, 1972).

A similar variety of designations is found with other combinations of dispenser and bomb (see table 5.12).

The SUU-30 has the external appearance of a conventional large bomb, and is released from the aircraft in the same manner. As it is released, an arming wire initiates a short delay fuze, blowing open the front of the casing, which is made in two halves. The halves are forced apart and the hundreds of small bombs fall out and are dispersed over a wide area. Other examples of free-fall cluster bombs include the Mk 20 Rockeye, containing 247 Mk 118 Mod 0 bombs, and the CBU-59/B containing 717 BLU-77/B bombs. Both of these are primarily designed for use against armoured vehicles, the bombs containing a shaped charged. However, when they hit soft targets, they explode to produce fragments. When the BLU-77/B hits a soft target it is first thrown up into the air by a propelling charge before fragmenting over a wider area, which allows it to hit more people.

A number of reusable bomblet dispensing systems have been designed for particular aircraft. Two SUU-24/A bomb, bomblet and grenade dispensers can be fitted into a B-52 heavy bomber, each dispenser divided into 24 cells containing three box-like cluster bomb adapters. Each adapter contains 74 BLU-3/Bs, 177 BLU-26/Bs or BLU-36/Bs, or 535 M40 grenades. Thus, a single B-52 bomber could disperse:

10 656 BLU-3/B bombs
25 488 BLU-26/B or BLU-36/B bombs, or
77 040 M40 grenades.[6]

With two NC-123X dispensers a C-123 military transport aircraft could be used to dispense half the above quantities of munitions. The B-57 Modular Bomb Dispenser for the B-57 bomber is divided into 22 cells, each of which contains one cluster bomb adapter, giving it a capacity of somewhat less than one-third that of the B-52 (US Departments of the Army, the Navy and the Air Force, 1970).

The BLU-3/B bomb is cylindrical in shape and weighs 0.78 kg and propels radially small steel balls at high velocity when it detonates. The BLU-26/B weighs 420 g and is spherical in shape and has steel balls embedded in the casing material. The surface is fluted, causing it to spin in flight with the dual purpose of dispersing the munitions and arming the fuze. It detonates on impact, propelling the steel balls in all directions at high velocity. The BLU-36/B is similar but has a random time-delay fuze. The BLU-63/B is also similar in appearance but consists of two hemispheres of fragmenting alloy steel. The M40 grenade weighs only 135 g and is made of a spherical, ribbed, steel case and high explosive filler; it is also used in the Honest John and Little John guided missiles (table 5.9).

Dispenser systems, such as the Tactical Fighter Dispenser, have been

Table 5.13. Non-US fragmentation cluster bombs

Producing country and designation	Dispenser type	Remarks
France		
Giboulée	12- or 24-tube, rearward ejection	60 or 120 shaped-charge/fragmentation bomblets; area coverage 300 by 20 m in anti-personnel mode; development began in 1966
Alkan cartridge launchers	Tubes	Launchers for anti-personnel cartridge
FR Germany		
Streuwaffen	..	'Dragon Seed'; 19 launcher tubes; 409 × 0.5 kg bomblets
Strebo/BD1/MW1	..	Various prototype systems; 4 600 kg bomb; 4 000 bomblets or mines
UK		
BL 755	Clamshell	1 471 kg shaped-charge/fragmentation bomblets; casing material and notched steel wire producing c. 2 000 fragments on explosion; area coverage less than 1 ha; feasibility studies began in 1964; entered service 1971

Sources: Jane's Weapon Systems 1974–75; International Defense Review (October 1973; August 1974); *Flight International* (14 February 1974); *British Defence Equipment Catalogue* (1974).

developed for a wide range of other aircraft and many kinds of bomb for them have been made, including not only anti-personnel and anti-tank bombs but also bombs containing incendiary, white phosphorus and other chemical and biological agents. Although US cluster bombs have been the most prominent, Britain, France and FR Germany have also developed cluster bombs (table 5.13), some of which have been supplied to other countries. A comprehensive range of Soviet cluster bombs has been referred to in the Western technical literature (*International Defense Review*, April 1976).

Clearly, with such a variety of munitions, no general statements can be made about such questions as the accuracy of delivery, area of coverage, and so on. The dispersion of the bombs released by cluster bombs and bomblet dispenser systems depends upon such factors as the height and speed of delivery, the height at which the cluster opens, prevailing winds, and structural aspects of the design of the bomblets and release system. Difficulties have been experienced in achieving an even dispersion from free-fall bombs, the bomblets tending to concentrate around the perimeter of an elliptical area.

A grenade or small bomblet might be designed to have a casualty radius of about 5–10 m. An effective distribution against personnel would be to place one bomb, say, in every 100 m². A single CBU-24/B containing 670 BLU-26/B bombs, could, therefore, cover an area of some 67 000 m² (6.7 ha). A B-52 loaded with 25 488 BLU-26/Bs could cover an area of 2 548 800 m² (254.8 ha).

IX. Summary and conclusions

Fragmentation weapons are the main source of battlefield casualties in the twentieth century. They often consist of a steel or iron case and a high explosive filler and may range in size from a few hundred grams to several hundred kilograms. In some designs the steel case is replaced or supplemented by steel balls, pieces of steel wire, or flechettes or other missiles.

Fragmentation warheads may be thrown by hand, propelled from a rifle or special grenade thrower, tube-launched from a mortar, howitzer, gun or recoilless rifle, propelled by a rocket, or dropped from a fixed-wing or rotary aircraft.

Modern designs seek to produce an optimum distribution of fragment sizes and velocities. At very high velocities, fragments less than 0.5 g may be sufficient to cause a casualty. However, since the density of fragments near to the point of detonation is invariably much greater than the density further away, fragments are never evenly distributed throughout the area of effect. As a result, persons close to the point of detonation will receive multiple severe injuries.

Fragmentation weapons are best regarded as *area* weapons, even if the area of effect is small in some cases. The reason is that they are intended to cause casualties by saturating an area with a concentration of incapacitating fragments, rather than being aimed at each enemy soldier individually, as is the case with point weapons. (Automatic point weapons may also be used to give area coverage.)

Cluster bombs and bomblet dispenser systems – and more recently bomblet-dispensing artillery shells and rockets – are designed to provide more effective area coverage. Some cluster bombs, particularly those designed for use against armour or mechanized infantry forces, cover an area approximately equivalent to that covered by a conventional artillery barrage, that is, about 1 ha. Bomblet dispenser systems used primarily against personnel can cover much larger areas, a single B-52 heavy bomber, for example, being capable of dispersing tens of thousands of bomblets or grenades over an area of several hundred hectares. The possibility of using such weapons for 'interdiction' far behind battle lines adds greatly to the danger of indiscriminate effects. Not only are inhabited areas likely to be within the area covered, but the presence of unexploded delayed-action bombs and duds presents a long-term danger (chapter 8).

Fragmentation weapons present a difficult challenge to international law. Grenades and shells under 400 g were the first category of anti-personnel weapon to be prohibited. There is no evidence that modern munitions in this category cause less injury today than those extant at the time of the St Petersburg Declaration of 1868 – on the contrary. Yet it is to be noted that an increasing number of grenades and shells under 400 g have been introduced.

Of even greater concern is the danger of indiscriminate uses of fragmentation weapons. This problem may partly be dealt with by means of strict procedures governing the use of the various weapons in order to avoid civilian casualties. In general, a munition with an area of effect of 10 m² which can be accurately placed can be used more discriminately than one with an area of effect of thousands of square metres. In each case a safety zone should be determined which takes into account both dispersion due to the delivery system and the dispersion of fragments. Such a safety zone should be several hundred metres for an artillery shell and up to several thousand metres for air-delivered cluster bombs.

Notes to Chapter 5

1. For a given munition exploding at a given height and a given angle of orientation, against a given target, for example, men in sitting and prone positions in hilly terrain, the 'lethal area' can be obtained by integrating the incapacitation probability over the area of effectiveness (i.e., the area within which there are effective fragments), as follows:

$$A_L = \iint_{A_E} P(H) \cdot P(I|H) \, dA$$

where A_L = lethal area, A_E = area of effectiveness, A = area, and $P(H)$ and $P(I|H)$ are the probability of a hit and the probability that a hit will be incapacitating.

2. One authority has contrasted an 'average' 4.2 g fragment from an old shell with an 'average' 0.1 g fragment from a modern, 'improved' munition (Copes, 1976). These figures suggest the magnitude of the change which has occurred since World War II.

3. The St Petersburg Declaration of 1868 prohibited the anti-personnel use of exploding projectiles under 400 g (chapter 9).
4. The method of calculation may be illustrated with a highly simplified example. It might be assumed that individual soldiers in the open offer a target of 0.4 m². To achieve a certain probability of hitting all the soldiers in an area of 1 ha it is necessary to shoot one 'moment of fire'. The number of shells in a moment of fire depends upon the calibre but might, for example, be taken as approximately 18 rounds from a 155 mm gun, 24 rounds from a 120 mm gun, 48 rounds from a 105 mm gun or 72 rounds from a 75 mm gun. For a greater area of coverage, the number of rounds must be multiplied by the number of hectares. For troops hidden in ditches or behind stones, the number of rounds might be doubled, and for troops dug into field fortifications it might be quadrupled or multiplied by an even greater factor. It might require 20 moments of fire to reach a 50 per cent incapacitation level for well-protected troops in shelters.
5. The protection of non-combatants in wartime could be greatly improved by the introduction of concept of a safety zone – at least as extensive as the risk zone of the weapons used – around civilians or civilian objects. This approach was adopted in the US Rules of Engagement in Viet Nam (see appendix 9D).
6. The B-1 bomber is designed to have about twice the carrying capacity of the B-52.

6. Blast and blast weapons

Superior numerals, thus [5], refer to notes on page 177.

I. Physical considerations

Only a few studies of the effects of blast on the human body were made up to World War II. The reason for this is twofold. Firstly, blast waves dissipate rapidly from the point of explosion and are only able to cause injuries over a very limited area. Injuries are much more likely to be caused by secondary missiles in the form of munition or stone fragments, glass splinters, and so on, which travel much further. Consequently, pure blast injuries are rarely seen. Secondly, pure blast injuries tend *either* to cause rapid death *or* to permit relatively easy recovery.

Experimental and clinical studies were initiated in both Britain and Germany during World War II. Following the war, the greater blast danger posed by the atom bomb led to further study of blast physics and biology.

Blast waves result from the rapid release of energy as a result of a chemical reaction or a change in mass (as in a nuclear explosion). In the chemical reaction the pressure wave results from the rapid expansion of a large quantity of gas. Unless confined in a container or other restricted space (such as a tunnel) or medium (such as water or soil) the pressure wave travels radially in all directions and dissipates in proportion to the third power of the distance from the point of explosion. This pressure wave is known as incident or local static pressure and is now measured in pascals (Pa). It is also known as the overpressure, the amount by which it exceeds the ambient pressure. The duration of the overpressure ranges from fractions or tens of milliseconds for high explosives, to tens of seconds for large nuclear explosions. While the overpressure decreases with range, the duration increases with range. Both the overpressure and the duration are important in determining the damaging effects of a blast.

In the open, the pressure wave may reach its maximum almost instantaneously, while in other circumstances – such as when a blast wave enters a building through doors and windows – the maximum pressure may be reached relatively slowly. Where the front of the pressure wave impinges upon a solid object, such as a wall, it may be reflected. The reflected pressure may be magnified 2–9 times the incident pressure, depending, *inter alia,* on the magnitude of the incident pressure. Therefore, in a confined space, such as a tunnel, the blast wave, rather than dissipating in three dimensions, is funnelled along the tunnel by the walls. Consequently, the damaging effect reaches much further. A similar effect occurs in underwater blasts, the pressure being reflected off the bottom of a lake, for instance, as well as from the surface downwards; at the surface, however, some of the blast may break through, causing the water to erupt into the air. The effect of the blast is less at the surface of the water than at a metre or so lower – a fact which has important consequences for persons floating in the water at the time of an explosion (see below, p. 168).

As the front of overpressure passes a given point it is followed by a brief period of underpressure, less in magnitude but of more extended duration. The passage of overpressure and underpressure is accompanied by winds, the force of which is sometimes called dynamic pressure. Thus, the blast of an explosion results in three types of increased pressure: *incident, reflected* and *dynamic*.

To give an indication of the force of these pressures it may be mentioned that hurricane force winds of 54 m/s have a dynamic pressure of 17 kPa, which may be compared with the pressures generated by explosions shown in table 6.1.

Table 6.1. Blast overpressures, duration and lethal range for various quantities of high explosive

Explosive *kg*	Maximum pressure *MPa*	Duration of overpressure *ms*	Lethal range[a] *m*
25	1.49	1.6	4.25
50	1.50	1.6	5.30
200	0.86	4.1	9.70
1 000	0.59	8.6	19.00
1 500	0.55	10.3	22.00
2 000	0.53	11.8	25.00

[a] The figures derive from experiments on dogs. According to the source, essentially 100 per cent mortality within a few minutes is to be expected within this range. Within a further 50–75 cm, irrespective of the size of the charge, about 50 per cent of the affected die within 30–60 minutes. Injuries, not immediately fatal, occurred in a further zone 3–4 m wide.

Source: Desaga (1950a).

Not only can the front of the pressure wave be reflected, but it can also be magnified. This explains certain apparent anomalies with regard to protective structures. Desaga (1950a) reports a case where two men, crouching by a telephone in an anti-aircraft emplacement, were killed from the blast of a bomb nearby, whereas other men in the same emplacement suffered varying degrees of injury, some of them minor. The explanation appeared to be that most of the men were by one wall which was in the lee of the blast wave. The two fatalities were near the other wall which caught the blast wave and reflected it downwards. Clearly, this has important implications for the construction of such fixtures.

Again, blast waves travel further through earth than through air. A man in a small foxhole may be protected from fragments. But if he crouches with his back against the wall of the foxhole, the blast wave travelling through the earth may be transmitted to his body, causing injury, and the walls may collapse, crushing and burying him. At the same distance from the blast in the open air he may have avoided blast injury (Desaga, 1950a). Even for the largest conventional high explosive bombs pure blast injury is unlikely beyond some 35 m. (An exception is the US BLU-82/B, described below, p. 171.)

Biological systems, including the human body, prove to be surprisingly resistant to the effects of blast. The danger is greater from flying stones, shattering glass or collapsing buildings. As a result, primary injuries due to blast, though well defined, are less likely than secondary injuries (by flying objects or crushing) or tertiary injuries (e.g., being hurled against a wall). Blast may also have a variety of other effects. Intense heat and hot gas may sear the body, while dust may lead to suffocation.

II. Primary biological effects of blast

Repeated reports of blast injuries during the Balkan Wars in the early part of this century led Rusca (1915) to perform a number of experiments on the effects of air blast on rabbits and underwater blast on fish. His descriptions and explanations coincide well with more recent studies but his studies 'seem to have fallen into complete oblivion' (Desaga, 1950a, p. 1274). World War I contributed very little to scientific knowledge of blast injuries, but Haldane and others wrote some reports on blast injuries in the Spanish Civil War.

The bombing of cities early in World War II led British and, later, German scientists to study the effects of blast more carefully (Zuckerman, 1940, 1941; Falla, 1940; Hadfield, 1941). The German work was kept secret during the war, some of it being performed more with a view to designing more effective weapons than to treating the wounded (Desage, 1950a). After the war, much of the German work was published under the auspices of the US Air Force (Benzinger, 1950; Rössle, 1950; Desaga, 1950a, b). Clemedson (1949), in Sweden, performed additional experiments and provided one of the most complete reviews of the subject. He and his colleagues have continued to study the physiological effects of blast up to the present.

After World War II considerable research was done in the USA on the effects of blast, primarily owing to interest in the effects of nuclear weapons (Glasstone, 1962; White & Richmond, 1959). As a result of all these studies, the syndrome of blast injury is now well described in the literature.

The most characteristic indication of blast injury is the bursting of the eardrums, which occurs at pressures of about 35 kPa. This indication is a useful one because other internal injuries are unlikely if the ear-drums are undamaged. With more powerful blasts, the inner ear may also be damaged. These injuries are painful but not normally threatening to life, although a case of fatal meningitis following ear injury has been reported (Desaga, 1950a).

At pressures above about 250 kPa, potentially fatal damage occurs to the lungs and other gas-containing organs in the body, such as the stomach and intestines. In simple terms, it is sufficient to describe the lungs as having been crushed or burst; indeed, Desaga (1950a) reports that the X-ray picture 'resembles that of the

166

thorax of a child run over by a vehicle'. There may be no external indication of injury, other than a bloody froth from the mouth and nose.

The actual mechanism of pulmonary injury has been described in considerable detail (e.g., Clemedson *et al.*, 1969; Rössle, 1950; White & Richmond, 1959). Svensson (1974) has developed a mathematical model of blast damage to the lungs which enables calculations of mortality (in per cent) to be made on the basis of transient pressure and duration. As the front of the blast wave comes in contact with the body, it is transmitted through the body fluids with the speed of sound in water (about 1 500 m/s) and reaches the air–fluid interfaces in the lung before the airborne pulse, travelling at near the speed of sound in air (about 340 m/s), can traverse the respiratory tree and counter the increased fluid pressure. The pressure differential between the fluids and the gas in the lungs is sufficient to rupture the membranes (White & Richmond, 1959).

This damage may be increased by spalling and inertia effects. Spalling occurs when a high pressure wave passes from a dense medium to a less dense medium. Particles of the dense medium are thrown off from the surface. (This phenomenon is seen in explosions under water, which create a fine spray of water at the surface, or in solid materials, where a layer at the surface appears to disintegrate into powder. A similar mechanism is suspected in the lungs.) Inertia effects arise where tissues of different densities, for example, the ribs and the surrounding muscles, are subjected to pressure. The less dense material is accelerated more rapidly than the more dense material, from which it may be torn away.

The rupturing of the membranes in the lungs has two potentially fatal effects: small bubbles of air may enter the bloodstream or there may be haemorrhage from the blood-vessels into the alveoli (sacs) of the lungs. The first effect, known as air embolism, appears to be the most likely explanation of rapid death following severe blast injuries. The bubbles of air, carried in the bloodstream, may effectively block the coronary arteries or arteries in important centres of the brain. Desaga (1950a) has demonstrated experimentally that a single small air bubble, the size of a pin's head, injected into the internal carotid artery of a cat, from where it is transported to the brain, results in a short series of spastic currents in the brain's electrical field, which remains deranged for 3–4 hours.

For obvious reasons it is not easy to locate small air bubbles in the bloodstream, and therefore it has proved impossible to demonstrate air embolism in every case of blast death. But in experimental studies, air embolism has been demonstrated in about 85 per cent of deaths (White & Richmond, 1959).

The presence of air emboli in the coronary arteries may cause almost immediate death but, more typically, death occurs after 2–10 minutes. Malfunction of vital centres of the central nervous system due to massive cerebral air embolism may also cause early death. In a few instances, direct damage to the heart (*commotio cordis*) is suspected as the cause of early blast fatalities.

In other instances of severe blast injury where rapid death does not ensue as a result of air embolism, bleeding in the lungs often leads to asphyxiation and death within some 30 minutes. In effect, the victim drowns in his own blood.

It is possible to survive less severe haemorrhage, particularly where the lungs are only partially affected. In such cases bleeding may cease within a few days and the prognosis for the patient is good. The main risk if the patient survives the first 24 hours is pneumonia.

Other gas-containing organs of the body may also suffer from haemorrhage. In some cases these injuries may be fatal, and there is a danger of peritonitis. Because concomitant damage to the lungs is likely, it is usually too risky to use anaesthetics and to operate on the patient, and therefore little can be done until the condition of the patient has stabilized. Neither are blood transfusions to be recommended since they add to the haemorrhage.

Abdominal injuries are relatively more common in underwater blast injuries. Because the pressure at the surface is less severe than at a metre or so deeper, a person floating in a vertical position will be subjected to more pressure on the abdominal region than on the thoracic region. The safest course is to float horizontally on the back, the abdominal organs being better protected from the back by bones and muscles than from the front (Benzinger, 1950; Clemedson, 1966).

III. Localized blast injuries

The injuries referred to above are the result of relatively large air blasts or underwater explosions affecting the whole body. Some weapons consist of small explosive charges which explode in contact with the body and cause local blast injuries, for example explosive bullets and some anti-personnel mines.

The explosive charges used in these weapons are usually too small to cause the kind of injuries referred to above. Inertia effects constitute the main cause of injury. The blast accelerates some parts of the body, usually the limbs or digits, much more than the body mass as a whole. As a result, the accelerated parts or tissues are literally torn off or blown apart. The proximity of the body to the charge may also lead to searing or burning.

In an experiment reported by Mendelson & Glover (1967), small explosive charges were detonated on the thighs of goats[1] and the wounds left untreated. All of the animals died from infection, while only some of the animals injured by high and low velocity projectiles died (table 3.3).

IV. Secondary and tertiary blast injuries

Secondary blast injuries are those that result from projectiles set in motion by the blast. Many types of material may act as missiles, including stones, splinters of wood or glass, and pieces of metal. The pieces may range in size from fine dust to large chunks. These projectiles may or may not penetrate the body. In principle, the severity of injuries due to penetrating projectiles is determined by the factors discussed in chapter 3 on bullet and fragment wounds; in practice, there are a number of additional problems, such as the great risk of wound contamination.

Non-penetrating projectile injuries may also be fatal. Studies have shown that a projectile of a few hundred grams hitting the chest at a relatively low velocity of 50 m/s may lead to death, and at lower velocities may result in rib fractures or lung haemorrhage (White & Richmond, 1959; see table 4.11).

A further type of secondary injury is due to crushing by falling masonry, or by a collapsing building or field fortification. Crushing may result in internal haemorrhage, broken bones and other injuries. Suffocation is also possible.

Tertiary blast injuries are those which result when a person is flung through the air by the force of the blast and hits a hard object. The forces of acceleration acting upon the whole body are not generally sufficient to cause severe injury. But if deceleration is instantaneous, as when the person hits a wall, a broken skull and bones and other injuries may result that may be fatal.

V. Additional pathological effects of blast weapons

Blast weapons may also lead to burn wounds (SIPRI, 1975a). The energy released by the explosion is partly in the form of heat, which – if a person is close enough – may cause searing or burns. Shaped-charge munitions produce a stream of particles of very high velocity which penetrate armoured vehicles or concrete fortifications and may burn people within (US Department of the Navy, 1970). Blast weapons frequently start secondary fires by igniting fuel in vehicles or buildings.

Occasional cases of suffocation by dust inhalation have been reported in civilian life. During World War II, autopsies showed a considerable number of victims of dust inhalation following bombing attacks on cities. From experimental studies it was estimated that the minimum density of dust required to suffocate a man is 100 g/m³ (Desaga, 1950b).

Dust may cause death within a shelter when a bomb explodes outside, owing to spalling effects on the inside walls. In one case, 25 children sheltering in the hallway of a school in Antwerp were suffocated by dust when a bomb hit a nearby house, even though the walls of the hallway were intact and there was no debris on the floor. Autopsies identified plaster dust in diminishing amounts as far down as the alveoli. In the cellar of the same building a nun died of suffocation but three children sheltering in her robes survived (Desaga, 1959b).

VI. Conventional high explosive munitions

As pointed out previously, the great majority of conventional munitions use high explosives, but for anti-personnel use the primary purpose of the high explosive charge is to propel solid projectiles, such as bullets or fragments, at high velocities. It is these projectiles, rather than the blast effect, which constitute the main source of injuries.

General purpose munitions. In some circumstances, however, the blast effect of general purpose munitions, such as artillery shells and aircraft bombs, is much more significant. Where enemy personnel are in prepared positions which protect them from bullets or fragments, munitions are fuzed to permit penetration of the ground or walls of fortifications. The explosion then transmits a blast through the earth or concrete, with the dual purpose of destroying the position and the men inside.

The depth of penetration of air-dropped bombs depends upon such factors as the height at which they are dropped, the density of the soil, and the weight of the bomb. The size of the crater is not indicative of the lethal range of the blast since the blast waves may travel further through the soil and cause death and injury to personnel in dug-out positions some metres further away.

Although it is now more common to bombard prepared positions with deep-penetrating bombs from high-flying aircraft, a much-used tactic in previous times was to dig a tunnel under the enemy positions and then blow them up from below. On one occasion during World War I, at Messines, British forces dug tunnels under German positions along a front of four kilometres and then detonated about half a million kilograms of explosives, destroying not only the German positions but killing thousands of men and obliterating several villages (Mullins, 1965). This type of mine appears to be the origin of the term 'mine', which is now more generally employed to refer to explosive devices emplaced in the ground or under-water (chapter 7).

Explosive charges, or explosive gaseous or liquid mixtures, may sometimes be placed or pumped into tunnel systems suspected of harbouring enemy forces or munitions (see p. 173). Special purpose blast munitions are used to damage or destroy armoured vehicles and their crews.

Offensive hand-grenades. Hand-grenades are usually of the fragmentation type and are described as 'defensive'; that is, they are used by troops in stationary positions against attacking forces. 'Offensive' grenades, on the other hand, may be used by troops in assault. They rely on blast, since – having a smaller and better-defined effective radius – they are safer for use by troops moving into the area of effect. Several modern designs consist of a basic blast grenade, often with a plastic case, over which a fragmentation 'sleeve' can be fitted if desired. For this reason, offensive as well as defensive grenades are included in table 5.1 in chapter 5 on fragmentation weapons.

Mines. Many anti-personnel mines rely on blast. Fragmentation mines have a greater area of effect, but metal fragments make such mines easier to detect with the aid of magnetic mine-detectors. Partly for this reason, the modern trend in anti-personnel mines is to make the case of plastic or other non-metallic material and to rely on blast as the casualty agent. Mines are discussed in more detail in the next chapter.

VII. Demolition or concussion bombs

It was pointed out previously that the damaging effects of blast depend not only upon the maximum pressure reached but also upon the duration. The effects of 'high' overpressure of 'short' duration may be exceeded by a 'low' pressure of 'long' duration. Where an explosive charge is primarily intended to impart a high velocity to fragments, then a high pressure of short duration is required. But where maximum blast effect is required, it may be better to maximize duration rather than peak pressure. Table 6.1 shows that the duration of the blast wave is related to the quantity of explosive.

Thus, whereas for fragmentation purposes a large number of small bombs may be more effective than the same weight of larger bombs, for blast purposes a larger bomb may be more effective than many small ones.

This is the explanation of the development during World War II of large 'block-busters' – bombs weighing one tonne or more, in some cases 5–10 tonnes. During World War II these bombs were used against built-up areas.

A modern development of the block-buster is the US BLU-82/B. This bomb, weighing some 6 800 kg, was first used, in Indo-China, in early 1970. It contains some 5 715 kg of a special dense blasting agent (DBA-22M) consisting of a gelled aqueous slurry of ammonium nitrate and aluminium powder (plus a binding agent). The energy yield is roughly 9×10^6 J/kg, about twice that of TNT. It produces a concussive blast greater than that of the smallest nuclear devices (cf. Glasstone, 1962). By means of a 97 cm long probe extending from the nose, it is fuzed to explode just above the surface of the ground.

It is reported that the BLU-82/B's radius of 100 per cent mortality for plant and animal life is 65 m (US Air Force press release, 10 January 1972) and that the radius of 50 per cent mortality for human beings is 71.6 m (Westing, 1972). The zone of death and injury, presumably mainly due to flying secondary missiles, falling trees, and so on, extends to nearly 400 m from the point of the explosion.

Perhaps several hundred of these bombs were dropped in Indo-China between 1970 and 1972. The primary purpose was said to be to produce instant clearings in the jungle so that helicopters could land troops and supplies. However, other uses were also reported. In some cases BLU-82/Bs were used to block roads by causing landslides. US diplomatic and military sources indicated to Westing (1972) that the bomb was also used on some occasions against suspected enemy troop concentrations. Anti-personnel use was also reported in the press (e.g., *New York Times,* 13 April 1971, 15 April 1971, 19 April 1971; Associated Press, 27 February 1972). The obliteration of a hamlet in Laos by a BLU-82/B was reported in Hanoi in 1971 (Westing, 1972).

VIII. Fuel–air explosives

Most military explosives are solids and contain an oxidizing agent. It has long been known, however, that some gas or aerosol clouds of small particles (Clague, 1972) or vapour droplets can become explosive when mixed with a certain proportion of air. Explosions in coal-mines are due to a mixture of methane gas and air. Many other gases as well as clouds of particles of, for example, aluminium, magnesium or even flour, may form explosive mixtures in air and have been responsible for some large industrial accidents.

Not surprisingly, this principle has been investigated for possible military application. There are a number of potential military advantages: (*a*) the air itself may provide the oxygen required for the combustion and therefore, weight for weight, a fuel–air explosive (FAE or FAX) is more efficient than a conventional explosive, which also has to contain an oxidizing agent (Blomqvist, 1976); (*b*) since the aerosol cloud spreads out over an area before detonating, a given quantity of explosive can produce a wider and more evenly distributed area of blast compared with conventional solid explosive, detonating at a point; (*c*) there is the possibility that the cloud can spread through vegetation, or follow the contour of the ground into, for example, foxholes or trenches, and thereby offer a more effective weapon against troops sheltered from fragmentation weapons; (*d*) the relatively well-defined area of effect makes FAEs attractive for use in certain situations, such as close support; and (*e*) the explosive substance itself is cheaper than conventional explosives (though the mechanical devices required to utilize it as a bomb may be more complicated).

In spite of these obvious advantages, fuel–air explosives have not been widely used in combat until recently because of the difficulties of devising an effective system for spreading and detonating the fuel–air mixture. These difficulties are now being overcome.

Some accounts describe a British attempt in 1944 to develop a bomb using compressed methane. This bomb consisted of a cylinder about 50 cm long, containing a mixture of petroleum and compressed methane, and weighing about 15 kg (Stettbacher, 1948). The liquid evaporated to form a cloud of gas which, when ignited, oxidized extremely rapidly with a combined fire and blast effect.

The US Navy tested a fuel–air explosive bomb at its China Lake test station in 1960 but did not begin extensive development until 1966. In 1967 the US Navy tested (i.e., used in combat) twenty 100 lb (46 kg) BLU-73 bombs in Viet Nam. The bombs, containing ethylene oxide, were implanted at the edge of minefields, and could detonate mines and defoliate trees over an area of about 15–30 m in diameter. At the same time the US Air Force tested a 2 500 lb (1 150 kg) bomb filled with liquid hydrocarbon fuel but operational tests were not successful. The two versions used in these tests, the BLU-72 (for use by A-1 aircraft) and the BLU-76 (for use by F-4s), were discontinued, as was the 450 lb (200 kg) BLU-64. Other fuels tested included propylene oxide and a liquid petroleum fuel, methylacetylene/propadiene/propene with traces of butane (MAPP). These fuels are produced in large quantities for civilian purposes and are relatively cheap. Development work focused on the CBU-55, a cluster bomb containing three of the smaller BLU-73 bomblets. By October 1970 an operational, air-dropped version of this bomb was shipped to Viet Nam, following further testing in tropical forests in Panama (Robinson, 1973).

The CBU-55 consists of an SUU-49 dispenser which, with the aid of an FMU-95 Mechanical Time Fuze, opens at a predetermined time to distribute the three BLU-73 bomblets. The three bomblets burst on contact with the ground by the action of an FMU-74 fuze, spreading out a cloud of ethylene oxide vapour. After a brief delay (usually 125 ms, though it may be up to 3–4 s) the cloud is detonated, producing a powerful blast.

This rather complex sequence of events meant that some difficulties were experienced before the technique was perfected. The bombs have to be retarded with a parachute to prevent too rapid contact with the ground and to enable the delivery aircraft to escape from the area. Early versions were designed to be dropped by helicopters and slow fixed-wing aircraft which could deliver the bomb at low speeds. The reason for this is that the fuel–air mixture is only explosive within certain limits: at higher or lower concentrations the mixture does not explode. Therefore the whole process of dispensing the cloud of gas has to be carefully controlled.

In 1974 the US Navy requested $6.2 million to buy 3 500 CBU-72 fuel–air explosive bombs during the fiscal year 1975 (1 July 1974–30 June 1975). These bombs are essentially similar to the CBU-55 but modified for use by jet aircraft flying at up to 450 knots. According to Admiral Gaddis:

> This weapon is designed to be an effective blast weapon against protected and concealed troops, land mines, booby traps and light material targets ... These weapons are more effective, as well as more sophisticated than the Southeast Asia mainstay the 500 pound (230 kg) MK 82 ... (US Senate Committee on Appropriations, 1974, part 3, p. 860).[2]

The US Army has modified the CBU-55 for use on helicopters in a system known as FAESHED (Fuel Air Explosive Helicopter Delivered). It is also developing a system called SLUFAE (Surface Launched Unit FAE System), which consists of an array of 30 rocket-launching tubes firing rockets equipped with FAE warheads (*Aerospace Daily*, 15 July 1974). Each warhead contains about 39 kg of propylene oxide and produces an explosive aerosol cloud about 4 m in thickness and 17 m in diameter. When all 30 rockets are launched simultaneously, an area of 8 × 100 m is affected at a range of up to 700 m (Dennis, 1975). The primary role is the rapid clearing of minefields (see chapter 7).

Some US reports suggest many possible future developments for fuel–air explosives. For example, the US Marine Corps has been reported as developing a system known as MAD FAE (Mass Air Delivery FAE). (MAD is also a common acronym for 'Massive Assured Destruction' by nuclear weapons.) MAD FAE consists of a pair of dispensers, each of which contains twelve 136 lb (62 kg) FAE warheads – that is, the equivalent of at least 8 CBU-55s. The whole device is suspended from a helicopter. This device could therefore destroy an area of several hectares in a single attack.

In another application of the fuel–air explosive principle, US forces in Indo-China destroyed tunnels and people sheltering in them by pumping in and detonating acetylene (Sayle, 1973). A special acetylene pack was produced for this purpose, as was a pack containing ammonium nitrate/nitromethane liquid explosive.

A wide range of other hydrocarbons have possible military applications, including those which (*a*) do not require oxygen for spontaneous combustion (e.g., ethylene oxide), (*b*) continue to burn without oxygen or air (e.g., propyl nitrate),

(c) contain a high proportion of oxygen and cause a violent reaction on contact with combustible material (e.g., peracetic acid), (d) explode on contact with moist air at ambient temperature (e.g. diborane), or (e) react violently on contact with oxygen-rich materials, and in addition, ignite spontaneously on contact with certain substances (e.g., anhydrous unsymmetrical dimethylhydrazine) (Johannsohn, 1977).

According to Johannsohn (1977), a 'third generation' of FAE weapons is already being developed. He estimates that the blast area of a 553 kg FAE charge of the new kind would exceed 400 m in diameter, and a 1 000 kg charge would cover an area with a diameter of 490 m at a peak pressure exceeding 0.42 kp/cm² (about 42 kPa). (A blast of this magnitude is sufficient to destroy parked aircraft and damage ships and other material.) As a result, it is possible to develop FAE warheads for many purposes, such as anti-ship cruise missiles and anti-ballistic-missile missiles, since even a 'near miss' of several hundred metres would still destroy the target.

When the cloud of vapour from an FAE bomb explodes it produces a powerful blast with a maximum peak pressure of some 2.5 MPa. This is about 25 per cent lower than that of TNT but the duration is much longer. As a result, the blast of FAE is some 2–5 times as effective, weight for weight, as TNT (Johannsohn, 1977). The blast level is 2–3 times that required to kill 99 per cent of the men in the area, according to experts at the Lucerne Conference of Government Experts (ICRC, 1974), or 10 times the level at which severe injuries may be expected. This overpressure is produced evenly throughout the cloud, which for a 35–40 kg load is typically several metres thick and about 15 m in diameter (Blomqvist, 1976).

Although the blast wave dissipates rapidly beyond the borders of the vapour cloud, it covers an area about 40 per cent larger than the blast wave from an equivalent weight of TNT (Johannsohn, 1977). The succeeding underpressure is also capable of causing injury to persons at some distance from the point of detonation.

In general, fuel–air explosive bombs differ from conventional munitions in that they are pure blast weapons. Therefore they produce few injuries via fragments, flying stones, glass, and so on, which are the most common causes of injury from conventional weapons. Rössle (1950) pointed out that 'neither in combat nor in aerial warfare in Germany has death by blast occurred frequently. Accordingly earlier literature does not contain any relevant data ... The external injuries resulting from hurling, entombment, shell fragments, etc. had attracted all the attention' (p. 1270). Fuel–air explosives may cause a very high proportion of pure blast injuries with few external symptoms, in marked contrast to conventional weapons. It seems most likely that this is the explanation of reports from Cambodia (*Le Monde,* 5 February 1974) and Viet Nam (AFP, 23 April 1975), which emphasize the asphyxiating effect of fuel–air explosive bombs. These and other press reports suggested that asphyxiation was due to the fact that an FAE bomb uses up all the oxygen in the area of effect.

While it is quite correct that a large amount of oxygen is consumed, it is promptly replaced by an inrush of air. It seems unlikely, therefore, that asphyxiation results from lack of oxygen. Rather it results, as described above, from physical damage to the membranes of the lungs.

In a confined space, shortage of oxygen following an FAE detonation might lead to the production of carbon monoxide. A concentration of only 0.5 per cent of carbon monoxide in the air can lead to death in a few minutes. But in a confined space, the blast effect of FAE is also likely to be the predominant effect.

When the cloud detonates it produces a rapid fire-ball which produces much heat. It is of too short a duration to have a notable incendiary effect, but it might cause searing and flash burns.

At some concentrations, fuel–air mixtures burn rather than explode. 'Chemical fire-ball' weapons causing third degree burns by means of thermal radiation have already been developed (SIPRI, 1975a). Research has been done on an intermediate category of 'flame-blast' weapons (US Army Munitions Command, 1973).

Again, if the correct concentration of the vapour in air is not attained, the mixture may not detonate at all. The explosive concentration is usually reached within 200 ms, and there are therefore great demands on the precision of the fuzing system. Ethylene oxide is toxic and only small concentrations in the air produce physical symptoms (Thiess, 1963; Thiess & Goldmann 1968).

Although the USA has been the main developer and user of fuel–air explosives, there are signs of proliferation. The USA supplied CBU-55 bombs to the Khmer Republic (*Le Monde,* 5 February 1975) and to the Saigon Government in Viet Nam (*The Times,* 24 April 1975), and it apparently offered them to Israel (Lescaze, 1976), although the offer was later withdrawn. The Soviet Union is reported to be testing FAE devices (Robinson, 1973b) and may well have a large arsenal of them (Johannsohn, 1977). Tests have been carried out in other countries, such as Sweden (Norrvi, 1975a, b).

IX. Summary and conclusions

Although most conventional weapons employ high explosives, pure blast injuries are seldom seen because secondary missiles and other effects extend further than the injurious blast wave. High explosive munitions are therefore more likely to cause death and injury by means of penetrating or non-penetrating missiles than by the direct effects of blast on the human body. Where blast injuries, in air or in water, do occur, they are characterized by very high lethality within a restricted area, due most frequently to air embolism in the heart or brain. In a further narrow band around the point of detonation, damage to the lungs and gas-containing organs of the abdomen may lead to haemorrhage.

Localized blast injuries, usually caused by anti-personnel mines, typically cause severe lacerations, fractures and often amputation of limbs or digits.

The most usual anti-personnel blast munitions are 'offensive' hand-grenades and anti-personnel mines. Recently, however, a number of blast munitions with a much wider area of effect have reportedly been used against personnel. These include large concussion bombs, such as the BLU-82/B, and fuel–air explosive bombs.

A wide-area blast weapon would completely clear an area not only of enemy forces but of obstructions, such as vegetation, which might obscure their presence, and with no danger to any troops subsequently landed in the area.

The very high mortality resulting from area blast weapons makes their use as anti-personnel weapons dubious from the point of view of humanitarian law. The possible public reaction to the use of large concussion bombs appears to have made military users more cautious in providing information about their effects (Westing, 1972).

Fuel–air explosives in particular raise a delicate point of law, particularly in relation to the Declaration of the Hague Conference of 1899, where it was stated:

> The contracting Powers agree to abstain from the use of projectiles the sole object of which is the diffusion of *asphyxiating or deleterious gases* (italics added).

There can be little doubt that the action of a fuel–air explosive is deleterious. It is also asphyxiating, but by physical rather than chemical means. The similar effects on the victim of chemical and physical asphyxiation can be seen from the following descriptions with regard to chemical asphyxiants and blast weapons respectively. The first quotation describes the effects of an asphyxiating gas on soldiers during World War I:

> ... The civilized world ought to have the truth fully brought before them in vivid detail, and not wrapped up as at present.
> ... It was a most appalling sight, all these poor black faces struggling for life, what with the groaning and noise of the effort for breath.
> ... There is practically nothing to be done for them, except to give them salt and water to try to make them sick.
> The effect gas has is to fill the lungs with a watery frothy matter, which gradually rises till it fills up the whole lungs and comes up to the mouth; then they die; it is suffocation; slow drowning, taking in some cases one or two days. (*The Times,* 7 May 1915)

The second quotation is taken from World War II studies of blast injuries:

> After the blast, most of the injured persons groan and scream continuously, they complain of severe pain in the chest when breathing and sometimes of pain in the whole trunk and extremities. ... As a rule dyspnea and expectoration of blood-containing froth appeared immediately even in cases of mild injuries ... Severely injured persons pant heavily, showing a labored respiration – particularly conspicuous in expiration – which may be very slow, *similar to toxic respiration ...*
> ... The patients discharge varying quantities of bloody froth from

176

mouth and nose during the first 5 to 6 hours. This is a typical symptom of blast injury. . . .

Severely injured or moribund individuals often have a bloody froth protruding like a mushroom from mouth and nose. (Desaga, 1950*a*, pp. 1285–86; italics added)

From these descriptions it is clear that asphyxiation is much the same whether the membranes of the lungs are destroyed by toxic chemicals or by blast pressure. This being so, it might be argued that the anti-personnel use of blast weapons should be subject to the same legal restrictions as chemical weapons.

A substantial argument for banning weapons of this kind (in addition to arguments depending on the high lethality, unnecessary suffering, and so on) is the threshold argument (SIPRI, 1976*b*). The weapons used so far may be only the beginning of a whole new area of military technology. Fuel–air explosives could be increased in size almost indefinitely. For example, it has been calculated that the liquefied natural gas (LNG) contained in a tank-ship could explode with the power of an atom bomb. It takes little imagination to conceive of the scale of possible proliferation – at a time when there is considerable concern about possible nuclear proliferation.

A further consideration is the fact that blast weapons are predominantly offensive weapons, mainly intended to overcome the defence. For example, compared with fragmentation weapons, they are hardly cost-effective against troops in the open, but they may be more effective against troops in defensive positions. Most accounts of FAE weapons emphasize their effectiveness for instantly clearing minefields, but minefields have hitherto had mainly defensive functions. Some press accounts suggest that fuel–air explosive bombs may be able to damage or destroy aircraft on the ground in protected positions. Partly for this reason, there was concern that the USA would supply these weapons to Israel. This could be tantamount to providing a 'first-strike capability', which could have very serious implications for the military balance of the region – a fear apparently shared by some US officials (Lescaze, 1976; Greenway, 1977).[3]

Notes to Chapter 6

1. This method was standardized and described by Ochsner, Jacob & Mansberger (1958).
2. In 1973 the US Navy budgeted for 468 600 MK 82 500-lb conventional high explosive bombs at a total cost of $172 762 000, that is, $368.67 each. The CBU-72s cost $1 771.42 each the following year.
3. The very first question put to incoming US President Carter at his first Presidential press conference concerned these weapons. The questioner, the doyen of the Washington press corps, was assured by the President that the bombs (referred to as concussion bombs, but later explained as meaning fuel–air explosives) were a matter of great concern. It was later announced that the United States would *not* export these bombs and that previous indications to the contrary had not been authorized at the highest levels.

7. Delayed-action weapons

Superior numerals, thus [5], refer to notes on pages 200–201.

I. Non-exploding devices

A variety of non-explosive, delayed-action weapons have been employed, probably throughout history, in many parts of the world. They may take the form of covered pits, perhaps with sharpened stakes at the bottom, an arrangement also used for trapping animals. Many other kinds of trap make use of mechanical energy. For example, a heavy stone may be propped up in such a way that when the intended victim disturbs the prop, the stone crashes down on him. A flexible bough or piece of bamboo may be bent and fixed in some way so that when it is released it catapults a projectile, such as a sharpened wooden or bamboo stake, at the victim.

Devices of this kind are often used in jungle warfare, since materials are readily to hand and they are easy to improvise and disguise. They can be very effective in putting a man out of action and may cause very unpleasant injuries.

Devices of this kind were used in some areas of Indo-China during the recent war there. A small percentage of US soldiers were wounded by them (Kovaric *et al.,* 1969; Rich, Johnson & Dimond, 1967) but none of these authors records any fatalities.

Although there is a possibility that primitive non-exploding devices may be indiscriminate in their effects, in that unsuspecting persons for whom they were not intended may inadvertently walk into them, they are often used in areas where the local population is small and fully aware of such defensive measures. There is only a minor long-term hazard, and once the device is detected it is usually very easy to dismantle.

The scatterable, non-explosive device constitutes a different approach. An example is the caltrop – a four-pronged piece of iron, so designed that, whichever way it falls, one prong always points upwards. Such objects can relatively easily be seen and avoided by foot-soldiers, but are more effective in injuring the feet of horses and other draught animals. Development of caltrops continued in the USA during the 1960s.[1]

II. Delayed-action shells and bombs

There is a great variety of delayed-action weapons, ranging from inert or explosive devices waiting for an unwary foot to tread on them, to munitions which explode after a given time or when detonated by remote control. They may consist of conventional projectiles fitted with a time-delay fuze or, as in the case of mines, be specially constructed. Some delayed-action devices are improvised in the field.

The wounding effects of delayed-action weapons are no different from those of the weapons with immediate effect already described. The legal and humanitarian problem raised by delayed-action weapons is due to their possible indiscriminate effects, both short-term and long-term. Since, in general, they depend upon the 'target going to the weapon' rather than vice versa, the user often has much less control over the effects of the weapon, as other persons or animals than those for whom the weapon was intended may inadvertently actuate it. For those categories of delayed-action weapon which do not detonate automatically or otherwise render themselves harmless, the hazard may remain long after the conclusion of hostilities unless difficult and expensive measures are taken to locate and dispose of them. All too often those who deploy the weapons fail to dispose of them at the conclusion of hostilities. As a consequence of World War II, for example, thousands of people have died from unexploded munitions left behind by passing armies, and casualties still occur every year.

Delayed-action fuzes are available for many types of conventional artillery shells and bombs. Time fuzes have several functions which should be clearly distinguished:

1. A time fuze may be used to detonate a shell or bomb in the air *before* it hits the target. The purpose is to maximize the distribution of fragments over the target.

2. A time fuze may be used to detonate a shell or bomb *after it penetrates* (rather than on impact with) the target. The purpose is usually to maximize the effects of blast on protected targets, on buildings or underwater.

3. A short-time fuze (or other delay device such as a drogue parachute) may be used to allow the delivering agent (often an aircraft) to escape from the risk zone.

4. A long-delay time fuze may be used to increase the duration of effect of the munition or of other munitions delivered simultaneously.

The present discussion is entirely concerned with the fourth category. The first three categories, though they use time fuzes, are essentially immediate impact munitions, plus or minus a few seconds, and are in this respect no different from the munitions described in the preceding chapters.[2]

Shells and bombs fitted with long-delay fuzes may be used in a variety of ways, some of which raise issues of humanitarian concern. During World War II it became common practice to mix bombloads of incendiary bombs with explosive bombs, some of which were fitted with delayed-action fuzes. This tactic was described as follows:

> The bombing of an already burning area with [high explosive bombs] serves to impede the efforts of local fire fighters ... Fragmentation bombs have been found to be reasonably satisfactory in restraining firemen without impeding the progress of the fires. These of course must be detonated while the firefighting is in progress. Delayed action bombs dropped at random throughout the area also add to the uncertainty and confusion of the defence. (Fisher, 1946, p. 9)

A British military directive suggests that the use of delayed-action bombs was learned from Germany:

> The use of approximately 10 per cent delay action bombs is recommended in view of the difficulties experienced by the railway authorities from the small number of similar bombs dropped in England, especially if set to explode at frequent intervals and so prevent or seriously interfere with firefighting, repair and general traffic organisation. (Directive, 9 July 1941, from Air Vice-Marshal N. H. Bottomley, Deputy Chief of Air Staff, to Air Marshal Sir Richard Peirse. In Webster & Frankland, 1961, vol. IV, p. 140)

Many of the anti-personnel fragmentation bombs dropped by the USA on Indo-China were of a kind which either remained inactive until disturbed (that is, they acted like mines) or they exploded after a random delay. The major purpose of using these over North Viet Nam was said to be to suppress anti-aircraft fire, permitting bombers to reach military, industrial and communications targets. Delayed-action fuzes were fitted in an attempt to force anti-aircraft artillery crews to take cover for a longer period of time, during which the bombers could reach their targets, deliver their loads and return to a safe distance.[3]

Harvey (1967) reports that delayed-action fragmentation bombs were also used against personnel in South Viet Nam:

> ... the deadliest weapon of all, at least against personnel, were CBUs – cluster bomb units ... Some types were fitted with delayed action fuzes and went off later when people have come out thinking the area was safe. (Harvey, 1967, p. 57)

III. Land-mines

Until World War I it was a standard procedure to dig shafts and tunnels ('mines') under enemy positions and blow them up with large quantities of explosives. The method had its drawbacks in that the attacking troops either could not cross the large crater formed, as at Messines during World War I (Mullins, 1965), or were trapped in it and massacred, as at Petersburg, Pennsylvania during the US Civil War (Pleasants, 1938).

The advent of the tank made this kind of mine obsolete by providing an alternative means of crossing the no man's land between the lines and breaching the defences of the other side (Kitching, 1975). But the presence of the tank on the battlefield promoted the introduction of a new type of 'mine', a small explosive device, intended to put tanks out of action. World War I mines for this purpose were often improvised from trench-mortar ammunition, buried with the contact uppermost. During the 1920s, specially designed anti-tank mines were developed and they have remained much the same up to the present day. They typically consist of a container about 30 cm in diameter, containing about 10 kg of explosive. Some modern types make use of a shaped charge or kinetic energy penetrator (US Department of the Army, 1964; Tresckow, 1975).

Initially, the purpose of anti-personnel mines was to prevent the removal of anti-tank mines, which, since they often required a pressure of several hundred kilograms to detonate them, could be handled comparatively safely by personnel. Anti-tank minefields, therefore, are typically 'seeded' with anti-personnel mines. Alternatively (or perhaps in addition), anti-tank mines may be booby-trapped – that is, equipped with additional fuzes which detonate the mine if it is disturbed. Some anti-tank mines are manufactured with wells for as many as three additional fuzes; other mines can only be booby-trapped by means of improvised or special devices (US Department of the Army, 1964).

Subsequently, anti-personnel mines were widely used independently to protect infantry positions from enemy foot-soldiers (Kitching, 1975) or to delay occupying forces after a retreat. These mines were usually actuated by foot pressure on pins projecting from the mine itself or by means of a trip-wire. Mines can also be rigged for remote detonation by a hidden observer.

There are several categories of conventional anti-personnel mine. *Non-directional fragmentation mines* are the simplest, so called because they detonate on or just below the surface of the ground and eject fragments in all directions. The effective casualty radius (i.e., the radius of the circle within which about 50 per cent of exposed persons can be expected to be incapacitated) is about 10 m, but individual fragments may travel 100–150 m. Much of the effect is lost in the ground surrounding the mine. This type of mine is not common nowadays.

Bounding fragmentation mines are equipped with a propelling charge which throws the mine about 2 m into the air before it detonates. The effective casualty radius is 30–50 m and the risk zone about 200 m. The German S-mine, introduced in 1935, was one of the first mines of this type. It ejected metal balls as well as steel fragments. During World War II most of the combatants made use of similar mines (table 7.1), and they have remained in service until recently. The high velocity steel fragments ejected at eye-level are particularly deadly.

Directional fragmentation mines, as the name implies, project fragments in a limited arc. The best-known mine of this kind is the US *Claymore* (M-18 and M-18A1). It was invented during the Korean War for use against the so-called 'human wave' infantry attacks and awarded US patent no. 2 972 949 in February 1961 (MacLeod, 1967). It is designed to project 700 steel spheres at high velocity in a 60° arc about 2 m high and about 50 m across some 50 m from the point of origin. Powerful C-4 explosive is packed behind a layer of steel spheres embedded in a glass fibre matrix. The blast is dangerous within a circle of 16 m radius and the spheres can cause casualties at distances up to 250 m. It is detonated electrically by trip-wire or remote control (US Department of the Army, 1964). Similar mines are now produced in other countries, for example, Sweden.

Blast mines rely primarily on blast rather than fragmentation for their effects. Some are quite small, have a plastic case, and are mass produced. Others are larger and may have a wooden, glass or concrete case, and in some cases are improvised in the field. The reason for dispensing with metal is that mines containing

Table 7.1. Examples of anti-personnel mines

Producing country and weapon designation	Total weight kg	Explosive	Explosive weight g	Type	Actuation	Approx. casualty radius m	Approx. risk zone m	Remarks
Belgium								
PRB-AP-BAC-H 28	0.165	TNT/RDX	65	Blast	Pressure	..	..	Plastic case
PRB-AP-M 35	0.158	TNT-KNO$_3$	100	Blast	Pressure	..	..	Plastic case
PRB-AP-M 409	0.183	Trialene	80	Blast	Pressure	..	..	Plastic case
PRB-413	0.640	Composition B	90	600 fragments	Trip-wire	14	30	Plastic with steel wire sleeve
Canada								
M-25 *Elsie*	0.86	..	10	Blast	Pressure (6–8 kg)	..	..	Hollow charge
C3A1	0.86	..	10	Blast	Pressure (6–8 kg)	..	..	Hollow charge
Czechoslovakia								
Na-Mi-Ba	2.4	TNT	..	Blast	Trip-wire	..	..	For use in booby traps
PP-Mi-Sr	3.2	TNT	325	Bounding, fragmentation	Trip-wire or pressure (3.5 kg)	..	..	
PP-Mi-Sb	2.1	TNT	75	Fragmentation	Trip-wire or pressure (1 kg)	..		Case of steel pieces embedded in concrete; for mounting on stake
PP-Mi-St	1.7	TNT	75	Fragmentation (cast iron)	Trip-wire	20	..	Same as Soviet POMZ-2

France

..	..	..	..	Bounding, fragmentation	Pressure or trip-wire	50	..	Adapted 60 mm mortar shell, World War II
Mle 53	..	..	..	Bounding, fragmentation	Pressure or trip-wire	50	..	
Mle 51	85	Trotyl	40	Blast	Pressure	..	..	Plastic case
Mle 59	0.130	..	56	Blast	Pressure	..	..	Plastic case; optional metal ring to permit electromagnetic detection

Germany (pre-1945)

S-150 Behelfs-Schützen Mine	0.35	Picric acid	149	Blast	Pressure	..	..	
S. Mine 35	4.0	..	280	Bounding, c. 350 steel spheres and fragmentation	Pressure (6.9 kg)	50	150–200	World War II
Glasmine 43	..	..	..	Blast	Pressure (18.4 kg)	..	..	
S. Mine 42	..	..	100	Blast	Pressure	..	..	Impregnated plywood or fibre case
S. Mine 43 (N)	..	..	..	Blast	Pressure	..	..	Impregnated plywood or fibre case
S. Mine 44	..	..	..	Fragmentation	Pressure (9.6 kg) or trip-wire (6.4 kg)	20	100	
Schützen-Dosenmine	..	..	..	Blast	Pressure	..	..	

Table 7.1 (*continued*)

Producing country and weapon designation	Total weight kg	Explosive	Explosive weight g	Type	Actuation	Approx. casualty radius m	Approx. risk zone m	Remarks
Germany, FR								
DM-11	200	..	..	..	..	..	..	Swedish L1AB
DM-31	..	..	..	..	..	..	..	
German DR								
SM-70	..	..	102.4	90 iron cubes	Trip-wire	..	..	Placed along border
K-2	50	..	..	Bounding, steel balls and fragments	Trip-wire	..	..	Placed along border
Hungary								
M-49	0.3	TNT	75	Blast	Trip-wire	..	..	Wooden or plastic case
..	3.6	TRI-II	800	Steel balls	Trip-wire	..	..	Can be mounted on stake
Israel								
IMI No. 10	0.120	TNT	50	Blast	Pressure (15–35 kg)	..	..	Supplied to Uganda
IMI No. 12	3.5	TNT	250	Bounding, steel balls	Trip-wire	40	..	Supplied to Uganda, Argentina
Italy								
..	0.45	..	150	Blast	..	..	..	Plastic case; World War II
SACI 56	..	..	..	Blast	..	..	..	
Valmara 69	..	..	..	Fragmentation	..	50	50	
VS 50	..	..	..	Blast	..	..	..	Similar to French Mle 51

Japan (pre-1945)								
Model 99	1.2	..	..	Fragmentation	..	..	..	4 magnets to hold it in place against metal target, e.g., vehicle
Netherlands								
M-2A3	..	..	..	Bounding, fragmentation	..	..	..	Modified French design
AP 22	85	Trotyl	40	Blast	Pressure	..	..	French Mle 51, plastic case
Sweden								
L1AB	..	..	..	Blast	..	..	..	Plastic case
AP-12	14	..	..	Steel spheres	Trip-wire or electrical	50	..	*Claymore* type
UK								
Mk II	4.6	Amatol	460	Fragmentation	Trip-wire (1.8 kg)	30	..	World War II
AP 6 MK 1	..	..	..	Bounding	..	50	..	World War II
AP 8 *Red Elsie*	..	..	..	Blast	..	..	..	Plastic case
	..	..	..	Blast	..	..	..	Hollow charge; modified Canadian M-25
Dingbat	..	..	..	Blast	..	..	..	Camouflaged
Ranger	..	..	..	Blast	..	..	..	1 296 scattered by 78-tube launcher
USA								
M-2	2.3	TNT	156	Bounding, steel fragmentation	Pressure (3.7–9.2 kg); trip-wire (1.4–4.6 kg)	10	150	Modified 60 mm mortar shell

Table 7.1 (*continued*)

Producing country and weapon designation	Total weight kg	Explosive	Explosive weight g	Type	Actuation	Approx. casualty radius m	Approx. risk zone m	Remarks
USA (*continued*)								
M-3	..	TNT	414	Non-directional, cast-iron fragmentation	Pressure (3.7–9.2 kg); trip-wire (1.4–4.6 kg)	10 on ground; 10+ above ground	100	3 fuze wells to permit booby-trapping
M-16/M-16A1	3.6	TNT	454	Bounding, steel or cast-iron fragmentation	Pressure (3.7–9.2 kg); trip-wire (1.4–4.6 kg)	30	200	
M-18/M-18A1 *Claymore*	1.6	C-4	690	Directional, 700 steel spheres (0.68 g)	Electrical (trip-wire or remote)	50–100	250	Fragments projected in 60° arc, 2 m high; blast effect to 16 m
M-14	0.09	Tetryl	28	Blast	Pressure (9.2–16 kg)	..	..	Non-metallic

USSR

PMD-6	0.4	TNT	200	Blast, wooden splinters	Pressure or trip-wire	..	..	World War II; wooden case
PMD-7/PMD-7ts	0.3	TNT	75	Blast, wooden splinters	Pressure (1–5 kg)	..	..	World War II
PMK-40	90	..	50	Blast	Pressure (9 kg)	..	..	Impregnated paper case
..	..	..	..	Bounding	..	..	..	World War II
POMZ-2	1.7	TNT	75	Fragmenting, scored-steel	Trip-wire	20	..	Resembles hand-grenade, mounted on stake
PMND-2-65	..	..	..	..	..	..	..	
PMN	0.6	TNT	240	Blast	Pressure	..	..	Plastic case; 4 wells for booby-trapping
OZM	18.6–45.4	TNT	1.8–6.3	Blast or fragmentation; bounding	Pressure, pull or electrical	..	..	Kit for converting 120 mm mortar bomb or 122 mm/152 mm artillery shell into bounding mine

Sources: Beyer (1962); US Department of the Army (1964); Tresckow (1975); Kitching (1975); Owen (1975).

187

metal are more easily detected with conventional magnetic mine-detectors. Small blast mines are detonated by direct contact as their area of effect is very limited. Those containing about 30 g of explosive cause mainly local injuries to the lower limbs. Those containing larger quantities may cause traumatic amputation of the limbs and other severe and often fatal injuries. There is a trend towards distributing larger numbers of smaller blast mines. Some mines, such as the British *Dingbat,* are covered in camouflaging materials.

IV. Mine delivery systems and scatterable mines

Most conventional mines are manually emplaced. This is time-consuming and requires much manpower. Increasingly, the trend is towards mechanical systems for distributing or burying mines, particularly anti-tank mines. Usually these systems, like the British bar-mine layer and the Soviet PMR-60 equipment, consist of a plough which digs a furrow, an arrangement for planting the mine, and a harrow to smooth the soil again afterwards. In this way a small crew can lay up to 600 mines per hour (Kitching, 1975).

A system of this kind may be supplemented with a means of scattering small anti-personnel mines to some distance on either side of the anti-tank mines. An example is the British EMI *Ranger* system. This consists of 72 mortar-like tubes, each of which fires 18 mines at a time (i.e., a total of 1 296) up to a distance of several hundred metres. The *Ranger* mines are small, pressure-operated blast mines containing enough explosive to injure the lower extremities (Kitching, 1975).

Remotely delivered mines are small blast or fragmentation mines that are distributed by fixed-wing aircraft, helicopter, artillery shell or rocket. A principal advantage is that they enable the rapid deployment of a minefield in front of an advancing enemy. Unlike conventional hand- or mechanically-emplaced landmines, but like delayed-action bombs or shells, they can also be used behind enemy lines.

Nunes-Vais (1974) records that the idea of remotely delivered mines first arose in the USA in the early 1960s but that 'a requirement did not materialize until impetus was provided by the conflict in Southeast Asia'. The notion that the supply of men and matériel from North to South Viet Nam through Laos and Cambodia could be stopped by 'seeding' the trails in mountain and jungle areas with air-delivered mines was adopted as early as 1961 (US Senate Committee on Foreign Relations, 1972). A variety of small anti-personnel mines were developed (table 7.2) and procured in large numbers (see table 2.7).

The *Gravel* mine is made of soft material, somewhat resembles a large tea-bag, and contains a small quantity of lead azide explosive. It can be coloured so as to match the terrain. It has a simple, chemical fuze system. In the moist tropical

Table 7.2. Examples of mine systems for remote delivery

Producing country and weapon designation	Remarks
Germany, FR	
LARAT 1/2	Light artillery rockets to deliver AT1 *Pandora* and AT2 *Medusa* anti-tank mines; being developed by consortium of Dynamit-Nobel, Diehl, Honeywell, Philips and Volvo
Italy	
DAT	Helicopter mine-delivery system
UK	
EMI *Ranger*	Anti-personnel mine-launching system made up of 72 mortar-like tubes, and firing 18 *Ranger* mines; vehicle-mounted
USA	
Deneye	Anti-personnel area denial mine
Dragontooth	Air-delivered from SUU-13 dispensers
Gravel (XM22, XM27, XM45E1)	'Tea-bag'-like, air-delivered from SUU-41 dispenser
Gator	Anti-personnel/anti-tank dual capability mine, delivered by rotary- or fixed-wing aircraft using SUU-54 2 000-lb (920-kg) dispenser
Grasshopper	Extremely sensitive, logic-gated (seismic/radio-frequency) mine which is air-delivered and can bury itself; bounding type; can be remotely activated and deactivated
Piranha	Air-delivered anti-tank mine for use in shallow water
M56	Delivery system for US-1H helicopter; dispenses 160 anti-tank mines from 2 SUU-13 dispensers
M483A1 155-mm ICM	Improved Conventional Munition; carries 88 M43 hollow-charge minelets
M692/M731 155-mm ADAM	Anti-personnel Area Denial Artillery Munition fired from 155 mm gun; contains 36 M43A1 anti-personnel grenades fitted with trip-wires and bounding mechanism

Sources: Kitching (1975); *International Defense Review* (April 1974; February 1977); *DMS Market Intelligence Report: Ships/Vehicles/Ordnance* (1976).

conditions of Indo-China, *Gravel* mines are believed to have deteriorated and become inoperative quite rapidly; it is not clear how long they would remain active in other conditions.

The BLU-43 and BLU-44 *Dragontooth* mines were designed to nest into each other when packed in large numbers in dispensers. The BLU-54 *Wide Area Anti-Personnel Mine* (WAAPM) is of the bounding type and contains 134 g of composition B explosive. The *Spider* mine is a modified anti-personnel bomblet fitted with trailing trip-wires.

These mines were primarily intended for use in remote areas under enemy control. They were dispersed from dispensing systems similar to (and in some cases identical with) those used for bomblets (see chapter 5).

More powerful mines were introduced for use against vehicles, and later, with anti-tank capability. The introduction of remotely deliverable anti-tank mines opened up the prospect of the tactical use of these mines in a large-scale conventional war situation, for example, in Central Europe. It was envisaged that, in the case of a sudden invasion by mechanized forces, remotely delivered mines could be rapidly deployed to delay the advance while a counter-attack was prepared. But the forces launching the counter-attack might then be faced with the problem of their own mines. For this reason it was decided that such mines would require a reliable self-neutralizing or self-destruct mechanism which made the mine inoperative after a predetermined period of time.

This concept was primarily developed in the Federal Republic of Germany, where the *Drachensaat* ('dragon seed') artillery-delivered mine system and the LARAT (Light Artillery Rocket Anti-Tank), carrying a load of *Pandora* Type AT1 or *Medusa* Type AT2 mines, have been produced. The USA and other countries are now developing artillery and rocket mine systems. The USA has already developed the M56 helicopter mining system, using the SUU-13 bomblet dispenser. The Italian company Valsella has developed VS 50 anti-personnel and VS 1–6 anti-tank mines for helicopter delivery.

V. Booby traps

A US military manual defines a booby trap as 'an explosive charge which is exploded when an unsuspecting person disturbs an apparently harmless object, or performs a presumably safe act' (US Department of the Army, 1964, p. 8). This definition formed the basis of considerable discussion at the Lugano Conference of Government Experts (ICRC, 1975), during which it became clear that the question of booby traps was more problematic than might at first appear.

Mining and booby-trapping of evacuated towns and of communications is said to be a defensive tactic of great importance. Such a tactic might include not only conventional minefields but, for example, mines placed in houses and fuzed to explode when the door is opened, or a charge attached to a motor vehicle so that it explodes when an attempt is made to start the engine. Such devices would force an invading enemy to proceed warily and could delay his advance.

A similar defensive tactic is the booby-trapping of anti-tank mines to prevent their removal (see above, p. 181) or of abandoned stocks of matériel to prevent their use by the enemy.

Booby traps may also be used more offensively in order to demoralize troops or spread terror among a civilian population. One means, reportedly used by Japanese forces during World War II, is to attach an explosive charge to a dead or wounded soldier which kills or wounds his comrades or rescue personnel (Beyer, 1962). Another means is to distribute harmless-looking objects, such as children's toys, pens or transistor radios, which explode when interfered with.[4] A third method – more discriminate than the others – is to send booby-trapped packets ('letter-bombs') by post to selected victims.

VI. Unexploded munitions

A final category of delayed-action munition is represented by those conventionally fuzed munitions that fail to detonate immediately and remain in the terrain as a potential hazard. This problem is perhaps greater than is sometimes appreciated.

The US Department of Defense provided the following information to a US Congressional committee:

> In late 1967, the [US] Army recognized that the North Vietnamese Army and the Vietcong were reusing U.S. Army dud munitions in the form of mines and booby traps. Although the average overall dud rate was low, in the order of 1 to 2 per cent, the number of rounds available to the hostile forces was significant due to the high volume of U.S. fire. The most frequently utilized point detonating (PD) fuzes used in SEA [South-East Asia] were the M-557 and M-51A1 series. Since 1965, these fuzes have reached an average dud rate of about 2.5 per cent in the superquick mode and from 5 to 50 percent in the delay mode. (US House of Representatives Committee on Appropriations, 1972, part 4, p. 198)

Swearington (1969) made a study of failure rates of a variety of US munitions used in Indo-China. He found that 40–50 per cent of US hand-grenades failed to function during the monsoon, compared with 15–25 per cent during other times of the year. The number of unserviceable grenades destroyed every month by ordnance personnel exceeded the number used in combat. The explanation was apparently that the fuzes of the US grenades were not waterproofed and were corroded. As was the case with hand-grenades, more M72 LAW light infantry rockets were destroyed every month than were used in combat. During the monsoon, 30 per cent or more of the US mortar rounds failed to function, compared with 10–20 per cent during the rest of the year. Less information was available with regard to aircraft munitions, but one ordnance-disposal unit destroyed 17 000 malfunctioning 2.75 in (70 mm) rockets in one year; in another example, 16 of 26 bombs dropped from a single aircraft failed to function. Observers report that large numbers of the small anti-personnel bomblets dropped over Indo-China failed to explode immediately, whether by design or mechanical failure.

According to Swearington, Soviet- and Chinese-produced munitions used in Indo-China were more reliable, due to simpler fuze designs, waterproofing and better packaging; indeed, these munitions were sometimes stored underwater to avoid detection. This suggests that it is not possible to generalize from US experience to other manufacturers and theatres of war. But it does indicate that in some areas the problem of unexploded munitions – not only during the war but also for many years afterwards – may be extremely great (see pp. 197–99).

VII. Wounding effects of delayed-action munitions

In principle, the wounding effects of delayed-action munitions are similar to those caused by the other munitions described previously.

Directional and bounding mines typically cause multiple, high-velocity fragment injuries. Blast and non-directional land-mines probably cause the maximum wounding effects through the agency of secondary missiles, such as sand, stones, and other materials immediately over or surrounding the mine. High velocity propellants are commonly used in mines, and the detonation usually occurs very close to the victim, so that the impact velocities attained by primary and secondary missiles are high, and wounding effects severe and multiple (French & Callender, 1962).

The fact that the land-mine is a lethal weapon was 'convincingly demonstrated' by findings during the Bougainville campaign of World War II (Beyer, 1962). Of seven cases autopsied, five had died instantly from many severe wounds, and the other two had died later later from shock and gas gangrene. Beyer (1962) records that in the surveys carried out during World War II, mines accounted for about 2 per cent of US casualties.

Modern scatterable anti-personnel mines usually contain much less explosive than older, hand-emplaced mines. This may decrease the number of fatal casualties and increase the number of living wounded, usually suffering from severe injuries to the lower extremities and additional injuries caused by secondary projectiles.

VIII. Precautionary measures

Because they are often hidden and remain active for a long time, mines and other delayed-action munitions may present a considerable hazard not only to the enemy but also to the side using them, as well as to the civilian population. In the Bougainville campaign of World War II, 33 of the 34 US mine casualties recorded were due to US mines (Beyer, 1962). Regarding the Korean War, Beyer writes: 'Because of fluctuations in battle – up and down the length of Korea – a large number of mine casualties were caused by mines planted by friendly personnel in the defense and during retrograde movements' (Beyer, 1962).

For this reason, as well as to avoid civilian casualties, it is necessary to take a number of precautionary measures when employing mines. These measures are of three types: (1) recording the positions of minefields; (2) marking the positions of minefields; and (3) fitting the mines with self-neutralizing mechanisms.

1. *Recording of minefields.* The principle that minefields should be recorded is well established in maritime law but is less well-established on land, where the problems are much greater. To record the exact placing of a single mine on land or, for example, in a stream may require the efforts of several men and take some time (US Department of the Army, 1964). The positions of hand-emplaced or mechanically emplaced mines can be more readily recorded than those of remotely emplaced mines.

The reliability of minefield records is greatly dependent upon the quality of the maps on which they are charted. Even if minelaying aircraft dropped the mines accurately according to given coordinates, recording these coordinates on large-scale or inaccurate maps would be of little help in locating the mines on the ground.

Geographical conditions may limit the reliability of minefield records in other ways. Small mines dropped in forest areas may lodge in trees, perhaps to fall to the ground later or create a hazard in subsequent foresting operations. Mines dropped in mountain areas may tumble, be carried in ice or streams, be hidden in snow for years only to surface later, be hidden behind boulders or in fissures, and so on. Again, recording on a map the general area in which the mines had been scattered would be of little help in locating and disposing of the mines subsequently.

2. *Marking of minefields.* Defensive minefields are often marked by means of stakes, cords and pennants around the perimeter. This method is effective so long as the minefield is of limited proportions and time is available in which to mark it. In many defensive situations it is no military disadvantage to mark the minefield in this way. Indeed, dummy minefields may be marked out in order to mislead the enemy. The USA has worked on the development of a marking system which can be dropped along with the mines from a helicopter (Nunes-Vais, 1974).

In other situations, however, it may be a military disadvantage to mark mines, particularly where they are used individually to disrupt communications or infantry patrols.

3. *Self-neutralizing devices.* The concept of self-neutralizing mines is of increasing importance, for both land-mines and naval mines. The mechanism may take several forms. A chemical, mechanical or electrical timing device may detonate the mine after a period of time. Other modern mines are electrically detonated using as a power source batteries which expire after a certain time so that the mine ceases to be operational. Mines of the self-destruct type have the advantage that they dispose of the explosive material as well as the fuze and prevent reuse by the enemy. They could cause considerable rural or urban environmental damage, particularly in the case of anti-tank mines.

The use of self-neutralizing mechanisms that do not detonate the mine may be preferable in inhabited areas, but they have the military disadvantage that they may, perhaps, be collected and reused by the enemy (who may simply need to change the batteries).

Thus, although precautionary measures are essential in order to reduce the indiscriminate effects of mines and other delayed-action munitions, none of the current measures is fully satisfactory from the humanitarian and environmental points of view.

IX. *Explosive ordnance detection and disposal*

In recent years there has been somewhat increased military interest in improving means of detecting and neutralizing mines and other delayed-action devices. The reason for this is that conventional mines and booby traps, which are mainly used for defence, have proved extremely costly to attacking forces and may prove more so in the future if scatterable mines are employed. According to Dennis (1976), mines and booby traps accounted for 33 per cent of US casualties in Viet Nam, and up to 70 per cent of tank and vehicle losses. The US capability to clear a minefield has been described as 'incredibly cumbersome' and 'methods have changed little since World War I' (*Aerospace Daily,* 15 July 1974). The USA has undertaken a programme of research and development to improve the tactical capability to breach a minefield.

British forces have experienced many problems in detecting and neutralizing explosive devices in Northern Ireland. Here again, research has been undertaken in recent years to find new methods (*New Scientist,* 9 May 1974).

Although the Soviet Union has not recently been directly involved in combat to the same extent as the USA and the UK, it has very large military capabilities in the field of conventional weaponry, including mine warfare and countermeasures. For example, the Soviet Union has issued mine-clearing rollers and ploughs which can be attached to armoured vehicles employed to breach minefields. This equipment detonates or renders mines inoperable in front of the vehicle and appears to be relatively successful. The USA has devoted several million dollars to studying similar systems (*Aerospace Daily,* 15 July 1974).

Traditional and new methods of mine detection and neutralization at present under development are briefly described below.

1. *Manual methods.* Probably the most common method is that of prodding the ground carefully with a long stake (see pp. 196–97).

2. *Mechanical methods* are used by armoured vehicles to breach minefields. They consist of devices attached to the front of the vehicle to clear mines from the path of the tracks only, or across the whole width of the tank.

3. *Burning.* In some types of terrain, mines can be detonated by burning off surrounding vegetation during a dry season.

4. *Explosive methods.* Mines can be detonated by means of an explosive charge placed near them. The USA has two special devices for breaching minefields in this way. One system consists of a long line of explosive charges held together by steel or aluminium plates, flexible in the vertical plane. This 'explosive snake' weighs some 5 tonnes and is towed to the minefield by an armoured vehicle. It is then unrolled, and the vehicle moves to the rear and pushes the 'snake' across the minefield, where it is detonated. It costs $10 800 and requires an eight-man team to operate it. When it explodes it forms a crater about 1 m deep and 4–5 m across. Slightly less cumbersome is the M173 system, which fires a rocket trailing an explosive cord (US Department of the Army, 1964; *Aerospace Daily,* 15 July 1974).

More recently, the USA has developed the use of fuel–air explosives (see chapter 6) for this purpose. The Surface Launched Unit Fuel Air Explosive (SLUFAE) Mine Neutralization System consists of a 30-tube rocket launcher mounted on an M548 tracked cargo carrier, a rocket-propelled fuel–air explosive round and a control system. The rocket contains 39 kg of propylene oxide. This forms an aerosol cloud in the air about 16 m in diameter and 4 m thick which explodes when detonated, destroying mines beneath the cloud. The rockets can be timed to impact systematically at ranges of 300 to 1 000 m (Dennis, 1976).

5. *Electromagnetic detection methods.* Devices containing iron or steel can be detected using a magnetic mine-detector. The latter is also sensitive to other pieces of steel or iron, which may or may not be a desirable characteristic. Some battlefields contain such huge quantities of shell fragments that a magnetic mine-detector is essentially useless in locating remaining explosive charges. Further, it is

not effective in locating mines not containing metal. Research is going on into the use of radar to detect buried pieces of metal. Other methods being investigated include the use of forward-looking infra-red imaging for aerial detection; rapid-sweep microwave detectors; and X-ray, gamma ray, and other nuclear methods. The US AN/PRS-7 metallic/non-metallic detector is sensitive to changes in the dielectric properties of the soil.

6. *Olfactory detection systems.* Most explosives contain nitro compounds which are somewhat volatile. One of the most effective means of detecting the vapour given off by an explosive compound is the specially trained dog (Krauss, 1971). Dogs are used for this purpose by military and other security forces, just as they are used to locate illicit narcotics. Dogs may be used in buildings as well as in the open. The dog must be specially selected for its stable personality, intelligence and obedience to the handler; Alsatians (German shepherd dogs) and Labradors are most commonly used.

A number of artificial 'explosive-sniffing' devices are now available (*International Defense Review,* 1973, no. 5). These devices pass a stream of argon over a radioactive source which ionizes the gas, which is in turn mixed with the vapour to be tested. A standing current passed through the gas decreases, and this decrease in the current activates an alarm, such as a buzzer or light. Some versions are only able to detect nitroglycerine vapours given off by gelignite and dynamite; others contain a heating unit which enables the detector to detect TNT, RDX and some other explosives. The devices have the disadvantage that they may also respond to some non-explosive vapours, including the Freon in aerosol sprays and the musk in perfume. For police work they have the advantage that they may be able to detect persons who have worked with explosives, or places where explosives have been prepared, for up to about 24 hours after the explosives have been removed.

Most of the devices described above have been developed for specific military and security needs, such as breaching a minefield during a battle to enable the passage of armoured vehicles, or locating booby traps. The problem of clearing minefields (as opposed to breaching them) and disposing of other unexploded munitions is of a quite different order of magnitude, and far too little attention has hitherto been paid to it

There is little doubt that mine technology has advanced considerably beyond mine detection and disposal technology. The commonest means of detecting mines and other unexploded munitions on land still appears to be to prod carefully with a long pole, rake or even rifle and bayonet. For this method to be effective it must be done extremely systematically. A recent Vietnamese account gives the following description:

> After the re-establishment of peace, it was necessary to clear Gio Le and other villages in the South from these explosives and to restore production; this is a job which can be done only by mass mobilization.
>
> Children at Gio Le made 8,000 pennants of coloured paper or linen to plant on the suspected places, while old people went in search of iron

and steel for the blacksmiths to forge into a sounding stick for each family to detect enemy bombs and mines.

When everything was ready, an energetic campaign began. Streamers, posters and slogans were displayed everywhere. The village was divided into lots to facilitate the search ... In this campaign, even the mines which had previously been laid by the French troops were spotted. The atmosphere became more and more tense. The work was carried out with great caution according to the instructions given on defusing lethal weapons.

After three days of work, twenty families were able to return for re-settlement ... (*Vietnam Courier*, No. 45, February 1976)

Another account, also from Viet Nam, states:

Mine-detectors have also been employed, but there are always mines that somehow escape detection. So, a primitive but also very effective measure has been taken: to divide the land in to 20cm by 20cm squares and probe them one by one with a sharp stick. (Yen Thanh, 1974*a*)

This method is relatively effective but very hazardous. Egyptian Army engineers lost 100 men in a year while clearing 700 000 mines from the banks of the Suez Canal (Graves, 1975).

Once the mine is located it still has to be disposed of. This may be done by carefully scraping away the surrounding soil and, where possible, removing the fuze. But mines and trip-wires may be booby-trapped to prevent removal in this way (US Department of the Army, 1964). Usually, therefore, the mine is deliberately detonated in place by firing at it with a heavy machine-gun; some remotely controlled equipment has been developed for this purpose. Where mines or other ordnance can be successfully removed it may be gathered together and detonated in a safe place.

X. Long-term hazards of delayed-action munitions

In a resolution adopted by the UN General Assembly, the United Nations Environment Programme (UNEP) was asked to undertake a survey of the extent of the problem of unexploded munitions.[5] Preliminary results indicated that the number of victims of unexploded munitions left over from World War II must be numbered in the thousands, and that the presence of these munitions is a continuing problem in some countries. Reports from Viet Nam and the Middle East also indicate a large number of victims.

Delayed-action munitions and unexploded ordnance create a long-term problem of considerable proportions. For example, in spite of the great efforts such as those described above, a Vietnamese hospital doctor reported in 1974 that 27 per cent of the patients during the previous year had been injured by war remnants, explosive or otherwise:

> The majority of cases ... concern people reclaiming fallow land wounded by unexploded steel-pellet bombs and mines left behind by the enemy and not yet entirely removed. In certain fields, rice is grown for one season, but peasants tilling the land during the next are injured by exploding munitions. There are cases where mechanical ploughs pass without incident but, subsequently, a peasant working with his buffalo is wounded by an exploding mine. (Dr Le Son, cited by Yen Thanh, 1974b)

This problem is a familiar one to people in North Africa, Central Europe and other parts of the world. But regrettably, no systematic information on the size of the problem is as yet available. Several examples indicate that the hazard is a long-term one:

1. In July 1976, 21 persons were killed and about 300 wounded when a World War II mortar shell exploded in a village near Mandalay (*United Press International,* Rangoon, 5 July 1976).

2. In May 1972, one person was killed, one was missing and 44 were injured after an explosion on a dredger in Niigata harbour, Japan, believed to have been caused by a World War II mine. Officials of the Maritime Safety Agency recalled that a total of 781 mines had been dropped in the harbour during the closing stages of World War II and only half of them had been deactivated in sweeping operations. It was believed that, as of 1970, more than 5 000 mines remained in or near major Japanese harbours (*Kyodo,* Niigata, 27 May 1972).

3. According to a Polish Government report, nearly 4 000 people – the great majority of them children – have died as a result of accidents involving World War II munitions. About 30–40 people are reported killed every year, and the task of munitions disposal continues.

Another problem is due to the extremely large numbers of unexploded munitions left behind by combatants. Again, there is as yet no systematic information available but some examples indicate the size of the problem:

1. During World War II Soviet local Civil Air Defence forces rendered harmless 430 000 unexploded bombs and nearly 2.5 million dud artillery and mortar shells. In the post-war years a further 225 000 bombs, over 1 million artillery and mortar shells and nearly 300 000 mines and other explosive devices were removed (Ryabchikov, 1977).

2. In West Berlin it was announced as recently as March 1977 that the search for unexploded munitions remaining in water-ways since World War II had formally ended. Since 1945, 7 013 bombs, 748 418 shells, 475 777 lesser explosive devices, such as grenades, and 83 584 weapons of all types had been disposed of

in West Berlin. A similar task had been performed in East Berlin (*Associated Press,* Berlin, 25 March 1977).

3. Although a major international effort was mounted to clear mines from the Suez Canal itself, huge numbers of mines are to be found in the surrounding terrain, estimates of the number varying from 1 million to 26 million (Mardell & Söderberg, 1975).

4. In Indo-China, it has been estimated that there were *at least* 400 000 unexploded bombs, 2 million unexploded artillery shells as well as 'untold numbers of dud mortar shells, rockets, grenades, mines and other time-delay munitions – all just below the surface' (Westing, 1975).

XI. Summary and conclusions

Delayed-action munitions include non-explosive devices, conventional shells and bombs fitted with long-delay fuzes, mines, booby traps and other unexploded munitions. The wounding effects of these munitions are similar to those of other blast, fragmentation and non-explosive munitions.

If a single rifle bullet is regarded as having an essentially 'one-dimensional' effect, the effects of area fragmentation and blast weapons can be seen as 'two-dimensional'. Proximity fuzes and the propelling charges of bounding munitions are ways of increasing effectiveness in a third dimension (though the purpose is usually to give increased area coverage). Delayed-action weapons are those whose effectiveness extends into the fourth dimension – time.

Delayed-action munitions have a high probability of indiscriminate effects, both in the short term and in the long term, even if special measures are taken. In some cases they have been used intentionally as indiscriminate weapons, in order to terrorize a civilian population, or to harass salvage- and rescue-personnel. In other cases, it is impossible for the user to avoid civilian casualties, even though they may not be intended. Marking minefields or issuing warnings may ease this problem, but does not solve the long-term problem of mine disposal. A reliable self-destruct or self-neutralizing mechanism fitted to all mines may solve the long-term problem of mine disposal but may not necessarily prevent civilian casualties during the period in which the mines are active.

Although a variety of new devices for detecting explosives have appeared in the past few years to supplement the traditional magnetic mine-detector (which is not effective against non-metallic mines), none of the new mechanical and electronic devices is as yet fully reliable. Specially selected and highly trained dogs and their handlers remain one of the best means for detecting unexploded munitions, but they are in short supply. Therefore the most commonly used method continues to be systematic manual prodding of the ground with a long stake or rake – a hazardous, time-consuming and labour-demanding task.

Although the use of fuel–air explosive munitions offers promise as a means for the tactical breaching of minefields during combat, it is out of the question for the systematic clearing of mines, except perhaps in some isolated areas with clearly defined minefields. Mines can be cleared from certain types of terrain by armoured vehicles fitted with special rollers, but this method is not feasible in other types of terrain.

Delayed-action munitions and other material remnants of war (such as barbed wire and sharp metal fragments) continue to cause indiscriminate injury and damage long after the cessation of hostilities. Often in the past, combatants have failed to dispose of their unexploded munitions and other remnants of war. In recent years, several important precedents have been established for international collaboration in the disposal of dangerous munitions and other remnants of war in the immediate post-war period. It is time to establish in international humanitarian law the duty of combatants not only to take every precaution to avoid civilian casualties during hostilities, including the marking and recording of minefields, but also to ensure that all dangerous objects are removed or rendered safe at the close of hostilities. It should be a guiding principle that no new munition be deployed until a means exists for locating it and disposing of it or otherwise ensuring that it is rendered harmless to man and the environment.

Notes to Chapter 7

1. A preliminary study by the US Army Engineer Research and Development Laboratories, Fort Belvoir, Virginia, suggested the following:

   > (1) Caltrops will penetrate footgear to inflict puncture injuries on all types and conditions of soil considered except in areas where walking would be difficult because of the depth to which a foot would sink. In these areas, penetration would initiate and the caltrop would remain in the footgear. Therefore, either injury will occur once firmer soil is reached, or delay will be caused because the caltrop will have to be removed from the footgear while personnel are walking through the unfavorable soil area. (2) The delay time caused by caltrops, applied as an obstacle within an integrated defensive perimeter with a density corresponding to a probability of injury of 40 percent, will exceed that created by triple standard concertina. (3) Incapacitation, resulting from swelling and pain approximately 30 minutes after injury, makes caltrops highly effective for impeding travel over escape routes by unfriendly forces, pocketed or partially trapped by friendly forces. (4) Caltrops, distributed at low densities, will inflict serious injury upon anyone who attempts to 'hit the dirt'. (Stanley, 1967; from author's abstract)

2. It should be added that the proportion of duds is always higher when time-delay fuzes of any kind are used and therefore they add to the long-term problem of unexploded munitions.
3. There is also the possibility that delayed-action bombs were dropped in Viet Nam, as in World War II, to harass rescue- and salvage-personnel and affect civilian morale.

200

Dellinger (1966), one of the first US observers to visit North Viet Nam, reports: 'According to the Vietnamese, the general pattern of most attacks is to drop heavy explosive bombs and *then to follow* a few minutes later with fragmentation bombs and strafing, so as to interfere with relief operations and to kill those who are trying to flee the bombed out area. From personal observation, I learned that the fragmentation bombs are equipped with timing devices so that they do not all eject their murderous barrage right away. When relief workers are trying to rescue the wounded, or later when the planes have departed and the all-clear has been sounded, hundreds of fragmentation bombs may explode, wounding or killing the innocent' (italics added.)

4. Allegations of the dropping of booby-trapped toys and the like may perhaps best be seen in the general context of psychological warfare operations and countermeasures. For example, if, as occurred in Viet Nam, one side drops children's toys and gift packages (US Commander in Chief Pacific, 1968) in order to 'win the hearts and minds of the people', an obvious countermeasure would be to spread the rumour that such gifts were booby-trapped, thereby effectively alienating the people from the donor. Allegations that Israeli aircraft had dropped booby-trapped pens and pencils were made by Damascus Radio (*Arab Report & Record*, 16–31 October 1973). Allegations in Beirut that booby-trapped toys had been dropped (*The Times*, 20 May 1974) were categorically denied by the Israeli Ambassador to the UK, who in turn accused the Palestinians of scattering innocuous-looking booby-trapped objects near Israeli schools and public places (*The Times*, 24 May 1974). Similar allegations were reported from Mozambique (*International Herald Tribune*, 20 September 1975).

5. UN Resolution 3435, 9 December 1975. The UNEP General Council discussed the preliminary report of the Executive Director (UNEP/GC/103 and Corr. 1) on 19 May 1977, and in decision 101 (V) it requested the Executive Director to pursue the matter further; this decision was endorsed by UN General Assembly resolution 32/168 of 19 December 1977.

8. Electric, acoustic and electromagnetic-wave weapons

Superior numerals, thus [5], refer to notes on pages 209–210.

I. Electric weapons

New developments in anti-personnel weapons derive from three main areas of physics: electricity, acoustics, and electromagnetic radiation.

In principle, electrical devices can be produced which can deliver powerful non-fatal shocks or lethal charges. Lethal electrical devices are used in slaughterhouses, and have been used for executing criminals, but they have found little application as military weapons.

In recent years a number of non-lethal electrical devices have been utilized by police and military forces. Weapons based on the high voltage Tesla coil were used 'apparently indiscriminately against blacks in several Southern states' of the USA in the mid-1960s but have 'largely passed from the public scene as a result of extremely adverse publicity' (Coates, 1972, p. 7). The same source reports that the West German police have an armoured personnel carrier with a 'gate-like prosthesis in the front which is charged to a high voltage'. It is used to clear people from streets.

The Shok Baton, made in the USA, imparts a high-voltage, low-amperage electric shock when applied to the skin, and is effective even through light summer clothes. It is powered by flashlight batteries. It is made in various lengths and can be used as a conventional wooden baton. It originated from military research to find an alternative to the bayonet in certain close-contact riot situations and has since been supplied to paramilitary police forces in various countries (Applegate, 1971). According to a report to the US National Science Foundation by the Security Planning Corporation (1972), it aroused 'widespread public outrage ... when it was used by control forces during early civil rights marches', when it was likened to a cattle prod (Applegate, 1971).

Electric generators, often of the kind used in field telephones, have been used as a means of torture during the interrogation of prisoners. This method was used, for example, by French forces in Algeria (Massu, 1972).

Another device produces an electrified water jet. This concept was patented in the USA in 1965. Two jets of water, one negatively charged and the other positively charged, are directed towards a point where they meet, closing the circuit. The device is intended as a barrier, or as a means of dispersing a crowd or disabling individuals. Although the technology is available, the device has not gained acceptance.

Patents for electric guns, spears, arrows and harpoons have been awarded over the past 100 years but few have come into operation. One of the more recent is the *Taser*, patented in 1974 (US Patent no. 3 803 463). More than 2 000 were sold in the USA in 1975 to private citizens as well as to security guards and policemen (Ferretti, 1976). It weighs 585 g and looks rather like a flashlight, and indeed the upper portion does contain a flashlight. Underneath are two triggers which set off a gunpowder charge which fires two small darts attached to wires about 5 m long. The darts stick into the victim and conduct a charge of 50 000 volts but of low amperage into his body. The effect is instant incapacitation, but in normal, healthy adults is without long-term effects. A cardiologist, cited by Ferretti, expressed concern about the possible effects on persons with heart trouble or under stress. The Security Planning Corporation (1972) pointed out that the Taser might involve risks of infection, which had not been properly evaluated.

The Taser received a considerable amount of publicity in the United States, particularly when it began to be used for crime. Because of this a study was conducted by the US Bureau of Alcohol, Tobacco and Firearms and it was subsequently classified as a firearm, requiring registration (Associated Press, Washington, 21 March 1976). In Canada it was made a criminal offence to buy, sell or possess the Taser (Associated Press, Ottawa, 13 January 1976).

Electric currents of high voltage and low amperage cause the muscles of the body to contract forcefully, and they may go into spasm. The contraction may fracture bones and an affected person may be further injured if he collapses. Repeated shocks from a Taser for 10 seconds are said by the manufacturer to render a man unconscious (*Business Week*, 29 July 1972).

At higher amperage the resistance of the body generates heat around the path of the current through the body. Electrical burns so caused are particularly difficult to treat because they may affect organs and tissues deep in the body.

II. Acoustic devices

Acoustic or sound waves have a mechanical mode of operation on the human ear. Vibrations transmitted through the air impinge upon the ear-drum (tympanic membrane) and set it in motion. This motion in turn stimulates the organs of the inner ear, generating nerve impulses which are interpreted by the brain as sound. The labyrinths of the inner ear are primarily concerned with registering the spatial orientation of the body, but very low frequency sounds (infrasound) of high intensity may affect the labyrinths, causing a feeling of vertigo, imbalance and other effects. It has also been suggested that at very low frequencies, resonances may be set up at other sites in the body, such as the heart, with various physiological effects, including possibly death, as a result. It appears that these phenomena have been investigated with a view to possible military applications.

As a result of the military demand for an extremely powerful amplifier, the Applied Electro-Mechanics Company of Alexandria, Virginia, produced the HPS-1

Sound System. It was used for airborne psychological warfare operations in Indo-China. With 350 W power it can project a voice nearly 5 km. It can be mounted on vehicles or helicopters. A number were purchased by the British Army for use in Northern Ireland (*New Scientist*, 20, 27 September 1973). An accessory, known as the *Curdler*, projects a scientifically designed shrill, shrieking noise at irregular intervals at a decibel level just below that which causes pain, and it is intended for use as a riot-control weapon (Applegate, 1969). The noise irritates people and interferes with collective activities, such as chanting or clapping.

It has been suggested that a device of this kind could be used to transmit through separate loudspeakers two slightly dissimilar sound waves which would interfere to produce high and low resonances in the ultrasound and infrasound ranges (*New Scientist*, 20 September 1973). Although these frequencies would respectively be above and below the audible range, it is known that both ultrasound and infrasound can have physiological effects.

Ultrasound (high frequency) devices are already marketed commercially as a means of clearing rodents from restaurants and other sites. The physical effects on rats and mice are sufficient to drive them from the area. Although intensity levels are selected to be relatively harmless to human beings, the manufacturers warn that headaches, queasiness and other discomforts can be felt if the device is left operating while the building is occupied. By making use of the Doppler effect, ultrasound devices are also used as alarm systems. Any movement in the area between a transmitter and a receiver causes a slight variation in the sound pattern received. This variation activates the alarm system. It is likely that this use of ultrasound will have great utility for military and other security purposes. It seems possible that at higher intensities, ultrasound could have more severe physiological effects.

Infrasound (low frequency) has several properties which could make it attractive as a weapon. Firstly, its attenuation in the atmosphere or in solid materials is limited, so that it is able to travel long distances and to penetrate buildings (Liszka, 1973). Secondly, experiments have shown that at intensities of about 100 dB, infrasound has certain adverse physiological effects (Händel & Jansson, 1974). These include disturbances to the nervous system, such as increased reaction times and impaired ability to perform simple sensory-motor tasks (Hood & Kyriakides, 1971), momentary feelings of sickness (Brüel & Olesen, 1973), and disturbed balance (Leventhall, 1973). At 130-150 dB the pain threshold is reached and feelings of sickness, vibrations of the chest, disturbances of breathing and digestion, and tiredness arise (Mohr *et al.*, 1965). At 170 dB, an experiment with dogs showed that breathing temporarily ceased (Johnson, 1973).

At a meeting of the British Association for the Advancement of Science, John Connell, Director of the [British] Noise Abatement Society, reported that at a research centre at Marseilles, France, an infrasound generator had been built which generated waves at 7 Hz. He said that when the machine was tested, people in range were sick for hours. The machine could cause dizziness, nervous fatigue and 'seasickness' and even death up to 8 km away (Associated Press, Leicester, England, 9 September 1972).

Mironov (1976) reports that intensive research is going on in the Soviet Union into possible peaceful uses of infrasound in medicine and engineering. Among the projects indicated is the possibility of using *directed* infrasound to break up polar sea-ice. Should a serviceable apparatus materialize it might also have military applications as an anti-personnel weapon.

Generators of random ('white') noise have been used, in combination with other measures, as a tool to break down the psychological resistance of prisoners during interrogation. The purpose of the noise in this case is twofold. Firstly, it is unpleasant and disturbing. Secondly, it prevents the hearing of other sounds enabling a person to orient himself, that is, it results in 'sensory deprivation' (Shallice, 1973).

It has been known for many years that the human brain is dependent for its normal functioning on a regular input of sensory stimuli. Sensory deprivation leads to hallucinations and finally to mental breakdown. The use of these sensory deprivation techniques by British forces in Northern Ireland (Wade, 1972) was the subject of an official investigation (Compton, 1971). This commission concluded that physical torture had not been used. But a commission set up by Amnesty International concluded that the technique 'clearly amounted to brutality' and was 'dangerous both to the immediate mental health of the individual subjected to this treatment and to the long-term health of some subjects' (Amnesty International 1971).[1]

III. Electromagnetic-wave devices

Electromagnetic waves form a spectrum ranging from very low frequency, long wavelength, to very high frequency, short wavelength. Radio waves are at the low frequency (c. 10^6–10^8 Hz) end of the spectrum and X-rays at the high frequency end (c. 10^{17} Hz). In between are the microwave, infra-red, visible light and ultra-violet ranges (see plate 14). The *laser* is a device that amplifies radiation of frequencies within or near the range of visible light.

The various parts of the spectrum of electromagnetic waves have enormous military significance, ranging from the use of very low frequency radio waves to transmit signals to and from nuclear submarines, to infra-red devices for night viewing, to the use of lasers for range-finding, mapping and guiding weapons. The increase in the power of transmitting devices has led to interest in the possible biological effects of electromagnetic waves and in possible new weapons utilizing these effects.

Light devices

Two categories of light weapons have been investigated, light-flash devices and stroboscopic devices (ICRC, 1975). Light-flash devices operate on the principle of the photographer's flash but at greatly increased power. They have been proposed for use at night by, for example, a guard at an isolated position who suspects the enemy is creeping up on him. The powerful flash of 0.1 s duration and with a light energy flux on the retina of 0.05–0.5 J/cm² could induce blindness for 5–10 min. Permanent retinal damage could ensue from an energy flux of 5–10 J/cm². Optical equipment, such as binoculars, would magnify the effect of the light-flash. Devices of this kind are known to have been the subject of research proposals, but there is as yet no indication of actual use in battlefield conditions (though, of course, conventional military illuminants are widely used). High-intensity lights which can be switched on and off to impair night vision have also been developed for police use (Security Planning Corporation, 1972).[2]

Stroboscopic flashing has also been considered for use against demonstrators in civil disturbances. At 5–15 Hz it can cause various physical symptoms and it is believed that it may initiate epileptic seizures in a small proportion of people. The fact that flashing lights can precipitate epileptic fits has been known for many years but it attracted more attention when it became fashionable to equip discothèques with 'strobes'. In 1972 the Greater London Council restricted the use of strobes to the range 1–8 Hz because of the problems associated with slightly higher frequencies. Possible military potential was investigated in the 1960s and a device known as the *Photic Driver* was developed by a British company, Allen International (*New Scientist*, 29 March 1973). The use of a Photic Driver by South African police during interrogation of prisoners has been reported. The stroboscopic effect may be enhanced by the use of infrasound.

Laser weapons

Lasers constitute a special category of light-emitting device. Since they were first described (Maiman, 1960), lasers have been developed for a remarkable range of uses in science, engineering, medicine and military technology. Although they are well established in many spheres of civilian life, it is believed that most – perhaps as much as 80 per cent – of the investment in laser research is for military purposes. It is outside the scope of the present study to describe laser technology and its military applications in detail. But a number of developments make laser weapons (as opposed to ancillary devices) an increasing possibility.

A laser is a device which uses energy to excite the molecules in a substance to the level where they emit a needle-thin stream of photons, small bundles of light energy travelling at about 300 000 km/s. Different substances are used for generating laser beams with different characteristics. Unlike most light sources, which contain a range of wavelengths, laser emissions are of a single wavelength, depending upon the substance used. The wavelengths produced range from the infra-red, through the visible part of the spectrum, to ultraviolet emissions. Attempts have been made to make an X-ray laser.

Solid-state lasers are the most common and use a solid substance, such as neodymium glass or ruby (chromium-doped aluminium oxide). They operate at relatively low efficiencies, but are convenient to use. The energy delivered in a single pulse, say 10 J, may not appear great. But power depends upon the *time* in which the energy is delivered. If 10 J is delivered in 0.0005 s, then the power is 20 000 W. If the same amount of energy is delivered in 100 ns (1×10^{-7} s) then the power is 100 million W.

The nearly parallel radiation can be focused into a very small spot, as small as a wavelength in diameter. For example, the beam from a 50 kW infra-red neodymium glass laser can be focused so that the radiant density is 10^{12} W/cm^2 – about 100 million times the power density at the surface of the Sun (Meyer-Arendt, 1968).

To achieve these levels of power, most lasers must emit the energy in pulses of very short duration. However, lasers have been produced which emit energy as a continuous wave (CW), and at increasing power levels. An example of a laser of this kind is the CO_2 gas laser, which can emit a continuous wave in the infra-red part of the spectrum and at high powers.

A laser of this kind has several characteristics which might make it attractive as a weapon. Firstly, infra-red radiation is invisible to the human eye and therefore more difficult to detect than visible light. Secondly, there is an 'atmospheric window' at this wavelength so that there is little or no attenuation of the beam in the atmosphere, which is otherwise a major limiting factor in the range of lasers. The infra-red laser transmits heat. It can be calculated that a 1 kW CO_2 laser beam will cause a localized soft tissue burn 1 cm deep over an area of 1 cm^2 within one second. If the beam is larger, or of greater power, the injury will be greater. If it is of longer duration, the injury will be deeper and may penetrate to vital organs, causing permanent injury or death. Clothing or nearby inflammable objects may be ignited at lower power levels and increase the hazard.

Laser beams, like other light phenomena, may be reflected or focused by lenses, including that of the eye. This fact has several implications of possible military significance. Firstly, it means that the human eye is particularly sensitive to laser beams, whether they are viewed directly or reflected from shiny surfaces. Exposure of the eyes of rabbits to a CO_2 laser beam at 5 W power for one second caused severe corneal burns which healed by secondary scar formation, leaving disabling opacity (Litwin *et al.*, 1969). However, because of the focusing ability of the eye, even radiation in the visible part of the spectrum may cause damage to the retina. It has been estimated that because of this effect, the retina may be damaged at power levels the order of one million times less than that required to damage the skin (Sliney & Palmisano, 1968).

Secondly, optical equipment may also have the effect of magnifying the intensity of the laser beam on the eye. Although somewhat simplified, it may be assumed that the radiation density level on the retina increases as the square of the magnification of the optical instrument (Sliney & Palmisano, 1968).

It may be added that optical systems themselves may be particularly sensitive to infra-red laser emissions. Not only do the lenses intensify the emission, but glass requires less heat to melt than metal. Glass will start to melt with a radiation intensity of 300 W/cm^2 for 0.1 s, whereas an aluminium sheet, for example, will require 40 kW/cm^2 before it starts to melt (Born, 1976). Optical appliances – binoculars, periscopes, television cameras, image intensifiers and infra-red viewers, as well as windscreens, portholes in ships and armoured vehicles, and aircraft canopies – are of increasing military importance and consequently so are means of putting them and the personnel using them out of action.[3]

At higher power levels it is suggested that the laser may be suitable for defeating incoming missiles, putting satellites out of action, and so on. It may also be possible to use a laser to initiate the fusion reaction in a hydrogen bomb without the need for fissile material.

There has been speculation on the use of lasers as weapons for some time (e.g., Meyer-Arendt, 1968; Foley, 1972; Born, 1976). It is known that large sums of money are now being spent on the development of laser weapons. But the actual status of such weapons is closely guarded information. From published sources it is known that the technology has progressed from the stage of 'research' to that of 'development' and possibly even to that of advanced engineering for field applications. The US Army, for example, has had for some years a vehicle-mounted laser weapon system for test purposes. The US Air Force, which is considering the use of lasers in the B-1 bomber (*US News & World Report,* 18 October 1971) and as an air-to-air weapon (*Aviation Week & Space Technology,* 9 September 1974) has an airborne version (airborne laser laboratory). The US Navy is studying the use of laser weapons on board ship; indeed, because of the greater power sources which it is possible to mount on large ships, naval applications may be the first to emerge. Research on laser weapons is also going on in the UK (Reuter, London, 22 May 1973), the Federal Republic of Germany (Born, 1976) and elsewhere. Very advanced research on lasers has been performed in the USSR and it seems likely that possible weapon applications are included, though published work is mostly on pulsed rather than continuous wave lasers, and is mainly theoretical and oriented towards understanding the chemical reactions involved (Ksander, 1971a, b).

The principal problem associated with turning lasers into usable weapons is that of the size of the power source.[4] The development of the gas-dynamic CO_2 lasers, and is mainly theoretical and oriented towards understanding the chemical great many operating hazards associated with high energy laser beams and equipment (Sliney & Palmisano, 1968) which may delay the introduction of laser weapons. But it seems likely that laser weapons will be developed as a result of current research and development efforts. It remains to be seen whether they will be cost-effective compared with alternative weapons.

Microwave devices

The proliferation of high-power radio transmitters and powerful radars employing microwaves has stimulated some research into the biological effects of such waves (Harrison, 1973; Lebowitz, 1972). Microwaves are already widely used for the rapid heating of foods, and the possibility of using them as weapons provoked some discussion at the Lucerne Conference of Government Experts (ICRC,

1974). Military research into the effects of microwaves on animals and materials is continuing (*US Army Research and Development News Magazine*, March–April 1977).

Masers (which are analogous to lasers but which utilize the microwave part of the spectrum rather than the light part) may, in the future, find applications as weapons.

IV. Summary and conclusions

Most of the candidates for new or future weapons rely on electricity or electronics and a variety of devices are reviewed. Apart from nuclear, biological and chemical weapons, they appear to offer the only possibilities for utilizing new scientific principles in the production of anti-personnel weapons. None of the devices discussed has at present any significant battlefield application. It is noteworthy that a high proportion of the devices described have been used for paramilitary and police purposes, ranging from dispersing crowds of demonstrators to interrogating prisoners.

Of the devices discussed, the laser seems to have most potential as a battlefield weapon, particularly lasers which emit radiation in the infra-red part of the spectrum, such as a high energy gas-dynamic CO_2 laser. The effects of such a laser on the human body are primarily a function of the generation of heat in tissues. They might therefore be comparable with incendiary weapons.

It is significant that during the Lucerne Conference of Government Experts (ICRC, 1974), a definition of incendiary weapons was promoted, particularly by the experts from the USA and the UK, which would *exclude* lasers from the category of 'incendiary munition'. Should this definition be retained in the subsequent international consideration of the legal status of incendiary weapons, then it may be necessary to consider laser weapons as a separate category. Conversely, a definition of incendiary weapons could be adopted which would include all weapons causing injury by means of thermal injury.

The prospect of weapons which not only burn people but, in particular, burn out their eyes, is one which may be difficult for international public opinion to accept.

Notes to Chapter 8

1. The use of this method by British forces in Northern Ireland was officially discontinued. In spite of subsequent repudiation of the method by spokesmen for the British Government, the Irish Government took the issue to the European Court of Human Rights. The case is of considerable legal interest since it is the first time one government has taken another to the Court.

2. In October 1977, the West German GSG-9 paramilitary unit defeated the hijackers of an aircraft in Mogadishu (Somalia). A British light-flash grenade, which temporarily immobilizes people for some six seconds by means of a blinding flash and a deafening report, played a vital role in the operation (*The Times*, 19 October 1977).

3. In fiscal year 1972 the US appropriated $5 million for a programme described as follows:

> The objective of this program is to develop techniques and equipment to degrade [deleted] optically directed weapons. Experience in Southeast Asia has shown that [deleted] aircraft losses resulted from automatic weapons and anti-aircraft artillery that were aimed by the naked eye or telescopically aided eye. [Deleted]. ... The following efforts are planned: development of a [deleted] system to degrade the visual tracking capability of a man; development of a [deleted] system to prevent tracking by visual means. (US Senate Committee on Appropriations, 1971, part 4, p. 828)

In an article in *Aviation Week & Space Technology* (26 June 1972) Brig. Gen. R. T. March, deputy for reconnaissance/strike/electronic warfare at the Aeronautical Systems Division of the US Air Force, is quoted as saying that 'more than 75% of aircraft losses are still attributed to optically-directed weapons. ... All the ECM in the world won't do any good if the enemy is tracking you with his eyeball. There is talk about lasers, but we don't have effective countermeasures against the direct optical threat'.

4. 'From a practical standpoint, laser countermeasures are not yet here, Gen. Marsh said, pointing out the constraints of weight, space, power, and cooling onboard the aircraft. Someday laser countermeasures could be practical, he said, but meanwhile other solutions are being looked at. ...' (*Aviation Week & Space Technology*, 26 June 1972.)

9. The development of the laws of war on anti-personnel weapons

Superior numerals, thus [5], refer to notes on pages 225–227.

I. Early history

Various attempts have been recorded in history to restrain the use of weapons of war. The Second Lateran Council, in 1139, attempted to outlaw the use of the crossbow, at least between Christians. According to Hogg (1970), it had some success; but the crusading English king Richard I subsequently failed to 'distinguish' between infidels and the French and effectively destroyed the ban.[1]

Manucy (1949) writes that 'at one time the Pope saw fit to excommunicate all gunners'. Again, however, there was singularly little impact on the use of guns.

It was not until the latter part of the nineteenth century that international legal agreements to prohibit certain weapons were reached. The prohibitions of explosive bullets (1868) and dumdum (expanding) bullets (1899) are of considerable historical interest since they represent two of the successes achieved in banning the use of certain weapons in war; and they are of contemporary interest since, in the absence of any substantive disarmament measures, a major effort has been launched by a number of countries in the 1970s to introduce new bans of a similar nature. For these reasons, the origins of these prohibitions are considered in some detail.

II. Explosive bullets and the Declaration of St Petersburg

By the mid-nineteenth century explosive bullets, or 'rifle shells', came into use for hunting very large game in Asia and Africa, and also for certain military purposes, such as blowing up the stout wooden boxes in which gunpowder was transported.

Several armies were experimenting with similar bullets at about the same time. They were used in the US Civil War (Lewis, 1956); the British used them in India (Fosbery, 1869); and some Prussian regiments were said to be armed with bullets containing 9.7 g of powder for their Dreyse rifles (Fosbery, 1869). The Russians developed an exploding bullet in 1863 for use against ammunition wagons. In 1867 a modification was suggested, allowing this bullet to explode on impact with a soft target.

The danger that bullets of this kind might be used against troops seems to have played a role in the Russian decision to summon an International Military Commission in 1868 (Holland, 1908) in response to what Fosbery called 'the repugnance which, reasonably or unreasonably, undoubtedly exists to their use as weapons of war'.

On 11 December 1868, the members of this Commission signed the Declaration of St Petersburg, to this day a cornerstone of the laws of war. This declaration stated, *inter alia:*

> That the only legitimate object which States should endeavour to accomplish during war is to weaken the military forces of the enemy;
> That for this purpose it is sufficient to disable the greatest possible number of men;
> That this object would be exceeded by the employment of arms which uselessly aggravate the sufferings of disabled men or render their death inevitable;
> That the employment of such arms would, therefore, be contrary to the laws of humanity.

The Declaration went on to forbid the use by the forces of the contracting parties of 'any projectile of a weight below 400 grammes which is either explosive or charged with fulminating or inflammable substances'.

This restriction is exceptional in that it is very specific. The effect of such light projectiles is to create large tissue wounds which, while not necessarily causing immediate death, render death (in the medical conditions of that time – similar to those found in many parts of the world today) virtually inevitable, owing to the complex physiological effects of shock, loss of body fluid, and infection.

It was presumably regarded at that time as sufficient for purposes of disablement to employ solid bullets (of low velocity), which either kill by penetrating a vital organ, or cause wounds sufficient in many cases to prevent the soldier continuing in battle, but from which he has a reasonable chance of recovery. Similar considerations apply to cutting or stabbing instruments, such as sabres, bayonets, arrows or spears.

This Declaration was reaffirmed in Article 13(*e*) of the Final Protocol of the Brussels Conference, held in 1874 on the initiative of the Imperial Russian Government. This document was signed but not ratified by all governments, but it formed a basis for the later Hague Rules of Land Warfare.

Although the St Petersburg Declaration itself referred to only one specific category of weapons, it is clear from the writings of international lawyers of that time that other categories of weapon were regarded as being inhumane; for example, Bluntschli (1874) writes that barbed arrows, lead shot and glass fragments were prohibited since they caused useless pain, and also that the use of chain shot on land was prohibited. De Martens (1858–61) asserted that the machine-gun and the firing of many bullets from a single gun were against the law, and Morin (1872) also suggested that machine-guns should be brought under international control.

Most contemporary international lawyers would probably agree with Meyrowitz (1968) that the preamble to the St Petersburg Declaration is now more important than the substantive prohibition. The Declaration enshrines a legal doctrine, derived from Rousseau, which states that war is not so much a matter of individual citizens fighting each other as a matter between States and hence defenders of States. Thus civilians and other non-combatants should be protected and among combatants it was sufficient to 'disable' rather than exterminate the opposing forces.

III. Dumdum bullets and the 1899 Hague Peace Conference

The high-velocity long-range rifle, the machine-gun and quick-firing artillery were to dominate the battlefield up to the present day. Although many people were slow to appreciate the implications, a Polish banker, I. S. Bloch,[2] published a book in 1897 which conjured up a frightening vision of a future great war in which these weapons would be used – a vision in which the deadly fire-power available from the military industries of both sides would lead to mass slaughter and inconclusive trench warfare. This book is said to have influenced the Russian Tsar Nicholas II in his decision to summon the first Peace Conference, held at The Hague in 1899, 'with the object of seeking the most effective means of ensuring to all peoples the benefits of a real and lasting peace, and, above all, of limiting the progressive development of existing armaments'.[3]

The Conference was attended by 26 governments, and although it failed to achieve its primary aim – the limitation or reduction of armaments – three Conventions and three Declarations were adopted. The Declarations, of particular interest here, are:

1. *The Declaration to prohibit the launching of projectiles and explosives from balloons or by other similar new methods*
2. *The Declaration to prohibit the use of projectiles, the only object of which is the diffusion of asphyxiating or deleterious gases*
3. *The Declaration to prohibit the use of bullets which expand or flatten easily in the human body, such as bullets with a hard envelope, of which the envelope does not entirely cover the core or is pierced with incisions*

The first Declaration, which was far-sighted but unsuccessful, presaged the coming of air warfare and was an effort to restrain the march of military technology. The second Declaration was the forerunner of twentieth century prohibitions of chemical and biological warfare.

The third Declaration, the prohibition of dumdum bullets,[4] provides the basis for much of the modern discussion on the prohibition of especially cruel weapons, and is therefore of considerable relevance to the subject of this book.

It is clear from the official record[5] that the delegates at the Hague Conference of 1899 saw the discussions on the dumdum bullet and other bullets causing similar massive wounds as a direct extension of the principles agreed to at St Petersburg. Indeed, an early Russian draft proposal stated that

> the use of bullets which expand or flatten easily in the human body, ought to be prohibited, *since they do not conform to the spirit of the*

213

Declaration of St. Petersburg in 1868. (Cited in Scott, 1920, p. 286; italics added)

Speaking in favour of a prohibition, the Netherlands delegate said:

> the dum-dum bullet whose point is very soft, whose projectile covering is hard, and whose interior is formed of a softer substance, makes, by exploding at the slightest resistance, enormous ravages in the body, its entrance being very small, but its exit very large. It is sufficient to disable a man for the rest of the campaign, and such ravages are not necessary. (Cited in Scott, 1920, p. 286)

The Russian and Netherlands delegates and others argued that 'there must be a specific limit and not a general limit'; that the proposed prohibition of dumdum bullets referred to bullets whose effects were known, although 'as to bullets which may be invented in the future, let them be taken up when the time comes' (cited in Scott, 1920, p. 84).

Against the proposal for a specific prohibition of bullets with known characteristics was the view represented by, among others, the delegate of the United States, who proposed a general formulation:

> The use of bullets inflicting wounds of useless cruelty, such as explosive bullets, and in general, every kind of bullet which exceeds the limit necessary for placing a man *hors de combat,* should be forbidden. (Scott, 1920, p. 80)

The arguments in favour of this general formulation are of considerable contemporary interest. The US delegate explained very clearly the advantages and disadvantages of the trend towards smaller calibres:

> The advantages of the small calibre are well known: flatter trajectory, greater danger space, less recoil, and particularly, less weight of ammunition. Now if any nation shall consider these advantages sufficiently great to wish to pass to a small calibre, which is to be regarded as quite possible, her military experts will at once occupy themselves with a method of avoiding the principal disadvantage of a small calibre, i.e. the absence of shock produced by the bullet. In devising means to increase the shock they will naturally examine the prohibitions which have been imposed, and they will find that with the exception of the two classes, explosive bullets and bullets which expand or flatten, the field is entirely clear. They will see that they can avoid the forbidden detail of construction by making a bullet with a large part of the envelope so thin as to be ineffective, and that they can avoid altogether the proscribed classes; first, by making a bullet such that the point would turn easily to one side upon entering the body, so as to cause it to turn end over end, revolving about its shorter axis (it is well known how easily a rifle projectile can be made to act in this way), secondly, by making a ball of such original form as, without changing it, would in-

flict a torn wound. It is useless to give further examples. A technical officer could spend an indefinite time in suggesting designs of bullets, desperately cruel in their effects, which, forbidden by my amendment, would be permitted under the [dumdum declaration]. (Cited in Scott, 1920, pp. 80–81)

Subsequently, at the commission stage, the US delegation voted for the more specific Russian formulation, which was agreed to by the Conference. However, in the end the United States did not sign the Declaration and never has. The British and the Portuguese did not agree to the dumdum prohibition until 1907.

The history of the development of small arms ammunition since 1899 largely bears out the predictions of the US delegate: to compensate for smaller calibre, bullets have been made to tumble, to disintegrate, and have been imparted with a very high velocity, causing large wounds similar to the dumdum bullet, but by other means (chapter 3).

The discussion of the dumdum prohibition at that time, both inside and outside the Hague Conference, makes it clear that considerable knowledge was already available about the effects of various bullets. The interest of the Conference in these bullets appears to have been aroused by the widely publicized studies of the German Professor von Bruns (1898, 1899). However, British medical writers (e.g., Ogston, 1899; Keith & Rigby, 1899) pointed out that von Bruns had used a hunting bullet with 5 mm (diameter) of the tip unjacketed, whereas the original dumdum military bullet had only 1 mm uncovered. The hunting bullet therefore caused a worse wound than the dumdum bullet, and it was unreasonable (or at least unscientific) to equate the two.[6]

Keith & Rigby (1899) commented that 'the fact remains that [the dumdum bullet] is immensely destructive' (p. 1499). Their experiments showed that the dumdum bullet caused larger wounds than fully jacketed bullets. However, this study also showed (as did others, e.g., Horsley, 1894; MacCormac, 1895; Nimier & Laval, 1899; LaGarde, 1900) that any of the high-powered bullets then in service in all major armies could cause 'explosive effects' if they hit the head or certain other organs, such as the liver, at ranges of up to about 500 m (chapter 3).

As a result, fears were expressed about the severity of the bullet wounds to be expected in a future war (MacCormac, 1895). Subsequently, however, as correspondent of the British Medical Association in the South African War of 1899–1902, MacCormac (1900a, b), reported that severe wounds were rare.

An examination of the case-studies recorded by MacCormac provides an explanation: the Boers were excellent shots at long range and most of the cases of shot wounds observed occurred at ranges beyond those at which 'explosive effects' may be expected. In the 37 cases reported by MacCormac, the ranges varied from 100 to 3 000 yards, the average being 805 yards; only seven of the cases were shot at ranges of less than 500 yards.[7]

It may be concluded that the 'explosive' effects of high velocity bullets were well known to military experts by 1899, but they did not prove to be a serious medical problem because of the long ranges at which combat took place, largely as a result of the introduction of the same bullets. Further, these bullets were so powerful that they were more likely to traverse the body than merely penetrate into it, thereby taking with them on exit a high proportion of the available energy. This in turn led to claims that they had insufficient 'stopping power'. But the dumdum prohibition, while ruling out one means of increasing the retardation of the bullet in the body, did not rule out other means, such as increasing the propensity of bullets to tumble by designing them with a pointed (*Spitzer*) tip, a hollow-point tip, or a tip filled with a light filler (chapter 4).

Although it did not achieve any success in this regard, the Hague Conference also approached the question of other new weapons, such as machine-guns.

Of particular interest were the proposals put forward by Colonel Gilinsky of the Russian delegation to restrict infantry weapons for a number of years according to the following criteria:

1. The minimum weight of the gun is fixed at four kilograms.
2. The minimum of the calibre at 6½ millimetres.
3. The weight of the ball shall not be less than 10½ grams.
4. The initial speed shall not exceed 720 metres.
5. The rapidity of firing be limited to 25 shots per minute.
6. Explosive and dilatable balls, as well as automatic loading, are prohibited. (Cited in Scott, 1920, p. 289)

Although this proposal was rejected at The Hague, it is interesting that the majority of military rifles, even today, have a weight of about 4 kg, a calibre of 7–8 mm and a bullet weighing nearly 10 g. On the other hand, the initial velocity of full-power ammunition may somewhat exceed 800 m/s, automatic loading is very common, and the rate of fire of automatic rifles may reach some 600 shots per minute.

Only with the development of rifles such as the US M-16, 60 years later, has the weight of the rifle and the calibre and weight of the bullet been substantially reduced below the suggested 1899 criteria, although the initial velocity has been markedly increased to some 1 000 m/s. It is weapons of this kind that have led to renewed interest in prohibitions of the dumdum bullet type because of the severe wounds which they may create (chapters 3 and 4).

A restriction on new small arms was also urged at the Hague Conference on financial grounds, some delegates even presenting cost estimates for re-equipping armies with new rifles. This aspect, too, is important now that NATO countries and others are considering replacing 7.62 mm weapons with 5.56 mm or some other calibre. This is a very expensive decision to make – but one which the industries producing the weapons have a great interest in encouraging.

The British delegate at the First Hague Conference, Sir John Ardagh, argued for the retention of the dumdum bullet for use against 'savage races'. As he explained:

> there is a difference in war betweeen civilized nations and that against savages. If, in the former, a soldier is wounded by a small projectile, he is taken away in the ambulance, but the savage, although run through two or three times, does not cease to advance. (Cited in Scott, 1920, pp. 286–87)

The Russian delegate Raffalovitch explained that the ideas expressed by Sir John Ardagh were 'contrary to the humanitarian spirit which rules this end of the nineteenth century' and went on to make the pragmatic comment that 'distinguishing between the enemies to wage war against and the projectiles to be used would necessarily induce complications of equipment' (cited in Scott, 1920, p. 287). The President of the commission expressed the belief that the opinion of the assembly was that 'there can be no distinction between the projectiles permitted and the projectiles prohibited according to the enemies against which they fight even in the case of savages' (cited in Scott, 1920, p. 287).

Nevertheless, it was pointed out that there was, indeed, 'a hiatus in the Declaration of 1868, a hiatus which permits the employment not only of the dum-dum bullets, but even of explosive balls, against savage tribes' (Colonel Gilinsky, cited in Scott, 1920, p. 287).

The reason for this hiatus is that the Declaration of 1868, like many others, refers to the regulation of relations between the contracting parties, and does not cover relations with non-contracting parties, such as savage tribes. Of course, by 'savage tribes' was meant the indigenous peoples who, often with desperate courage and determination, opposed the voracious invading armies of the colonial powers in the decades before the 1899 Conference.

Something of this hiatus remains to this day. Although international humanitarian law now applies to 'all peace-loving nations' rather than only to a small self-appointed group of 'civilized nations', it still applies only to armed conflicts between States. It offers little protection to colonial peoples or minority groups who find themselves in conflict with a State. However, for the first time, some attempt is being made to improve the situation. The International Committee of the Red Cross (1973*a*, *b*) proposed two Additional Protocols to the signatories of the four Geneva Conventions of 12 August 1949, and after much modification they were adopted by the Diplomatic Conference. The first Protocol further regulates the conduct of *international* armed conflicts, while the second regulates *non-international* armed conflicts (i.e., where there is fighting within a country).[8] Because the colonial era is rapidly drawing to a close, these legal efforts are too late for most colonial peoples. On the other hand, many States, made up of diverse cultural groups, are faced with internal conflicts, the control of which is a major challenge to humanitarian law.

It should be apparent from the discussion above that there are, indeed, many parallels between the debates at The Hague in 1899 and the current debates on the prohibition and restriction of certain weapons.

In addition to the discussions on specific weapons, the 1899 Conference drew up a number of Conventions regulating the conduct of warfare. Convention II with Respect to the Laws and Customs of War on Land included a chapter 'On Means of Injuring the Enemy, Sieges and Bombardments' where it was stated, *inter alia*, that the following were 'especially prohibited':

— to employ poison or poisoned arms (article 23[a])
— to employ arms, projectiles, or material of a nature to cause superfluous injury[9] (article 23[e]).

In addition, it was especially forbidden to kill or wound treacherously.

In 1907 a Second Peace Conference was held at The Hague. This second Conference drew up a considerable number of conventions on other aspects of the conduct of war but restricted itself to reaffirming the previous agreements on the question of specific weapons, with one exception. In Convention VIII, rules were agreed to regulate the laying of automatic submarine contact mines. In addition, in Declaration XIV, the discharge of projectiles and explosives from balloons or by other new methods of a similar nature was again prohibited – this time for a period extending to the close of the Third Peace Conference. Since such a Conference has never been held, this prohibition still holds; but it did not prevent the development of air warfare, any more than the prohibition of poison prevented the use of chemical weapons during World War I.

Whatever the practical effect of the agreements reached at the two Hague Peace Conferences, they had the important legal effect of reaffirming the principle established at St Petersburg that weapons which cause unnecessary suffering were prohibited.

In the discussion of chemical weapons, however, the Conference went further. It was not denied that gases could be very effective as military weapons. But gases were regarded as too repulsive or too cruel to be justified *even if* they had military utility in a particular situation.

Thus, two principles were adopted at that time and they are still valid (cf. SIPRI, 1976*a*):

1. Weapons which cause injury which has *no military utility* are prohibited.

2. Weapons which are too cruel or repulsive even though they may *have military utility* may be prohibited.

In the current legal discussions, the first of these principles – which requires an assessment of the military utility of the weapon – has been emphasized to the detriment of the second.

IV. Testing the Hague Rules in World War I

World War I provided the first major opportunity to test the scope and effectiveness of the Hague Rules. The two most clear-cut prohibitions – that on poison and poisoned weapons and deleterious gases, and that on the dropping of projectiles from balloons and by similar methods – did not prevent extensive use of both these methods of war. During the war most of the major participants accused each other of using prohibited anti-personnel weapons, although, generally, these accusations were rejected (see Garner, 1920; Fauchille, 1921). In some cases rejection took the form of a denial that the objectionable weapon had been employed, thereby supporting the interpretation that such use was illegal. In other cases, no attempt was made to deny the use; rather the law was interpreted in such a way as to allow the weapon concerned.

218

For example, as a result of accusations that its troops were using explosive bullets, the Austro-Hungarian Government first denied that this was the case; then admitted that some such bullets were indeed in use for purposes of range-finding; and finally, served an order that such bullets were not to be issued to troops except upon an order of the General Staff (Garner, 1920). The Austro-Hungarian Government, for its part, accused the Allied forces in Serbia and Montenegro of using cartridges filled with nails and bits of copper, and the like. This is an example of an interpretation of the 'unnecessary suffering' clause. Similarly, Oppenheim (1955) states that 'rifles must not be loaded with bits of glass, irregularly shaped iron, nails, and the like' (p. 340).

Shot-guns provide an example of differences in legal interpretation. In September 1918, the German Government through the Swiss legation at Washington protested against the use of shot-guns by the US Army. The protest was based on Hague Article 23(e) prohibiting the use of arms 'calculated to cause unnecessary suffering'. On 23 September 1918, the US Secretary of State stated the opinion of his government that the provision of the Hague Convention did not prohibit the use of the shot-gun; that in comparison with other approved weapons its use could not be made the object of a reasonable protest; and that the United States would not abandon its use. The US publicist Garner (1920) supports this view, adding that 'the use of the shot-gun is analogous to the employment of the shrapnel shell or a machine-gun and is certainly less condemnable than the flame-thrower or the poisoned gas shell' (p. 271).

This particular example of a difference of interpretation continues to this day. The West German manual of military law[10] regards shot-guns as an illegal means of warfare offering no real military advantage while causing unnecessary suffering. The US military legal manual DA PAM 27–161–2 (p. 45) quotes an opinion of the Office of the Judge Advocate General of 1961 that while there is no conventional law prohibiting shot-guns, certain restrictions are implied by international law. According to the author of this manual this means that while an unjacketed lead bullet is considered illegal, a fully jacketed bullet or chilled (surface-hardened) shot regular in shape is considered legal.[11]

The difficulties of leaving the job of interpreting the meaning of international legal provisions to the individual States are even more obvious in the case of ammunition which, as pointed out by the US delegate in 1899, may cause wounds similar to the prohibited dumdum bullet, but in a somewhat different manner.

Garner points out that one explanation for the many accusations and counter-accusations of the use of dumdum and exploding bullets during World War I was that the wounds diagnosed as having been caused by dumdum were made by 'a substitute for the dum-dum, the so-called *Spitz* or *Spitzer* bullet, which though not expressly forbidden by the Hague convention, is equally as objectionable as the one condemned' (Garner, 1920, p. 269).

At one time the British Government appears to have had a similar view, since in 1914, in reply to German charges that British troops used the dumdum bullet, it accused Germany of using not only this type of bullet, but also a bullet which was even more objectionable, although not expressly forbidden by the Hague Convention. This bullet was described as one which turns over completely when it strikes, traversing the body with the rear end foremost. The base, having no cover, permits the core to spread out in a manner similar to the dumdum, and with equally deadly results (Garner, 1920, p. 266).

By contrast, a British projectile was described as 'probably the most humane projectile yet devised, for the long, solid point, with the core completely covered, prevents it from breaking up into fragments and thus makes a clean incisive wound' (cited in Garner, 1920, p. 266).

These are just a few examples which demonstrate that at the time of World War I, there was fairly general agreement that ammunition causing severe lacerated wounds was illegal. While differences of opinion or practice arose with regard to certain weapons, and many accusations of abuses of international law were made by the opposing parties, in general, the ammunition adopted was in accord with the accepted principles.

In addition to the deliberate use of gas there were several developments which contravened previously accepted conventions. The extensive use of chemical weapons overshadowed these other developments in the post-war disarmament and legal discussions, which led, *inter alia,* to the Geneva Protocol of 1925.

One of these developments was the use of grenades, whether projected by hand or rifle, that weighed less than the 400 g stipulated by the Declaration of St Petersburg. This trend has continued up to the present.

A second development was the use of small explosive and incendiary projectiles against aircraft, which were, as offensive weapons, a most dangerous result of World War I. This development was recognized in the draft Hague Air Warfare Rules of 1922 and the Draft Disarmament Convention of 1933. The first of these allowed the use of the prohibited projectiles 'by or against aircraft'. The second allowed the projectiles 'for defence against aircraft'. The intention of these provisions is clear: to allow these weapons for defence against aircraft, but to maintain the prohibition of their use against troops on the ground.

Since aircraft could, on this basis, be legitimately equipped with weapons to defend themselves against (or to attack) other aircraft, military aircraft were fitted with the larger cannons capable of firing explosive or incendiary ammunition, as soon as their increasing power and size permitted. During World War I the use of aircraft to strafe targets on the ground became standard practice, and since World War II, the use of high-explosive–incendiary shells in the 20 mm class for this purpose has been common.

There is no doubt that these developments seriously undermined the specific provisions of one of the cornerstones of international humanitarian law, the St Petersburg Declaration.

At the same time, the high velocity bullet, which is apt to tumble and even disintegrate and thereby cause a wound similar to that caused by explosive or dumdum bullets, undermined the second cornerstone, the Hague Declaration Concerning Expanding Bullets.

V. Testing the laws of war in World War II

Systematic war crimes were committed on a large scale during World War II and gave rise to international war crimes tribunals after the war. The use of various weapons in infringement of international law does not seem to have been raised in these trials (SIPRI, 1976a). Nevertheless, there were occasional allegations of the use of explosive bullets and other prohibited weapons. For example, Beyer (1962) reports instances of the use of high-explosive incendiary bullets by the Japanese in the closing stages of the battle of Iwo Jima, though he adds that this may have been a result of salvaging ammunition from grounded aircraft. High-explosive and armour-piercing bullets were available to most of the combatants for use against aircraft and vehicles, and no doubt sometimes hit personnel.

Beyer also reports that 6.5 mm Japanese bullets, especially those made with a jacket of copper and zinc alloy (gilding metal), had a tendency to break up on impact with explosive effect, scattering small globules of lead core which embedded themselves elsewhere in the flesh. This effect was apparently due to the thinness of the jacket in the rear part of the bullet. The bullet was unstable, perhaps because of its design and perhaps also owing to worn or inferior weapons, and caused an unusually large exit wound. (Similar effects have been reported for the M-16 rifle used by the US in Viet Nam, particularly before the barrels were plated to reduce wear; see chapter 4.)

VI. The ICRC Draft Rules of 1956–58

In the years following the Korean War, the International Committee of the Red Cross made a further effort to extend the legal protection of the civilian population in time of war. In 1956 it circulated a set of Draft Rules to the parties to the four Geneva Conventions of 1949 and these rules were the subject of discussion and amendment at the XIXth International Conference of the Red Cross in New Delhi in 1957 (ICRC, 1958a). In 1958 the ICRC published, with a commentary, a revised version of these rules (ICRC, 1958b).

In the revised version, Article 14 covered 'Prohibited methods of warfare'. Paragraph 1 stated:

> Without prejudice to the present or future prohibition of certain specific weapons, the use is prohibited of weapons whose harmful effects – resulting in particular from the dissemination of incendiary, chemical, bacteriological or other agents – could spread to an unforeseen degree or escape, either in space or in time, from the control of those who employ them, thus endangering the civilian population.

Paragraph 2 of Article 14 stated:

This prohibition also applies to delayed-action weapons, the dangerous effects of which are liable to be felt by the civilian population.

Article 15 stated in Paragraph 1:

> If the Parties to the conflict make use of mines, they are bound without prejudice to the stipulations of the VIIIth Hague Convention of 1907 to chart the minefields. The chart shall be handed over, at the close of hostilities, to the adverse Party, and also to other authorities responsible for the safety of the population.

In Paragraph 2, Article 15 read:

> Without prejudice to the precautions specified under Article 9, weapons capable of causing serious damage to the civilian population shall, so far as possible, be equipped with a safety device which renders them harmless when they escape from the control of those who employ them.

These proposals focus upon the important fact that the user of the weapon cannot control the effects if they spread or persist in time.

The efforts of the ICRC in the 1950s led to nothing and 20 years later the issues raised are still unsolved. Some elements proposed by the ICRC in 1958 reappeared in the proposals put forward at the Lugano Conference of Government Experts in 1976, where much attention was given to delayed-action weapons such as mines and booby traps (see appendix 9C).

VII. Recent efforts to ban specific weapons

In the United States and elsewhere, the US arsenal of anti-personnel weapons became a target for opponents of US intervention in Viet Nam. The American Friends Service Committee, for example, established a study group called NARMIC (National Action/Research on the Military–Industrial Complex) which published a number of studies of US anti-personnel weapons (e.g., Kanegis *et al.*, 1970; Prokosch, 1972), bringing them to the attention of churches, anti-war groups, etc. The question of the morality and legitimacy of the new weapons led to some debate among US lawyers, politicians and others.[12] Various activities were directed against US arms manufacturers, such as Honeywell (largest producer of cluster-bomb components) and Dow (major producer of napalm).

Outside the USA, public attention was drawn to the new anti-personnel weapons by Bertrand Russell (1967) and the International Tribunal named after him.[13] In two sessions of the Tribunal, experts from various countries testified to the working and effects of various US anti-personnel weapons. The Tribunal was instrumental in provoking the concern which has given rise to international negotiations to prohibit or restrict the use of such weapons. It is therefore of historical interest to cite the original findings of the Russell Tribunal:

The Tribunal has received all necessary information on the diversity and power of the engines of war employed against the Democratic Republic of Vietnam and the circumstances of their utilization (high-explosive bombs, napalm, phosphorus and fragmentation bombs, etc.) ... Its attention in particular has been drawn to the massive use of various kinds of anti-personnel bombs of the fragmentation type, also called in American parlance, CBU, and in Vietnamese parlance, pellet bombs. These devices, obviously intended to strike defenceless populations, have the following characteristics.

Containers, called by the Vietnamese the 'mother bombs' release hundreds of small oblong or spherical bombs (pineapple or guava bombs) which in turn release hundreds of small pellets. A single mother bomb can therefore cause the dispersion of nearly 100 000 pellets: these pellets cause no serious damage to buildings or defence workers behind their sandbags. They are therefore intended solely to reach the greatest number of persons in the civilian populations.

The Tribunal has had medical experts study the consequences of attacks with these pellets. The path of the particles through the body is long and irregular and produces, apart from cases of death, multiple and various internal injuries.

The Hague Convention No. 4 of 18 October 1907 laid down the principle that belligerents may not have an unlimited choice so far as the means of injuring an enemy are concerned (Article 22); the said Convention specially prohibits the use of arms, projectiles and material deliberately designed to cause pointless suffering (Article 23) ...

... the Tribunal makes a point of declaring that fragmentation bombs of the CBU type, which have no other purpose than to injure to the maximum the civilian population, must be regarded as arms prohibited by the laws and customs of war. (J.-P. Sartre, in Coates, Limqueco & Weiss, 1971, pp. 183–84)

It is possible that these public campaigns had some inhibiting effect on the use by US forces of anti-personnel weapons, particularly napalm (see SIPRI, 1975a), and may have influenced the formulation of stricter rules guiding US combat activities (see appendix 9D). These rules are of some interest for the current international debate on the question of inhumane and indiscriminate weapons, discussed below.

Subsequently, the question of the legality of some of the new weapons was raised at the United Nations General Assembly and in the context of the continuing efforts of the International Committee of the Red Cross to update the Geneva Conventions (appendices 9A and 9B).

The question of inhumane and indiscriminate weapons is now firmly placed on the agenda of work of the international diplomatic community. Nevertheless, the question is one which raises complex legal, philosophical and political problems, and various States have taken different approaches to the issue – some of which are negative.

The two major lines of approach may be summarized as follows: Firstly, there is the approach that, in principle, all weapons are inhumane but, unfortunately, in the present world, they are necessary for national defence. Therefore, priority should be given to balanced disarmament measures rather than to arbitrary humanitarian limitations related to specific weapons.

Secondly, against this view is another which supports the need for real measures of disarmament but, in the absence of significant progress in this field, emphasizes the need to limit as much as possible the human suffering resulting from the continuing use of weapons that kill and maim. It is argued that the prohibition or restriction of use of particularly cruel weapons would be an important means of improving the legal protection of both combatants (soldiers) and non-combatants (civilians) and might indeed contribute to a better climate for disarmament measures.

The result of these differences of approach is a debate between States which has been pursued at a number of levels for several years. At the diplomatic level the matter has been raised at the committees of the UN General Assembly and at the Diplomatic Conference on the Reaffirmation and Development of International Humanitarian Law Applicable in Armed Conflicts – a conference of States which has been engaged upon the task of updating the four Geneva Conventions of 1949. A number of UN resolutions have urged the Diplomatic Conference to take up the question of specific weapons and the Conference responded by establishing a special *ad hoc* Committee (in addition to three regular commissions on various other aspects of its work) to do this. In the final session (1977) the Conference passed a resolution calling upon the UN to hold a special conference on the subject not later than 1979.

At a second level the UN Secretary-General and the ICRC have been authorized to convene a number of groups or conferences of experts to report on the military, medical and legal issues involved. In 1973 the UN Secretariat published a report on napalm and other incendiary weapons (United Nations, 1973*a*) and a two-volume survey of the current laws of war with respect to specific weapons (United Nations, 1973*b*). In the same year the ICRC published the report of a group of experts entitled *Weapons that may Cause Unnecessary Suffering or Have Indiscriminate Effects* (ICRC, 1973*c*). In the final remarks accompanying this report it was stated that:

> The facts compiled in the report . . . speak for themselves and call for intergovernmental review and action. Such action might be justified particularly in respect to two types of weapon apart from incendiaries, namely, high-velocity small arms ammunition and certain fragmentation weapons. The risks involved in their rapid proliferation and use would seem to constitute good reasons for intergovernmental discussions concerning these weapons with a view to possible restrictions upon their operational use or even prohibition. (ICRC, 1973*c*, pp. 71–72)

Some of the major military powers chose not to send their experts to participate in the writing of these reports and therefore their views were not well represented. In two subsequent Conferences of Government Experts, held in Lucerne in 1974 and Lugano in 1976, the views of these military powers were put by strong teams of experts. Consequently, the resulting reports (ICRC, 1974, 1976) tend to give more emphasis to the military utility, or even 'necessity', of some of the weapons which in the earlier reports had been regarded as possible candidates for restrictive measures.

In so doing they largely obscured the fact that some of the weapons discussed (particularly napalm and phosphorus) may be so cruel and repulsive as to justify a ban even if they have military utility.

During the Lugano Conference a number of proposals for restrictive measures were discussed and the discussion continued (though with little progress) at the Third and Fourth Sessions of the Diplomatic Conference in 1976 and 1977.

It is clear that agreement has not yet been reached at the inter-State level on the fundamental problems, namely:

1. In the absence of real measures of disarmament, is it desirable to single out certain particularly cruel weapons and restrain their use by legal means?

2. If such a course of action is desirable, is it feasible to draw up adequate criteria for distinguishing between the weapons to be restricted and those to be condoned?

These problems are of a philosphical as well as a pragmatic and political nature. How much human suffering is 'acceptable' is, in the last resort, a question of *norms* which may vary from one culture or historical period to another. It is not at all clear at the present time that universal norms on these matters can be said to exist – although the publicity given to the weaponry used in Indo-China seemed to contribute to the emergence of norms which were rather widespread.

In order for universal norms to develop it is essential that the world public be informed of the issues raised. Although the government experts at the Lugano Conference concluded that, on the whole, sufficient information was now available to governments to enable them to make up their minds about whether or not to prohibit the use of certain weapons, the public at large has not been told of this information. Consequently, there is a danger that government policies will continue to be determined by narrow military and political interests rather than by concern for the progressive development of international humanitarian law.

Notes to Chapter 9

1. The French chronicler William Le Bruton (1170–1230) records that Richard himself died from a crossbow.

2. See note 5, chapter 1.

3. Russian note of 30 December 1898–11 January 1899.

4. For the origin of the dumdum bullet, see pp. 14 and 55–57.

5. An English translation is to be found in Scott (1920).

6. The same criticism can be directed at studies carried out in 1975 by US experts and reported at the Lugano Conference of Government Experts (ICRC, 1976). These experiments were designed to show that dumdum bullets cause much worse wounds than 7.62 mm or 5.56 mm military bullets, but the bullets used were hunting bullets with a greater area of lead exposed.

7. 1 yard = 0.914 m. However, since the ranges quoted can only be imprecise estimates, yards and metres can here be taken as equivalent.

8. It seems likely that the non-international armed conflicts the ICRC had in mind included 'wars of national liberation' as well as civil wars. However, a majority of States, both at the UN General Assembly (Resolution 3103 [XXVII], 12 December 1973) and at the Diplomatic Conference on the draft Additional Protocols has expressed itself in favour of regarding 'armed conflicts involving the struggles of peoples against colonial domination and racist regimes' as international conflicts, thereby giving combatants the full protection of the Geneva Conventions.

9. The authentic French text reads *maux superflus*. The 1907 version is usually translated into English as 'calculated to cause unnecessary suffering' which, as several authors (e.g., Meyrowitz, 1968) have pointed out, has somewhat different semantic connotations.

10. Bundesministerium der Verteidigung Z Dv 15/10, *Kriegsvölkerrecht, Leitfaden für den Unterricht (Teil 7), Allgemeine Bestimmungen des Kriegsführungsrechts und Landkriegsrechts,* March 1961.

11. US forces are issued with shot-gun ammunition of several types, including cartridges which fire flechettes (US Defense Supply Agency, 1971).

12. The US Senate Committee on Foreign Relations (1970) held hearings on *Moral and Military Aspects of the War in Southeast Asia.* The American Society of International Law sponsored a series of anthologies on legal aspects of the Viet Nam War (e.g., Falk, 1968). Other books raising legal and moral issues of US involvement in Indo-China include Falk, Kolko & Lifton (1971) and Trooboff (1975). The question of the legality of the M-16 rifle was discussed by Paust (1974), cluster bombs by Krepon (1974) and the electronic battlefield by Fried (1972).

13. The International War Crimes Tribunal initiated by Bertrand Russell was composed of distinguished scientists and intellectuals from a number of countries who received testimony from witnesses, including scientists and medical doctors who had made investigations in Viet Nam and Vietnamese victims of the war. Russell explained the role of the Tribunal as follows: 'War crimes are the actions of powers whose arrogance leads them to believe that they are above the law. Might, they argue, is right. The world needs to establish and apply certain criteria in considering inhuman actions by great powers. These should not be the criteria convenient to the victor, as at Nuremberg, but those which enable private citizens to make compelling judgements on the injustices committed by any great power. It was my belief, in calling together the International War Crimes Tribunal, that we could do this . . .' (B. Russell, in Duffett, 1968, p. 4). The Tribunal was constituted in London in November 1966 and two sessions of the Tribunal were held, the first in Stockholm, Sweden, during 2–10 May 1967, and the second in Roskilde, Denmark, during

20 November – 1 December 1967. Several versions of the proceedings have been published (Dedijer, 1967; Duffett, 1968; Coates, Limqueco & Weiss, 1971); a Vietnamese commentary on the Tribunal was published in Hanoi by the Juridical Sciences Institute under the Viet Nam State Commission of Social Sciences (1968).

Appendix 9A

Chronology of events related to the prohibition of inhumane and indiscriminate weapons, April 1968–December 1977

22 April–13 May 1968

The International Conference on Human Rights at Teheran in its resolution XXIII calls upon the Secretary-General of the United Nations, in consultation with the International Committee of the Red Cross (ICRC) and other appropriate international organizations, to study:

(*a*) steps which could be taken to secure the better application of existing humanitarian international conventions and rules in all armed conflicts; and

(*b*) the need for additional humanitarian conventions or for other appropriate legal instruments to ensure the better protection of civilians, prisoners and combatants in armed conflicts and the prohibition and limitation of the use of certain methods and means of warfare.

19 December 1968

The UN General Assembly adopts resolution 2444 (XXIII) authorizing the Secretary-General to undertake the studies recommended by the Teheran Conference (above).

September 1969

The XXIst International Conference of the Red Cross held at Istanbul urges the International Committee of the Red Cross to draw up concrete rules to supplement the international humanitarian law of armed conflicts now in force and to hold consultations with government experts on those proposals.

20 November 1969

The first report of the United Nations Secretary-General on Human Rights in Armed Conflicts (Document A/7720) is published.

16 December 1969

The UN General Assembly adopts resolution 2597 (XXIV) in which the Secretary-General is requested:

To continue the study initiated under General Assembly resolution 2444 (XXIII), giving special attention to the need for protection of the rights of civilians and combatants in conflicts which arise from the struggles of peoples under colonial and foreign rule for liberation and self-determination and the better application of existing humanitarian conventions and rules to such conflicts.

Further, the Secretary-General is requested to submit a second report on respect for human rights in armed conflicts.

18 September 1970

The second report of the UN Secretary-General on human rights in armed conflicts (A/8052) recommends, *inter alia,* that he be authorized to commission a report on napalm and other incendiary weapons.

28 December 1970–4 January 1971

The UN General Assembly adopts five resolutions (2673 (XXV)–2677 (XXV)) on human rights in armed conflicts. Resolution 2677 (XXV), reaffirming previous resolutions, welcomes the decision of the ICRC to convene at Geneva in 1971 a conference of government experts on the reaffirmation and development of the international humanitarian law of armed conflicts. The resolution expresses the belief that one or more plenipotentiary diplomatic conferences of states parties to the four Geneva Conventions of 1949 and other interested states might be convened at an appropriate time, after due preparation, in order to adopt international legal instruments for the reaffirmation and development of international humanitarian law applicable to armed conflicts. The resolution also expresses the hope that the ICRC conference would consider specific recommendations in this respect.

24 May–12 June 1971

The First Conference of Government Experts on the Reaffirmation and Development of the International Humanitarian Law Applicable to Armed Conflicts is held in Geneva under the auspices of the ICRC.

2 September 1971

The UN Secretary-General submits a report on the Conference of Government Experts and on some other recent developments to the General Assembly (A/8370 and Add. 1).

20 December 1971

The UN General Assembly adopts resolution 2852 (XXVI), in which the decision of the ICRC to hold a second conference of government experts in 1972 is welcomed. The ICRC is invited to continue its work and to devote special attention to measures designed to ensure the better application of existing rules relating to armed conflicts; to measures to improve the protection of the civilian population and the protection of persons struggling under foreign or colonial occupation or racist régimes; to the protection and humane treatment of combatants in international and non-international armed conflicts and to questions of guerrilla warfare; and to additional rules for the protection of the wounded and sick. Further, the Secretary-General is requested to submit two reports, one on the second conference of government experts, and one on napalm and incendiary weapons and all aspects of their possible use, with the aid of qualified governmental consultant experts.

In resolution 2853 (XXVI), also on 20 December 1971, the General Assembly expresses the hope that the second conference of government experts would make recommendations for the further development of the international humanitarian law applicable in armed conflicts, including, as appropriate, draft protocols to the Geneva Conventions of 1949, for subsequent consideration at one or more plenipotentiary diplomatic conferences. The Secretary-General is requested to report to the 27th session of the General Assembly on the progress made.

3 May–3 June 1972

The Second Conference of Government Experts on the Reaffirmation and Development of International Law Applicable in Armed Conflicts is held in Geneva under the auspices of the ICRC.

20 September 1972

The UN Secretary-General submits a report on the second conference of government experts (A/8781 and Corr. 1).

9 October 1972

The UN Secretary-General submits a report entitled *Napalm and Other Incendiary Weapons and all Aspects of their Possible Use,* prepared by a group of qualified governmental consultant experts (A/8803).

29 November 1972

The UN General Assembly, in resolution 2932 (XXVII), 'deplores the use of napalm and other incendiary weapons in all armed conflicts', and calls upon the Secretary-General to publish the report on napalm for wide circulation and to report on the comments of governments at its 28th session.

18 December 1972

The UN General Assembly adopts resolution 3032 (XXVII) urging all governments to seek consultations in order that the forthcoming (1974) diplomatic conference on international humanitarian law applicable to armed conflicts would adopt rules which would 'contribute significantly in the alleviation of suffering' brought about by modern armed conflicts. Further, the General Assembly requests the Secretary-General to prepare as soon as possible a survey of existing rules of international law concerning the prohibition or restriction of the use of specific weapons.

26 February–3 March 1973

A meeting of military, medical and legal experts on the use of such conventional weapons as may cause unnecessary suffering or have indiscriminate effects is held in Geneva under the auspices of the ICRC.

11 October 1973

The UN Secretary-General publishes a report on the replies received from 21 Member States on the question of napalm and other incendiary weapons and all aspects of their possible use (UN document A/9207).

7 November 1973

The UN Secretariat publishes a Survey of *Existing Rules of International Law Concerning the Prohibition or Restriction of Use of Specific Weapons* (UN document A/9215 Vol. I–II).

8–15 November 1973

The XXIInd International Conference of the Red Cross, in resolution XIV, welcomes the expert report, published by the ICRC (1973), on *Weapons that may Cause Unnecessary Suffering or Have Indiscriminate Effects*, including, *inter alia*, high velocity projectiles, blast and fragmentation weapons, time-delay weapons and napalm and other incendiary weapons; urges the Diplomatic Conference to begin consideration of the prohibition or restriction of use of such conventional weapons; and invites the ICRC to call a conference of government experts in 1974 to study in depth the question of prohibition or restriction of use of such weapons.

6 December 1973

The UN General Assembly, in resolution 3076 (XXVIII), acknowledges resolution XIV of the International Conference of the Red Cross calling upon the Diplomatic Conference to take up the question of weapons and the ICRC to convene a conference of government experts.

20 February–29 March 1974

The plenipotentiary Diplomatic Conference on the Reaffirmation and Development of International Humanitarian Law Applicable in Armed Conflicts is held in Geneva at the invitation of the Swiss Federal Council to consider two draft additional protocols to the four Geneva Conventions of 12 August 1949. The Conference establishes an *ad hoc* Committee to examine the question of the prohibition or restriction of use of conventional weapons which may cause unnecessary suffering or have indiscriminate effects.

24 September–18 October 1974

A Conference of Government Experts on Weapons that may Cause Unnecessary Suffering or Have Indiscriminate Effects is held at Lucerne, Switzerland, under the auspices of the International Committee of the Red Cross with the participation of experts from 49 states as well as from international organizations.

15 October 1974

The UN Secretary-General submits a report to the General Assembly on the work of the Diplomatic Conference on inhumane and indiscriminate weapons (UN document A/9726).

9 December 1974

In two resolutions (3255 A and 3255 B (XXIX)), the UN General Assembly condemns the use of napalm and other incendiary weapons in circumstances where it might affect human beings or cause damage to the natural environment and/or natural resources, and urges all governments to compile without delay such supplementary data as may be required to enable them to focus upon specific proposals for prohibitions or restrictions of use of specific conventional weapons which may be deemed to cause unnecessary suffering or have indiscriminate effects. The Secretary-General is invited to report on the progress of the work to the XXXth session of the General Assembly.

3 February–18 April 1975

A second session of the Diplomatic Conference on International Humanitarian Law is held in Geneva. Agreement is reached on the prohibition of: area bombardment of populated areas; destruction of dykes, nuclear power stations and other facilities holding back dangerous forces; destruction of crops necessary for the survival of the civilian population; and attacks which might be expected to incur widespread, long-term or severe damage to the natural environment. The *ad hoc* Committee on specific weapons draws up a plan of work for a second Conference of Government Experts.

25–30 August 1975

The Conference of Ministers of Foreign Affairs of Non-Aligned Countries, held in Lima, Peru, condemns colonialist powers which have neglected to remove the material remnants of wars, such as mines, thereby impeding the development of certain developing countries.

24 September 1975

The UN Secretary-General reports to the General Assembly the responses of 15 governments, as well as the responses of the ICRC and the World Health Organization, to the request contained in resolution 3255 B (XXIX) to provide further information on napalm and other incendiary weapons (UN document A/10223).

18 September 1975

The UN Secretary General reports to the General Assembly on the work of the *ad hoc* Committee of the Diplomatic Conference (UN document A/10222).

9 December 1975

Taking note of the resolution of the Conference of Foreign Ministers of Non-Aligned Countries, the General Assembly of the United Nations calls upon the colonialist powers to assist in the removal of the material remnants of wars, particularly mines, and requests the Governing Council of the United Nations Environment Programme to undertake a study of the environmental problem posed by such remnants (resolution 3435 (XXX)).

11 December 1975

The UN General Assembly invites the Diplomatic Conference to continue its search for agreement on rules for the prohibition or restriction of use of conventional weapons having excessively injurious or indiscriminate effects.

28 January–26 February 1976

A second Conference of Government Experts on the Use of Certain Conventional Weapons is held at Lugano, Switzerland, during which a number of draft proposals for the prohibition or restriction of use of certain specific weapons are discussed.

9 April 1976

The Governing Council of the United Nations Environment Programme welcomes the efforts of the Diplomatic Conference and authorizes the Executive Director to proceed with the study requested by the General Assembly on the problem of the material remnants of wars, particularly mines, and to submit an interim report to the XXXIst Session of the UN General Assembly.

21 April–11 June 1976

A third session of the Diplomatic Conference on International Humanitarian Law is held in Geneva, Switzerland. The *ad hoc* Committee on weapons discusses the proposals put before the Lugano Conference as well as some new ones.

10 December 1976

The UN General Assembly invites the Diplomatic Conference to accelerate its consideration of specific conventional weapons and to do its utmost to agree on rules prohibiting or restricting their use.

17 March–10 June 1977

A fourth session of the Diplomatic Conference on International Humanitarian Law is held in Geneva, Switzerland. In the two Additional Protocols to the Geneva Conventions adopted no reference is made to specific weapons. A resolution is passed calling upon the United Nations to convene a conference on weapons not later than 1979.

19 December 1977

The UN General Assembly decides to convene a UN Conference in 1979 with a view to reaching agreements on the prohibition or restriction of use of specific conventional weapons.

Appendix 9B

Resolutions of the UN General Assembly on inhumane and indiscriminate weapons and related topics

The question of inhumane and indiscriminate weapons has been raised on many occasions at the United Nations. In a series of resolutions of the General Assembly, attention has been drawn to the use of such weapons and the international community has regularly been urged to undertake serious efforts to prohibit or restrict the use of such weapons.

In this appendix, the relevant resolutions of the UN General Assembly are listed, together with a summary of the substantive text and the voting data.

Resolution no. and date of adoption	Subject and contents of resolution	Voting results
2674 (XXV) **9 December 1970**	Considers that air bombardments of civil populations and the use of asphyxiating, poisonous or other gases and of all analogous liquids, materials and devices, as well as bacteriological (biological) weapons, constitute a flagrant violation of the Hague Convention of 1907, the Geneva Protocol of 1925 and the Geneva Conventions of 1949.	*In favour* 77 *Against* 2: Brazil,[a] Portugal *Abstentions* 36: Argentina, Australia, Austria, Belgium, Cambodia, Canada, Central African Republic, Colombia, Costa Rica, Denmark, Dominican Republic, El Salvador, Finland, France, Guatemala, Guyana, Haiti, Honduras, Iceland, Ireland, Israel, Italy, Lesotho, Luxembourg, Malawi, Netherlands, New Zealand, Norway, Paraguay, Spain, Sweden, Thailand, UK, Uruguay, USA, Venezuela *Absent:* Albania, Bolivia, Botswana, Ceylon, Equatorial Guinea, Fiji, Laos, Maldives, Malta, Mexico, South Africa, Trinidad and Tobago
2677 (XXV) **9 December 1970**	Calls upon all parties to any armed conflict to observe the rules laid down in the Hague Conventions of 1899 and 1907, the Geneva Protocol of 1925, the Geneva Conventions of 1949 and other humanitarian rules applicable in armed conflicts, and invites those states which have not yet done so to adhere to those conventions; expresses the hope that the conference of government experts to be convened in 1971 by the International Committee of the Red Cross will consider further what development is required in existing humanitarian laws applicable to armed conflicts and that it will make specific recommendations in this respect.	*In favour* 111 *Against* 0 *Abstentions* 4
2852 (XXVI) **20 December 1971**	Invites the International Committee of the Red Cross to continue the work that was begun with the assistance of government experts in 1971 and to devote special attention, among the questions to be taken up, to the need to ensure better application of existing rules	*In favour* 110 *Against* 1 *Abstentions* 5

relating to armed conflicts, particularly the Hague Conventions of 1899 and 1907, the Geneva Protocol of 1925 and the four Geneva Conventions of 1949; and to the need for a reaffirmation and development of relevant rules, as well as other measures to improve the protection of the civilian population during armed conflicts, including legal restraints and restrictions on certain methods of warfare and weapons that have proved particularly perilous to civilians, as well as arrangements for humanitarian relief.

Requests the Secretary-General to prepare, as soon as possible, with the help of governmental qualified consultant experts, a report on napalm and other incendiary weapons and all aspects of their possible use.

**2918 (XXVII)
14 November 1972**

Condemns the continuation by Portuguese military forces of the indiscriminate bombing of civilians, the wholesale destruction of villages and property and the ruthless use of napalm and chemical substances in Angola, Guinea (Bissau) and Cape Verde and Mozambique.

In favour 98
Against 6: Brazil, Portugal, South Africa, Spain, UK, USA
Abstentions 8: Belgium, France, Guatemala, Honduras, Italy, Luxembourg, Uruguay, Venezuela
Absent: Bolivia, Colombia, Costa Rica, Democratic Republic of Yemen, Dominican Republic, El Salvador, Equatorial Guinea,[b] Gambia, Guyana,[b] Haiti,[b] Lesotho,[b] Malawi, Maldives, Mali, Malta, Nicaragua, Niger,[b] Paraguay, Sri Lanka, Togo[b]

**2932 A (XXVII)
29 November 1972**

Deplores the use of napalm and other incendiary weapons in all conflicts; welcomes the report of the Secretary-General on napalm and other incendiary weapons and all aspects of their possible use; takes note of the views expressed in the report regarding the production, development and stockpiling of these weapons; requests the Secretary-General to circulate the report to the governments of member states for their comments and to report on these comments to the 28th General Assembly.

In favour 99
Against 0
Abstentions 15: Australia, Belgium, Canada, France, Greece, Israel, Italy, Japan, Luxembourg, Netherlands, New Zealand, Portugal, South Africa, UK, USA
Absent: Albania, Botswana, Dahomey, Equatorial Guinea, Gabon, Gambia, Guinea, Haiti, Honduras, Malawi, Morocco, Nepal, Nicaragua, Saudi Arabia, Sierra Leone, Somalia, Trinidad and Tobago,[b] Yemen

Resolution no. and date of adoption	Subject and contents of resolution	Voting results
3076 (XXVIII) 6 December 1973	Invites the Diplomatic Conference on the Reaffirmation and Development of International Humanitarian Law Applicable in Armed Conflicts to consider the question of the use of napalm and other incendiary weapons, as well as other specific conventional weapons which may be deemed to cause unnecessary suffering or to have indiscriminate effects, and to seek agreement on rules prohibiting or restricting the use of such weapons.	*In favour* 103 *Against* 0 *Abstentions* 18: Belgium, Bulgaria, Byelorussian SSR, Central African Republic, Czechoslovakia, France, German Democratic Republic, Greece, Hungary, Israel, Italy, Mongolia, Poland, Saudi Arabia, UK, Ukrainian SSR, USA, USSR *Absent or not participating in the vote:* Bahamas, Chile, Ecuador, Equatorial Guinea, Gambia, Guyana, Iceland, Kenya,[b] Lebanon, Malawi, Maldives, Mauritius, Nigeria, Swaziland
3255 A (XXIX) 9 December 1974	Notes with appreciation the expressed readiness of the International Committee of the Red Cross to convoke another Conference of Government experts and urges all Governments to compile without delay such supplementary data as may be required by them to focus upon specific proposals for prohibitions or restrictions.	*In favour* 108 *Against* 0 *Abstentions* 13: Bulgaria, Byelorussian SSR, Czechoslovakia, France, German Democratic Republic, Hungary, Israel, Mongolia, Poland, UK, Ukrainian SSR, USA, USSR *Absent or not participating in the vote:* Bahamas, Bhutan, Chad, Equatorial Guinea, Gabon, Grenada, Guinea,[b] Guinea-Bissau, Jamaica, Lesotho, Maldives, Mali, Mauritius, Saudi Arabia, South Africa, Swaziland, Togo
3255 B (XXIX) 9 December 1974	Deeply disturbed at the continuing use of napalm and other incendiary weapons, condemns, the use of napalm and other incendiary weapons in circumstances where it may affect human beings or may cause damage to the environment and/or natural resources; urges all States to refrain from production, stockpiling, proliferation and use of such weapons, pending conclusion of agreements on the	*In favour* 98 *Against* 0 *Abstentions* 27: Australia, Austria, Belgium, Bulgaria, Byelorussian SSR, Canada, Czechoslovakia, Denmark, France, German Democratic Republic, Germany (Federal Republic of), Greece,[b] Hungary, Ireland, Israel, Italy, Japan, Luxembourg, Mongolia,

prohibition of these weapons; invites all Governments, the International Committee of the Red Cross, the specialized agencies and the other international organizations concerned to transmit to the Secretary-General all information about the use of napalm and other incendiary weapons in armed conflicts; and requests the Secretary-General to prepare a report on this subject.

Netherlands, Norway, Poland, Turkey, UK, Ukrainian SSR, USA, USSR

Absent or not participating in the vote: Bahrain, Chad, Gabon, Grenada, Guinea,[b] Guinea-Bissau, Jamaica, Lesotho, Maldives, Mali, Saudi Arabia, South Africa, Swaziland

3435 (XXX)
9 December 1975
(Resolution on the UN Environment Programme)

Recognizes that the development of certain developing countries has been impeded by the material remnants of wars, the most important of which are mines, which continue to be present in their territories; condemns the colonialist powers which have neglected to remove the remnants of wars, particularly mines, and considers them to be responsible for any material and moral damage suffered by the countries in which such mines were placed; calls upon states which took part in those wars to make available forthwith to the affected state all information on the areas in which such mines were placed, including maps indicating the position of those areas, and on the types of mines; calls upon those states which created this situation to compensate forthwith the countries in which mines were placed for any material and moral damage suffered by them as a result, and to take speedy measures to provide technical assistance for the removal of such mines; requests the Governing Council of the United Nations Environment Programme to undertake a study of the problem of the material remnants of wars, particularly mines, and their effect on the environment, and to submit a report on the subject to the General Assembly at its thirty-first session.

In favour 100
Against 0
Abstentions 21
(States are not specified, because the votes were not recorded)

3464 (XXX)
11 December 1975

Invites the Diplomatic Conference on the Reaffirmation and Development of International Humanitarian Law Applicable in Armed Conflicts to continue its consideration of the use of specific conventional weapons, including any which may be deemed to be excessively injurious or to have indiscriminate effects, and its search for agreement for humanitarian reasons on possible rules prohibiting or restricting the use of such weapons.

Adopted without vote

Resolution no. and date of adoption	Subject and contents of resolution	Voting results
3500 (XXX) **15 December 1975**	Calls upon all parties to armed conflicts to acknowledge and to comply with their obligations under the humanitarian instruments and to observe the international humanitarian rules which are applicable, in particular the Hague Conventions of 1899 and 1907, the Geneva Protocol of 1925 and the Geneva Conventions of 1949; calls the attention of the Diplomatic Conference on the Reaffirmation and Development of International Humanitarian Law Applicable in Armed Conflicts, and the governments and organizations participating in it, to the need for measures to promote on a universal basis the dissemination of and instruction in the rules of international humanitarian law applicable in armed conflicts; and urges all participants in the Diplomatic Conference to do their utmost to reach agreement on additional rules which may help to alleviate the suffering brought about by armed conflicts and to respect and protect non-combatants and civilian objects in such conflicts.	Adopted by consensus
31/19 **24 November 1976**	Noting the report of the Secretary-General on the third session of the Diplomatic Conference and on the Conference of Government Experts at Lugano, calls upon all parties to armed conflicts to observe international humanitarian rules, in particular the Hague Conventions of 1899 and 1907, the Geneva Protocol of 1925 and the Geneva Conventions of 1949; calls the attention of the Diplomatic Conference to the need for measures to promote on a universal basis the dissemination of and instruction in the rules of international humanitarian law applicable in armed conflicts; urges all participants in the Diplomatic Conference to do their utmost to reach agreement on additional rules which may help alleviate the suffering brought about by armed conflicts.	Adopted by consensus

31/64
10 December 1976

Noting that the discussions and proposals regarding prohibition or restriction of use for humanitarian reasons have focused on napalm and other incendiary weapons, on indiscriminate methods of using land mines, on perfidious weapons and weapons which rely for their effect upon fragments invisible on X-ray, on certain types of small calibre projectile which may be especially injurious and on certain blast and fragmentation weapons; invites the Diplomatic Conference to accelerate its consideration of the use of specific conventional weapons, including any which may be deemed especially injurious or to have indiscriminate effects, and to do its utmost to agree for humanitarian reasons on possible rules prohibiting or restricting the use of such weapons.

Adopted without vote

32/152
19 December 1977

Decides to convene in 1979 a United Nations conference with a view to reaching agreements on prohibitions or restrictions on the use of specific conventional weapons, including those which may be deemed to be excessively injurious or have indiscriminate effects, taking into account humanitarian and military considerations, and on the question of a system of periodic review of this matter and for consideration of further proposals. Decides to convene a UN preparatory conference for the conference referred to above and requests the Secretary-General to transmit invitations to all states and parties invited to attend the Diplomatic Conference on the reaffirmation and development of international humanitarian law applicable in armed conflicts.

In favour 115
Against 0
Abstentions 21: Belgium, Bulgaria, Byelorussian SSR, Canada, Cuba, Czechoslovakia, France, German Democratic Republic, Germany (Federal Republic of), Hungary, Israel, Italy, Japan, Luxembourg, Mongolia, Poland, Turkey, UK, Ukrainian SSR, USA, USSR
Absent or not participating in the vote: Albania, Burma,[b] Cape Verde, China, Democratic Kampuchea, Djibouti, Gambia, Grenada, Guinea, Lao People's Democratic Republic, Seychelles, South Africa, Viet Nam

Resolution no. and date of adoption	Subject and contents of resolution	Voting results
32/44 **8 December 1977**	Welcomes the successful conclusion of the Diplomatic Conference on the reaffirmation and development of international humanitarian law applicable in armed conflicts which has resulted in two Protocols additional to the Geneva Conventions of 12 August 1949, adopted by the Diplomatic Conference on 8 June 1977, namely, Protocol I relating to the protection of victims of international armed conflicts and Protocol II relating to the protection of victims of non-international armed conflicts. Notes the recommendation, approved by the Diplomatic Conference, that a special conference be called on the issue of the prohibition or restriction of the use for humanitarian reasons of specific conventional weapons. Urges states to consider without delay the matter of signing and ratifying or acceding to the two Protocols additional to the Geneva Conventions of 1949; and calls upon all states to take effective steps for the dissemination of humanitarian rules applicable in armed conflicts.	Adopted by consensus

[a] Later indicated it had intended to abstain. Japan, which had voted in favour, indicated the same.
[b] Later indicated it had intended to vote in favour.

Appendix 9C

Superior numerals, thus [5], refer to notes on pages 255–256.

A review of recent developments related to the prohibition of inhumane and indiscriminate weapons

I. Developments in 1975–76[1]

The report of the Lucerne Conference of Government Experts on the use of certain conventional weapons (ICRC, 1975; Kalshoven, 1975; *SIPRI Yearbook 1975*) was examined at the Second Session of the Diplomatic Conference on Humanitarian Law. There it was agreed that more work at the government expert level was required before further progress at the diplomatic level could be expected, and it was decided to convene a second Conference of Government Experts, which was held in Lugano, Switzerland, in 1976. The report of this conference (ICRC, 1976), in turn, was examined at the Third Session of the Diplomatic Conference.

During 1975 the international community took several steps, with implications for the restriction of use of certain specific weapons, to limit the hazardous and indiscriminate ecological consequences of modern warfare. The Second Session of the Diplomatic Conference reached agreement on two articles (33.3 and 48 *bis*) which would prohibit 'methods or means of warfare which are intended or may be expected to cause widespread, long-term, and severe damage to the natural environment'.

At the same time a draft convention was put before the Conference of the Committee on Disarmament, which aims at the prohibition of 'military or any other hostile use of environmental modification techniques having widespread, long-lasting or severe effects as the means of destruction, damage or injury.'[2]

In resolution IV of the Conference of Ministers for Foreign Affairs of Non-Aligned countries, held at Lima, Peru, from 25 to 30 August 1975, colonial powers were condemned for having neglected to remove the material remnants, such as mines, of wars and of acts of aggression. This was noted by the UN General Assembly in resolution 3435 (XXX) of 9 December 1975, which not only placed responsibility for the removal of such remnants of war upon the Powers concerned but went on to request the Governing Council of the United Nations Environment Programme to study the problem of the material remnants of war, particularly mines, and their effect on the environment, and to submit a report on the subject to the General Assembly.[3]

In a further resolution related to the question of the restriction of the use of certain specific weapons, the General Assembly, in resolution 3464 (XXX) of 11 December 1975, took note of the fact that 'the proposals and suggestions which have been advanced have regard not only to napalm and other incendiary

243

weapons but to a number of other specific kinds of conventional weapons, such as various small-calibre projectiles, certain blast and fragmentation weapons, as well as some delayed action weapons and perfidious weapons' and invited the Diplomatic Conference to continue its 'search for agreement for humanitarian reasons on possible rules prohibiting or restricting the use of such weapons'.

During 1975–76 SIPRI published three books related to these issues. The first of these books (SIPRI, 1975a) provided a thorough study of incendiary weapons, including napalm and white phosphorus. It pointed out that not only was fire (like biological weapons) liable to propagate, thereby being particularly likely to cause indiscriminate effects, but that burn wounds of individuals were also likely to constitute unnecessary suffering in the legal sense. The reason for this is that burn wounds may not necessarily be immediately effective in incapacitating a human being (for which reason, flame weapons are of limited utility on the battlefield), but the areas of the body most likely to be affected – the hand and the face– are the areas which are (a) most susceptible to disabling, long-term contractions, (b) most difficult to reconstruct surgically, and (c) most essential for normal social and economic activity.

The second book (SIPRI, 1976a) examined the legal basis for the re-examination of specific categories of weapons in the light of both traditional and new principles of international humanitarian law. The traditional principles may be summarized as follows: (a) the prohibition of superfluous injury, (b) respect for civilians, (c) the principle that the demands of humanity may prevail over the demands of warfare, and (d) the principle that the demands of peace (including cease-fires and armistices) may prevail over the demands of warfare (prohibition of treachery).

The book further suggests that – in view of technological developments in weaponry – new principles with respect to the laws of war concerning the prohibition of specific weapons should be added to the traditional ones. The new principles include the following:

1. a recognition of the principle of *proportionality* which includes not only the number of persons affected by a military operation but also the amount of suffering caused to these persons, relative to the military advantages to be expected from disabling them; that, 'there may be room for the principle that specific cruel injuries may be disproportionate to the military advantage of disabling a soldier' (SIPRI, 1976a, p. 42);

2. the principle that the *survival of mankind* prevails over any national interest should be expressly stated and taken into account when examining specific means and methods of warfare;

3. the protection of the *environment* has become a basic concern which should also be taken into account when assessing the legality or otherwise of specific weapons or methods of warfare;

4. total prohibition of some classes of weapons may be justified where relatively innocent uses may represent a *threshold,* opening the way to general use (examples include the use of tear-gases in relation to chemical warfare in general, or 'mini' nuclear weapons in relation to standard tactical or strategic nuclear weapons).

The third book examines the impact of the recently concluded war in Indo-China on the environment (SIPRI, 1976*b*). It points out that the massive use of conventional munitions, combined with the extensive use of 'unconventional' measures, such as spraying crops and forests with chemical anti-plant agents and clearing vegetation with mechanical equipment, causes a severe degradation of the natural environment, with both short- and long-term consequences. This, together with the problem of unexploded munitions and other war remnants, greatly complicates the task of rehabilitation in the post-war period.

II. The Second Session of the Diplomatic Conference on Humanitarian Law in Armed Conflicts (Geneva, 3 February–18 April 1975)

Specific weapons and methods of warfare were discussed in Commission III and in the *ad hoc* Committee. The latter contented itself with examining the report of the Lucerne Conference – without progressing significantly in making specific proposals – and drawing up the mandate for a second Conference of Government Experts on inhumane and indiscriminate weapons.

The achievements of Commission III were much more notable. The Commission arrived at new rules which, if followed in war, could have a significant effect on the conduct of war. Briefly, these new rules amount to a prohibition of the following methods of warfare: (*a*) area bombing in populated areas; (*b*) 'starvation warfare'; (*c*) destruction of dams, nuclear power stations, and similar facilities containing 'dangerous forces'; (*d*) relocation of the population; and (*e*) destruction of the environment.

Nearly all these methods of warfare have been employed by major powers during the last third of this century. It represents a considerable step in the development of the rule of law that prohibitions of this kind have been put forward and widely accepted even though it has required over 20 years of effort by the ICRC and even though advances in military technology may make these methods largely obsolete as far as major military powers are concerned.[4]

III. The Second Conference of Government Experts on Certain Conventional Weapons (Lugano, 28 January–26 February 1976)

During the Lugano Conference of Government Experts (ICRC, 1976) a number of additional proposals were tabled which would either prohibit or restrict the use of certain specific weapons.[5] Comparison of these proposals gives some indication of the present state of thinking within the international community on this question. However, the complex structure of the Report of the Lugano Conference (in which the reader is directed first to the plenary proceedings, then to the General Working Group report and then to Special Working Groups) makes it difficult for the non-participant to grasp the main trends which developed at the Conference.

Incendiary weapons

The subject of incendiary weapons generated the greatest number and the widest variety of proposals.

Protection of civilians

All proposals would rule out the use of incendiary weapons against the civilian population as such and would insist in precautions being taken if incendiary weapons were to be used against military objectives within populated areas.

The first area of divergence is *whether or not to restrict the use of incendiary weapons against military targets in populated areas outside the battle zone.* Proposal COLU/207, presented by 11 Western nations including the USA,[6] would not accept restrictions, whereas COLU/205, presented by the Netherlands delegation and given a sympathetic reception by a number of Western delegations (including some sponsors of COLU/207) proposed to restrict the use outside the battle zone of certain incendiary weapons, namely, those based on a gelled hydrocarbon (including napalm).

All other proposals would restrict the use of incendiary weapons to a greater extent. COLU/211, put forward by Spain, would prohibit the use of incendiary weapons against military objectives outside the battle zone, whereas COLU/208 (Indonesia) would prohibit the use of incendiaries against military objectives in populated areas even within the battle zone. The remaining proposals would also prohibit use of incendiaries against military objectives in populated areas.

Thus, it can be concluded that there was general agreement that incendiary weapons should be prohibited for use against the civilian population as such. Many States would be prepared to go further and accept restrictions on the use of some or all incendiary weapons against military objectives in populated areas, particularly in rear areas.

Protection of combatants

The second area of divergent views was *whether or not to restrict the use of incendiary weapons against military personnel.* Some delegations – notably those sponsoring COLU/207 – were not prepared at Lugano to accept restrictions on the battlefield use of incendiaries. COLU/205, put forward by the Netherlands experts, restricted the use of napalm on the battlefield to military objects (such as airfields, fortified positions and armoured targets) except where troops were engaged in close combat. COLU/211, submitted by Spain, went further and would ban any use of incendiary weapons against personnel. Anti-personnel use would, of course, also be prohibited by those formulations seeking a more or less total ban on incendiaries.

246

It would seem that there is wide support for restriction of the use of incendiary weapons against military personnel except among the experts of some States with highly mechanized forces who argued – with some justification as far as such forces are concerned – that a distinction between anti-personnel and anti-matériel uses is somewhat artificial.

Protection of the environment
None of the proposals put forward at Lugano specifically referred to the protection of the environment from the effects of incendiary weapons, though this aspect was referred to in a number of supporting statements.

Outstanding issues with regard to incendiary weapons
The main outstanding issues with regard to incendiary weapons have to do with the question of the scope of the definitions adopted. The working definition arrived at in Lucerne (ICRC, 1974) has been accepted as a basis for further discussions and is found, for example, in CDDH/IV/201 and in COLU/205. However, COLU/205 then introduced a restriction of use of a subcategory of incendiary weapons, namely, those employing a gelled hydrocarbon as the incendiary agent.

It is clear that this formulation is intended to apply to the case of napalm bombs and flame-throwers. However, the additional definition put forward would result in the anomaly that small incendiary bombs employing gelled hydrocarbons (such as those used against Japanese cities during World War II) would be subject to greater restrictions than would similar bombs using, for example, magnesium or thermite (as were used in particular against Finnish and German cities during World War II), or thickened pyrophoric agents, such as triethyl aluminium (TEA).[7] Conversely, the Netherlands proposal would not cover other scatter-type agents, such as white phosphorus or, presumably, flame-throwers using unthickened fuel.

Thus, it may be said that the intention of COLU/205 is well taken, but that it needs some further consideration from the technical point of view.

A further issue requiring clarification is the use of *white phosphorus*. Evidence presented by US specialists indicates that burns from white phosphorus may take as much as 40 per cent more time to heal than other burns (Curreri, Asch & Pruitt, 1970). In addition, a number of recent studies have brought to light the possibility of toxic effects from white phosphorus.[8] For these reasons, there is a strong case for prohibiting at least its anti-personnel use. However, some experts would argue that the working definition of incendiary weapons would not cover white phosphorus munitions since they are *primarily* designed for producing smoke. If this is so, then it is essential to introduce a further rule prohibiting the use of white phosphorus munitions as incendiaries or as anti-personnel munitions.

Small calibre weapons

Protection of combatants
As recognized in the 1868 Declaration of St Petersburg, the legal problem of

small calibre weapons relates primarily to the protection of combatants (rather than civilians). Although the proposal included in document CDDH/IV/201, put before the Second Session of the Diplomatic Conference, was discussed in some detail in Lugano, no new proposals were presented. On the other hand, the subject of small calibre projectiles gave rise to a considerable amount of technical discussion (see chapters 3 and 4 above).

The main points underlying these discussions seemed to be as follows:

1. Many experts advocated standard tests to compare the effects of various projectiles, for example, by firing them into blocks of soap, but no agreement was reached.

2. If it is assumed that standard tests can demonstrate that some projectiles cause larger cavities than others, the question arises as to whether it is possible to determine what size of cavity satisfies military demands without being unacceptable from a humanitarian standpoint. Those experts who advocated agreement on standard test procedures had in mind the possibility of demonstrating that certain bullets caused larger cavities than others, but also, at a later stage, of reaching agreement on a prohibition of those bullets that caused the larger cavities.

This prospect – rather than technical problems – may explain the reluctance of other experts to agree to standard test procedures. These experts emphasized the great technical complexities of testing bullets. This is remarkable in view of the advance of technology since the Hague Conference of 1899, at which time similar experiments were used to compare the dumdum bullet with other bullets (Keith & Rigby, 1899); these experiments were repeated in the United States in 1975 with apparently similar results.[9]

There is very little reason why technical experts, given the opportunity, could not agree on the parameters which determine such factors as the tumbling of bullets or the forces which the jacket of a bullet can withstand before breaking up. What is much more difficult to achieve is agreement that wounds of a certain size are adequate to incapacitate a man whereas other wounds would amount to superfluous injury. In the last resort this requires a subjective or political judgement. Positions taken at the Conference of Government Experts were often influenced by political rather than scientific considerations, with the result that the report still does not present the international community with any agreement on the facts.

Outstanding issues with regard to small calibre weapons
The earlier report of a group of experts (ICRC, 1973) pointed out that the legal position on the military use of smooth-bore shot-guns was ambiguous. Some countries regarded these weapons as contrary to existing law while others did not.

A resolution of this ambiguity is important because of the development of other multiple projectile small arms systems. One arrangement – which is reported to have already been used in combat, at least on a trial basis – is to replace the lead shot in a shot-gun cartridge with up to 20 flechettes. Because of their ballistic characteristics, the flechettes are said to maintain their velocity better and thereby have greater range and wounding effect than spherical shot.

A number of other systems fire multiple projectiles, intended to improve the probability of hitting the target. By the same token they also increase the probability of causing multiple wounds.

Blast and fragmentation weapons

Since most conventional weapons rely on blast and fragmentation for their effects, this topic is potentially the most important with regard to the protection both of the civilian population and of combatants. Yet, hitherto, it has received the least satisfactory analysis.

Protection of civilians
The only proposal presented so far with a view to protecting non-combatants from the effects of specific blast and fragmentation weapons is paragraph II of CDDH/IV/201. Though the text of the proposal makes no reference to the civilian population, a memorandum accompanying it explains that the wide area of coverage of certain anti-personnel cluster warheads makes them a particular threat.

Although no other proposal has been put forward with respect to specific weapons, important progress had been made at the Second Session of the Diplomatic Conference, where Articles 43–51 of draft Additional Protocol I and Articles 24–29 of draft Additional Protocol II, as adopted in Commission III, would have the effect of prohibiting certain tactical and strategic uses of blast and fragmentation weapons.

There would appear to be a widespread view that the problem of restricting the use of conventional blast and fragmentation weapons is so complex that only the most general rules are feasible. However, the publication of some of the Rules of Engagement applicable to US forces in Viet Nam at some periods of the recent war in Indo-China (appendix 9D) indicates that it is possible to draw up much more specific guide-lines where a reduction of civilian casualties is perceived to be important.

The US Rules were based to some extent upon the Hague and Geneva Conventions. It is of great significance that it was necessary to elaborate these rules in considerable detail in order to ensure that field commanders could apply them in their tactical planning.

Although the US Rules are very complex, restrictions on the use of blast and fragmentation weapons (including artillery and aircraft munitions) are based on two simple principles:

1. When attacking a military target in an inhabited area, only direct-fire weapons should be used and the target should be positively identified.

2. Between the target and the inhabited area there should be a 'safety zone', its size depending upon the characteristics of the specific weapon used.

In order to ensure the safety of their own troops and civilians in peace-time it is usual for armed forces to issue safety regulations regarding the use of weaponry for training purposes.

In combat conditions, where greater risks may be warranted, it is usual to reduce the safety zone to perhaps one-half. The novelty about the US Rules is that they applied this concept to the protection of the civilian population in combat conditions. In so far as the safety zones applicable to such standard weapons as artillery and aircraft bombs are relatively constant, it might well be feasible to adopt such an approach in international regulations.

Protection of combatants

The meagre proposals put forward at the Lugano Conference were more related to the protection of combatants than to the protection of civilians, though prohibitions or restrictions of the use of certain weapons would, of course, also benefit civilians.

Two proposals were put forward which would prohibit or restrict the use of fuel–air explosives. Fuel–air explosives cause a powerful blast of relatively extended duration, evenly spread throughout the cloud. These characteristics make them effective in certain roles, such as detonating minefields. However, the well-defined area of effect and exceptionally high immediate lethality may make them attractive weapons also for use in close support or other anti-personnel roles. It is this possibility – reinforced by reports that such uses have already occurred on the battlefield – that has aroused some concern.

Of the two proposals put forward, that of Switzerland and Mexico would amount to a total prohibition, while that of Sweden would only rule out use against personnel.

Several proposals and amendments were put forward on the question of munition fragments that cannot be detected by common procedures, such as X-rays. There appeared to be widespread agreement on the acceptability of a ban on such non-detectable fragments, at least where they were intended to be the primary means of injury. Initially, attention was drawn to this problem because of the reported use of plastics in the construction of munitions. However, because of the low density of plastic fragments – and hence low range and penetrativity – it is unlikely that they will be used as the primary wounding agents. The formulations at present being discussed, however, would allow plastics to be used in munitions so long as they were not intended to be the primary cause of injury. On the other hand, these formulations would also rule out the use of materials, such as wood, bamboo or glass, which have been used as field expedients and in some cases in manufactured munitions, where wooden or glass splinters were a primary cause of wounds (see chapters 5 and 6). These formulations would tend to rule out more primitive weapons but to permit sophisticated ones.

Finally, Norway put forward a proposal about especially injurious pre-fragmented elements, although it is not clear to which munitions such a formulation was intended to apply. The main merit of the proposal is that it may eventually generate further discussion of the wounding effects of various fragments, including not only steel fragments but also cubes, spheres, flechettes, pieces of wire, and the like.

On the subject of flechettes, there was some discussion of the proposals made in CDDH/IV/201 (which would prohibit the use of flechettes and the like) but no new proposals were put forward. There were conflicting opinions about the casualty effects of flechettes, but clearly the effects depend upon the ballistic characteristics, such as the impact velocity and the stability and strength of the flechette in the wound (chapters 3 and 4).

Delayed-action weapons

A great deal of attention was paid at Lugano to proposal COLU/203, presented by the Netherlands, the United Kingdom and France, on the subject of mines and booby traps. But only limited time was devoted to the question of other kinds of delayed-action weapon, such as those referred to in COLU/213, sponsored by the experts of Mexico and Switzerland.[10]

Protection of the civilian population

Delayed-action weapons are particularly liable to cause indiscriminate effects (chapter 7). Mines and booby traps, for example, are characterized by the fact that the target comes to the munition rather than the other way round. But the user cannot be sure that the 'target' is a military person or vehicle rather than a civilian or other protected person.

On the whole, the discussion in Lugano resulted in general agreement (*a*) on the military necessity for mines, and (*b*) on the need for certain rules to protect the civilian population, such as a requirement to record the location of minefields. There was greater divergency of opinion on the question of booby traps, in part because of differences of understanding as to what was covered by the term. (In later versions of COLU/203, the term booby trap only appeared in a heading but not in the substantive paragraph.) Representatives of some great powers said they were prepared to accept a total prohibition of booby traps, whereas experts from some smaller countries claimed that some kinds of booby traps were essential to their defence against invasion by a more powerful army. A final consensus on this subject was not achieved.

In one area, however, there is cause for considerable concern. This is the problem of remotely delivered mines. Whereas the sponsors of CDDH/IV/201 proposed a total prohibition of air-dropped anti-personnel land-mines, the sponsors of COLU/203 contented themselves with two restrictions on the use of such mines (viz., that *either* they would be fitted with a self-neutralizing mechanism *or* that the areas in which they are dropped should be marked). This proposal was discussed at an early meeting of a special military working group and only a few objections were made. The discussion brought to light the following possibilities:

1. Remotely delivered mines open up the possibility of *offensive* mine warfare behind enemy lines.

2. Anti-personnel and anti-armour mines are usually spread together in order to prevent or complicate the disposal of the anti-tank mines.

3. Although various forms of neutralizing device are technically feasible, there is a military preference for the kind which detonates the mine, in order to prevent the reuse of the mine by the enemy.

4. If remotely delivered mines are scattered across the countryside, enemy forces may be expected to redeploy to the cities. *Therefore* (it was argued) *it is necessary to be able to spread remotely delivered mines in urban areas as well.*

Clearly, in these circumstances, the scattering of markers in an urban area which is covered with remotely delivered mines is not an adequate means of protecting the population. Neither is a self-destruct device which detonates the mines after a period of hours, days or weeks. For adequate protection of the civilian population either of these means requires that the mines are dropped in well-defined 'barrier' areas which it is possible for civilians to avoid.

As it is, the Anglo-Dutch proposal in effect invited the international community to legitimize the use of remotely delivered mines in urban areas for the purpose of 'harassment and interdiction'. When some experts claimed that such tactics would be ruled out by Articles 43–51 of draft Additional Protocol I, this was denied by a British expert who asserted that existing definitions of 'attack' would not cover the use of mines. If this is so, it is clearly an ambiguity which it is imperative to eradicate.[11]

Protection of combatants

COLU/203 also contained a proposal to prohibit certain kinds of non-explosive device, namely, any booby trap or similar device 'designed to kill or injure by non-explosive means which stabs, impales, crushes, strangles, infects or poisons the victim'. It was argued that devices of this kind caused excessive suffering, in some cases being designed to cause a long-drawn-out and painful death, and were unnecessary in modern military operations.

These arguments may well be valid, but unfortunately the sponsors did not choose to present any of the kind of evidence which had previously been made available with regard to other weapons, such as napalm. Such information would have been of considerable interest in throwing further light on various conceptions of 'superfluous injury'. Without evidence to the contrary it is difficult to see that, for example, *punji* stick wounds cause excessive suffering, even if the legs become infected, compared with having the legs blown off by an explosive device, or having the face and hands severely burned by an incendiary device – both of which weapons would also be likely to cause a variety of other injuries simultaneously. It is also unlikely that resort would be made to primitive, non-explosive means, if modern explosive means were available; if this were the case the users might well lay claim to the 'military necessity' argument.

Nevertheless, this proposal was important in marking the first time that certain delegations had been prepared to indicate that they felt some additional categories of inhumane weapon could be added to those already specified in international law.

Protection of the environment

None of the proposals on delayed-action weapons took up the question of environmental effects. There is, however, little doubt that mines, other unexploded munitions and other material remnants of war can constitute a serious threat to the human and the natural environment. It is to be hoped that the study being under-taken by the United Nations Environment Programme at the request of the General Assembly will throw further light on the extent of this problem.

Conclusion

It may be concluded that the work of the Lugano Conference was useful in broadening the scope of the discussion in some areas, and in focusing the discussion on more concrete problems in others. But a great deal still remains to be done towards attaining a significant international instrument of law. In particular, closer examination should be made of the three main considerations: protection of the civilian population; protection of combatants; and protection of the environment. For each and every category of weapons it would be desirable to draw up rules specifying how these considerations were to be taken into account. The fact that some proposals put before the Lugano Conference explicitly took such an approach is a welcome sign indicating the possibility of further progress.

IV. The Third Session of the Diplomatic Conference on Humanitarian Law in Armed Conflicts (Geneva, 21 April–11 June 1976)

The question of the prohibition or restriction of certain weapons was considered at the Third Session of the Diplomatic Conference on Humanitarian Law in two commissions. In Commission I the subject arose in the context of Article 74, 'Repression of Breaches of the Present Protocol' (i.e., Draft Additional Protocol I). A revised text submitted by the International Committee of the Red Cross would include as a 'grave breach of the present Protocol' *the use of means and methods of combat prohibited by the present protocol.* In diplomatic language 'means and methods' includes certain specific weapons (the subject of a special *ad hoc* Commission) as well as certain military operations with particularly indiscriminate effects as far as the civilian population is concerned.

This formulation was not acceptable to two groups of States. One group refused to accept the implication that the use of certain specific weapons might be regarded as a war crime (grave breach), while a second group found the ICRC formulation too vague. Sweden proposed an amendment which attempted to be more specific about the methods of warfare included, such as 'systematically making foodstuffs, food producing areas, crops, livestock and drinking water supplies indispensable to the survival of the civilian population the object of attack . . . .' The Philippines put forward a more specific proposal with regard to certain weapons:

253

... the use of weapons prohibited by the law of war, such as asphyxiating poisonous or other gases and analogous liquids, materials or devices, dum-dum bullets, and those weapons that violate traditional principles of international law and humanitarian rules, such as biological weapons, blast and fragmentation weapons.

A formulation of this kind was supported by a number of other delegations, including Indonesia, Yugoslavia and Romania. It was strongly opposed by the United States and the Soviet Union. The USA argued that such a formulation could jeopardize the whole article, indeed even the whole Protocol – by which was meant that the USA would not sign it. The Soviet Union, on the other hand, repeated its contention that the Diplomatic Conference was not the competent forum to deal with issues related to armaments.

As a result of these objections and the inconclusive results of the work of the *ad hoc* Committee on weapons, it was decided to put off further consideration of the issue until the Fourth Session of the Conference, which was held during April–June 1977.

For its part, the *ad hoc* Committee did not proceed much beyond the work of the Lugano Conference. After some delays caused by translation problems, the Lugano report was discussed. A number of new or revised proposals were put forward. These included Mexican, Norwegian and Netherlands proposals on incendiary weapons, a Venezuelan proposal on booby traps, and a Mexican and Swiss proposal on mines. It was clear, however, that governments had had too little time to digest the results of the Lugano Conference and this, together with the delays and other frustrations of the work, 'helped to create a feeling of drift' (Suckow, 1976).

V. The Fourth Session of the Diplomatic Conference on Humanitarian Law in Armed Conflicts (Geneva, 17 March–10 June 1977)

The fourth, and final, session of the Diplomatic Conference adopted two Additional Protocols to the Geneva Conventions. The first, on international conflicts, is notable in that it prohibits area bombing in inhabited areas and some other indiscriminate means of warfare. However, in explaining their vote, some States claimed that this prohibition did not apply to nuclear weapons.

The second Protocol, on non-international conflicts, was a greatly watered-down version of the original draft. Clearly, in a period when the majority of armed conflicts are the result of attempts to consolidate centralized state systems, States are not prepared to forgo the methods of 'pacification' previously employed by colonial powers.

The *ad hoc* Committee on inhumane weapons was again convened but it produced no concrete results. In the final plenary session an attempt was made to add a provision to Protocol I for the future consideration of inhumane weapons. This amendment failed by a few votes to achieve the necessary two-thirds majority.

As a result, the Additional Protocols contain no restrictions on the use of specific weapons. In spite of regular urging from the UN General Assembly to reach agreement on such restrictions, it must be concluded that the years of effort to this end have again been thwarted by the forces of militarism.

In a separate resolution – opposed by a majority of the NATO and Warsaw Treaty Organization countries – the Conference suggested that a special conference on the subject of weapons might be held not later than the spring of 1979.

Notes to Appendix 9C

1. Previously related events were reviewed in *SIPRI Yearbook 1973* and *SIPRI Yearbook 1975*. The developments referred to mainly relate to the Diplomatic Conference on the Reaffirmation and Development of International Humanitarian Law Applicable in Armed Conflicts (CDDH). This Conference has held four sessions to draw up a set of extensions and modifications to the four Geneva Conventions of 12 August 1949. As a basis for its work, the Conference took the two Draft Additional Protocols put forward by the International Committee of the Red Cross (ICRC, 1973*a, b*), the first relating to international armed conflicts and the second to non-international armed conflicts. It is these texts and the proposals which might form the basis of amendments and additions which are referred to below. The legal background has been examined by Baxter (1973), Blix (1974), Cassese (1975), Fleck (1973), Joenniemi & Rosas (1975), Kalshoven (1975), Kussbach (1977), Malinverni (1974), Sandoz (1975) and SIPRI (1976*a*).
2. See CCD/472, 21 August 1975, Article 1. For a discussion of this document, see *SIPRI Yearbook 1976*. The terms of a treaty on hostile environmental modification have since been agreed and the treaty has been opened for signature.
3. As a result of this resolution, the Governing Council of UNEP authorized the Executive Director to initiate the study required. A preliminary report was submitted to the General Council at its meeting in early 1977.
4. Reference is here made to the fact that new precision-guided munitions (PGMs) greatly reduce the military demand for area attacks in populated areas.
5. The proposals, tabled in the form of documents identified as COLU/201–221, are to be found in ICRC (1976). The proposals have been presented and analysed from a legal point of view by Kussbach (1977).
6. With regard to incendiary weapons, the US Rules of Engagement in Viet Nam stated: 'The use of incendiary type munitions in inhabited or urban areas will be avoided unless friendly survival is at stake or is necessary for the accomplishment of the commander's mission.' Elsewhere it was stated with regard to the use of direct-fire, flat-trajectory weapons in urban areas: 'All types of munitions, *except incendiary (white phosphorus)*, may be used in direct fire weapons including flechette (beehive), HEAT, and canister rounds' (italics added); see appendix 9D.
7. For details, see the Report of the Secretary-General on *Napalm and Other Incendiary Weapons and All Aspects of their Possible Use* (United Nations, 1973*a*) or SIPRI (1975*a*).
8. For an extensive review of the literature of white phosphorus burns and an examination

of the question of possible toxic effects, see SIPRI (1975*a*).

9. Statement of the US experts at the Lugano Conference (ICRC, 1976).

10. This proposal would prohibit the fitting of fuzes with a time delay of more than 24 hours to bombs and all other dropped munitions, to projectiles, shells, grenades, rockets and all other projected munitions, and to all other 'remotely delivered' munitions.

11. Article 44 ('Field of application') of Draft Additional Protocol I (ICRC, 1973*b*) stated that the provisions regarding the protection of the civilian population 'shall apply to any land, air or sea warfare which may affect the civilian population, individual civilians or civilian objects on land. They further apply to all attacks from the sea or air against objectives on land . . . .' 'Attacks' were further defined as 'acts of violence committed against the adversary whether in defence or offence'. It was claimed that the dropping of mines by air would not constitute an 'attack' in this sense, since the mine requires that the 'target' go to the mine rather than vice versa. Be that as it may, it is difficult to argue that the dropping of mines is not an act of 'land, air or sea warfare which may affect the civilian population . . . .'

Appendix 9D

Superior numerals, thus [5], *refer to notes on pages 266–267.*

The US Rules of Engagement in Viet Nam as they relate to certain specific weapons: a brief survey and analysis

I. Rules of engagement

On 6 June 1975, extracts of the Rules of Engagement applicable to US forces in Viet Nam were published in the *US Congressional Record* (pp. S 9897–9905). They comprised the following documents:

1. US Military Assistance Command, Vietnam, Directive Number 525–13, Dated May 1971 (Unclassified contents), including the following Annexes:
   – Rules of Engagement – Surface Weapons Excluding Naval Gunfire;
   – Rules of Engagement – Fixed Wing Air Operations;
   – Rules of Engagement – Rotary Wing Air Operations;
   – Rules of Engagement – Naval Gunfire.
2. Excerpts from various directives concerning rules of engagement and operating authorities for Southeast Asia.
3. Regulation Number 525–4, 16 March 1968, Headquarters, American Division, APO San Francisco, Combat Operations, Rules of Engagement.
4. Regulation Number 525–1, 30 January 1968, Headquarters, 11th Infantry Brigade, APO San Francisco, Combat Operations, Rules of Engagement.
5. Change 1, Regulation 525–1, 10 April 1968, Headquarters, 11th Infantry Brigade, American Division, Combat Operations, Rules of Engagement.
6. Change 1, Regulation Number 525–1, 9 February 1968, Headquarters, 11th Infantry Brigade, APO San Francisco, Combat Operations, Rules of Engagement.

This was the first time these Rules had been published. Since the Geneva Diplomatic Conference on International Humanitarian Law has been engaged in discussing the laws of war – in particular, those designed to protect the civilian population – these Rules of Engagement are very interesting, but, the published versions are incomplete and originate from various periods of the Viet Nam War and must accordingly be interpreted with some care.

II. General principles

The directives state that indiscriminate effects of fire-power on the civilian population are to be avoided (e.g., document 1, paragraph 3(a)). This principle is fostered by an introductory comment to the excerpts from various directives (document 2) where it is said that these excerpts 'show a consistent national policy of concern for humanity, and for the institutions of the people of Indochina during the many years of war.'[1]

The excerpts cited refer to instructions, such as taking 'due precaution against the possibility of bombing noncombatants', 'prevention of noncombatant casualties must be a continuing objective', and so on. At one point it is stated that 'indiscriminate fire into populated areas is prohibited', while elsewhere certain weapons are prohibited for use within stated ranges of inhabited places.

Taken at face value, therefore, the documents present considerable evidence for an underlying norm intended to minimize civilian casualties.

Of particular interest in the documents are the more explicit instructions to military commanders intended to ensure that military operations are carried out as far as possible according to the general principle of avoiding indiscriminate effects. These explicit instructions are of considerable relevance to the international discussion of specific weapons.

III. Instructions regarding the use of specific weapons

Incendiary munitions

Document 1, dated May 1971, introduced under 'General Rules' an instruction that

> The use of incendiary type munitions in inhabited or urban areas will be avoided unless friendly survival is at stake or is necessary for the accomplishment of the commander's mission. (Paragraph 6 (*d*) (1))

Annex 1 of the same document states, with regard to direct-fire, flat-trajectory weapons that

> All types of munitions, except incendiary (white phosphorus), may be used in direct fire weapons including flechette (beehive), HEAT, and canister rounds. (Paragraph 3 (*e*) (2) (*c*))

A directive issued on 16 March 1968 (document 3) states:

> The employment of any ordnance which would cause intentional burning of dwellings will be avoided, unless absolutely necessary in the accomplishment of the commander's mission. (Paragraph 5 *b* (3) (*b*))

258

A regulation of 30 January 1968 (document 4) states with regard to attacks on villages and hamlets:

> The use of incendiary type ammunition will be avoided unless absolutely necessary to successful accomplishment of the mission. (Document 4, paragraph (5) (*d*))

Thus, it is clear that it was considered necessary to introduce special restrictions on the use of incendiary weapons in order to reduce civilian casualties.[2] It is also of interest to note that white phosphorus was included as an incendiary weapon.[3]

The General Rules refer to no other categories of specific weapons with the exception of 'riot control' agents (which were permitted for use; see below).

Chemical munitions

The General Rules provided in document 1 state that

> Riot control agents will be used to the maximum extent possible. CS agents can be effectively employed in inhabited and urban area operations to flush enemy personnel from buildings and fortified positions, thus increasing the enemy's vulnerability to allied firepower while reducing the unnecessary danger to civilians and the likelihood of destruction of civilian property. (Paragraph 6 (*d*) (2))

Clearly US practice on this point differed from that regarded as acceptable by most members of the international community. Nevertheless, while mention is made of 'increasing the vulnerability' of the enemy, reference is also made to reducing civilian casualties or destruction.

Small arms

A regulation of 30 January 1968 states with regard to the employment of individual and crew-served small arms and automatic weapons (including the M-16 rifle, the M-60 machine-gun, the M-79 grenade launcher, the M18A1 Claymore anti-personnel mine, the M-26 grenade, the .50 calibre machine-gun, and the 90 mm and 106 mm recoilless rifles) that they may be used against:

> (1) Enemy personnel observed with weapons who demonstrate hostile intent either by taking a friendly unit under fire, taking evasive action, or who occupy a firing position or bunker.
> (2) Targets which are observed and positively identified as enemy.
> (3) Point targets from which fire is being received. (This will not be construed as permission for indiscriminate firing into areas inhabited by non-combatants.) (Paragraph 4*a*.)

A change was introduced into the wording on 9 February 1968 (document 6) where paragraph (2) (above) was superseded by the following:

> (2) Commanders will exercise utmost care to insure minimum non-combatant casualties and property damage.

The regulations of 16 March 1968 (document 3) state:

> Conduct of fire. (*a*) Individual and crew served weapons: (1) Pistols, rifles, grenade launchers, hand grenades, claymores, machine guns, and recoilless rifles *may be employed by* commanders under the conditions indicated below:
> (*a*) Against targets that are *observed and positively identified as enemy.*
> (*b*) Against point targets from which fire is being received. (*Indiscriminate fire into populated areas is prohibited.*)
> (*c*) *Against suspected enemy locations when non-combatants would not be endangered.*
> (2) Personnel positively identified as enemy who demonstrate an intent to surrender should not be engaged by fire. (Paragraph 5 (*c*); original italics)

Surface weapons

Surface weapons include artillery, mortars, tank guns, and guns fired from river patrol boats. The US Rules include separate regulations for naval artillery fired at shore-based targets.

The Rules for surface weapons are complex and to a large degree reflect specific conditions of the Viet Nam War. For example, different rules applied according to whether the target was located within a 'special strike zone' (SSZ; previously referred to as a 'free fire zone'); within an uninhabited area outside an SSZ; within an inhabited area, defined as including 'any group of dwellings as well as established hamlets and villages that do not qualify as an urban area' (document 1, paragraph 5 (*e*)); or within an urban area. Few restrictions applied to the use of munitions in SSZs, other than a requirement to notify an appropriate 'clearance authority'. Attacks against targets in urban areas, on the other hand, were subject to a number of restrictions.

A distinction is made between 'unobserved fires' and 'observed fires'. Observed fires, in turn, may be of two kinds: they may be observed by the gunner (direct fire) or by a forward observer (observed indirect fire). A forward observer may be situated on the ground or in an overflying aircraft and in each case must be in communication with the gunner in order to report on the accuracy of the fire. In general, unobserved fire is the more indiscriminate, and direct (observed) fire the more discriminate.

Of particular interest are the 'safety ranges' specified for particular weapons to be used against targets in inhabited areas. Document 4 of 1968 states:

> (*e*) Following criteria will be used against known or suspected enemy targets in areas occupied by non-combatants:

105 mm fires – no closer than 500 meters plus 4 range PEs (prob errors)[4]
155 mm fires – no closer than 800 meters plus 4 range PEs (prob errors)
8″ & 175 mm fires – no closer than 1 000 meters plus 4 range PEs (prob errors).

(*f*) Fires will be placed no closer than 200 meters of any main paved road. When targets are located on or near a road VT[5] fuze will be used to the maximum extent possible.

Document 5 adds an additional restriction in the case of unobserved fire:

Unobserved fires will not be fired closer than 1 000 meters to non-combatant or friendly troop locations when engaging known or suspected targets. (Paragraph 4*b* (5) (*e*))

Document 4 states, as do several others, that:

Villages and hamlets ... will not be fired upon without prior warning by leaflet and/or loudspeaker systems or by other means, even though fire is received from them. (Paragraph 4*b* (5) (*b*))

However, this paragraph is followed by another which significantly modifies its effect:

(*c*) Villages and hamlets may be attacked without prior warning if the attack is in conjunction with a ground operation involving maneuver of ground forces through the area, and if in the judgement of the ground commander, his mission would be jeopardized by such warning as specified in (*b*) above.

Air-delivered weapons

Similar restrictions were applied to air attacks by fixed-wing and rotary aircraft. Thus document 1, annex 2, states, for example:

Air attacks directed against urban areas must always be controlled by FAC ....[6]
Prior to subjecting urban area to an air attack, even when fire is being received from the area, the inhabitants must be warned by leaflets, loudspeakers, or other appropriate means prior to the attack and given sufficient time to evacuate the area. (Paragraph 2 (*i*) (3))

However, two important exceptions were made to this policy:

If the attack on an inhabited area from which enemy fire is being received is deemed necessary, and is executed in conjunction with a ground operation involving the movement of ground forces through the area, and if in the judgement of the battalion or higher commander his mission would be jeopardized by prior warning, the attack may be made without such warning or delay. (Paragraph 2 (*h*) (1))

Further,

An exception may be made for herbicide missions in cases where prior warning may jeopardize the safety of the spray aircraft. (Paragraph 2 (*h*) (2))

Additional rules for armed helicopters operated in urban areas state:

Further, only point targets, e.g. specific buildings, will be engaged and these targets must be positively identified to the pilot. The engagement of area targets in urban areas is prohibited. (Document 1, annex 3, paragraph 3 (*c*))

In document 2, 7th Air Force Operations Order 71–17 (Rules of Engagement), states with regard to 'Barrel Roll East'[7] operations in Laos:

Strikes may be conducted within 500 meters of an active village or non-combatants only when ground fire is being received from the location or when in close air support of friendly troops . . . .
No all weather strikes (except LORAN[8]) will be conducted within 3 000 meters of a known village or friendly position.
No LORAN strikes will be made closer than 1 000 meters to a known village or friendly position.

Regarding areas of cultural value in Cambodia, the same document states:

Except during SAR[9] operations, no US air strikes will be made within 1 000 meters of any of the areas of cultural value (nearly 100 other [in addition to Angkor Wat] sites specifically listed in the directive).

Naval gun-fire against land targets

Analogous rules were applied to the use of naval guns against land targets. Few restrictions were placed on such use in uninhabited areas or areas defined as 'special strike zones'. Conversely, fire in inhabited or urban areas required permission by a senior commander, control by an observer, and a warning to the population unless the fire was called for to support an ongoing ground operation.

IV. Criticisms of the US Rules of Engagement

The Rules of Engagement were provided to Senator Goldwater by the Secretary for Defense and entered into the *Congressional Record* by the Senator. In doing so, the Senator said he wished to draw the attention of the Congress, the press and the public to the restrictions placed upon US forces. In his words:

> It is absolutely unbelievable that any Secretary of Defense would ever place such restrictions on our forces. It is unbelievable that any President would have allowed this to happen . . . .
>
> I am ashamed of my country for having had people who would have allowed such restrictions to have been placed upon men who are trained to fight, men who were trained to make decisions to win war, and men who were risking their lives. I dare say that these restrictions had as much to do with our casualties as the enemy themselves . . . .
>
> I pray, Mr. President, that if we ever have to go to war again – and I pray that we never will – that such foolish restrictions never be formed again and applied to our troops. (Senator Goldwater, *Congressional Record*, 6 June 1975, pp. S 9904–905)

Senator Goldwater's action and reasoning were commended by Senator Thurmond, who stated that, as a member of the Senate Armed Services Committee, he had known about the Rules earlier and protested about them to the President. In his view, if the US public had known about the Rules, they would not have approved of them: 'They would not approve of sending their men into battle with their hands tied behind their backs to fight that way, to make gun fodder, so to speak, out of them' (Senator Thurmond, *Congressional Record,* 6 June 1975, p. S 9905).

While these critics argued that the Rules handicapped US forces and thereby contributed to combat losses, others have argued that the rules did not succeed in offering sufficient protection to the civilian populations of the countries of Indo-China.

An interesting account of the operation of the rules of Laos (which were apparently similar in many respect to those applied in Viet Nam) was written by two staff members of the US Senate Foreign Relations Committee. A 'sanitized' (i.e., censored) version of their report was published by the Committee (1971).

According to this report, the Rules 'seem to make it impossible for villages or other nonmilitary targets to be bombed . . . . Given the apparent stringency of these rules of engagement, it is difficult to see how roads with civilian traffic, villages and groups of civilians could have been bombed, rocketed, or napalmed . . . .' (pp. 10–11). Nevertheless, the report goes on: 'There are plenty of instances known to American civilian employees who have been in Laos for some years in which civilian targets have been bombed' (ibid.).

The report then indicates several reasons for this discrepancy which may be summarized by the following excerpts from it:

(*a*) mistakes do happen (especially when Forward Air Controllers begin flying missions as soon as they arrive in Laos);

(*b*) some pilots have deliberately violated the rules of engagement expending ordnance against unauthorized targets (the town of Khang Khay being a notable example);

(*c*) the effort to provide in the rules of engagement for every contingency appears to create obvious loopholes;

(*d*) the system itself is so complicated that it cannot possibly be foolproof.

(*e*) The Royal Lao Air Force is not bound by the same rules of engagement and is theoretically free to do what it wishes .... Lao Air Force Pilots .... are paid a bonus for each sortie so that there is an incentive not to adhere too strictly to rules of engagement.[10]

V. *Comments on the criticisms*

Criticisms of the second kind appear more credible than those of the first kind, which appear to derive partly from a lack of understanding of the type of warfare involved and partly from a lack of study of what the Rules actually state – not to speak of the lack of respect for international law.

The US Rules themselves state their own justification, not in terms of obligations derived from international law, but in terms of winning the war. Thus, document 3 states:

> The use of unnecessary force resulting in non-combatant casualties and property loss will embitter the population and make the long term goal of pacification more difficult and costly.
>
> *b.* The VC/NVA[11] exploit incidents of non-combatant casualties and destruction of property ... to foster resentment and to alienate the people against the Government.
>
> *c.* The circumstances of the conflict call for restraint not normally required of soldiers on the battlefield. (Paragraph 4)

Nevertheless, in spite of this reasoning, the US Rules were not prohibitions but restrictions, which in no case prevented the commander using a particular munition, for example napalm, if it were judged necessary for the accomplishment of his mission, or if not using it would jeopardize the success of his mission. Similarly, precautions, such as warning the civilian population of impending attack, were only obligatory where they could be carried out without jeopardizing the success of the operation. For example, document 3 states:

> *f.* Nothing shall infringe on the inherent right of a commander to exercise self-defense. The commander may take immediate action

against an attacking force with all means available; however, every possible safeguard short of endangering life will be used to avoid non-combatant casualties and the destruction of private property. Firepower will be brought to bear on enemy in populated areas only to the extent necessary to accomplish an assigned mission. (Paragraph 4)

It is difficult to see that rules of this kind reduce the freedom of action of the military commander so long as the actions of the troops under his command are restricted to accomplishing a specific mission as economically and effectively as possible. Unnecessary civilian casualties and property damage do not contribute to winning a war – indeed, as pointed out in the rules, they may make such a goal more difficult to achieve.

Criticisms of the second kind are of more interest to the international lawyer. For, on the one hand, the lawyer prefers to codify rules in such a way that they are both comprehensive and susceptible to only a single interpretation. On the other hand, the complexity which characterizes most legal documents makes them difficult for the non-lawyer – such as the military commander in the field – to interpret and apply. The question arises, Is it possible to draw up rules which are adequate to the task of protecting the civilian population, comprehensive enough to apply to all conceivable situations (without providing loopholes), and yet specific enough to be applied by field commanders in a tactical situation?

It is not possible within the framework of this short commentary to evaluate the extent to which the US Rules meet such criteria. Whatever their success in this respect, there can be little doubt that they do represent a rather ambitious attempt to go beyond the general formulations of the Hague Regulations and the Geneva Conventions and to draw up more specific rules applicable in a field situation.

VI. The US Rules and the modernization of the law of armed conflict

The very fact that it was deemed necessary to draw up such additional regulations suggests in the strongest possible way that, in the opinion of the military authorities of a State with perhaps the most extensive experience of military operations in the post-World War II period, the existing Hague and Geneva Conventions are not adequate to the task of protecting the civilian population. This raises the question of whether the approach adopted in the US Rules is one which could be applied in international law.

Clearly, there can be no question of making use of the entire body of the US Rules in an international document. Indeed, many aspects would be entirely inappropriate, both because of the specific circumstances of the war in Indo-China, and because of the nature of the US involvement in that war.

Nevertheless, there are many interesting sides to the US Rules which do merit consideration in the international context. Of particular interest are the rules with respect to 'blast and fragmentation weapons'. This category makes up the bulk of conventional weapons and causes about 70 per cent of battlefield casualties and probably at least as many civilian casualties. Yet it is the category which has so far been treated in the least satisfactory manner by the Conferences of Government Experts (ICRC, 1975; 1976).

The reason for the cursory treatment given to these weapons by the government experts is no doubt that, these weapons being the most commonly used conventional weapons, there is no question (at present) of their general prohibition. But, so far, hardly any attempt has been made to examine restrictions of specific weapons.[12]

But this is precisely what the US Rules have, to some extent, attempted. They make use of two simple principles, derived from extensive military practice, which could well be made use of in an international document. These principles may be summarized as follows:

1. In attacks against military objects in inhabited and urban areas the target must be specifically identified and fire against it aimed from direct-fire weapons or controlled by a forward observer on the ground or in the air.

2. In planning an attack, account should be taken, in order to ensure the safety of the civilian population, of the danger zone – ranging from 500 to 3000 m, depending on the weapon system – around the point at which conventional aircraft bombs or artillery shells are aimed.

VII. Conclusion

Although the general applicability of the US Rules of Engagement is limited in various respects, they are well worth study by international lawyers. In particular they point to one way in which the state of international law with regard to the use of conventional blast and fragmentation weapons might be improved, namely, by emphasizing the use of observed-fire and direct-fire weapons, and by taking account of the danger zone resulting from the dispersion and casualty radius of specific munitions.

Notes to Appendix 9D

1. It is beyond the scope of this appendix to enquire whether national practice consistently followed such a policy.
2. These rules were introduced at a time when there was considerable public concern about civilian casualties resulting from the use of napalm and phosphorus. After 1968 there appears to have been a reduction in civilian napalm casualties (see SIPRI, 1975a).
3. Some military experts would claim that white phosphorus munitions are primarily smoke munitions and are therefore not covered by the definition of incendiary munitions drawn up by the working group of the Conference of Government Experts

at Lugano in 1974 (ICRC, 1975) and which forms the basis for the prohibition proposed by nearly 20 States at the Second Session of the Diplomatic Conference on Humanitarian Law (Conference document CCDH/IV/201).

4. The 'probable error' refers to the radius of a circle within which 50 per cent of the projectiles can be expected to fall at a given range. In the case of a 105 mm shell fired at a range of 10 000 m it is about 100 m. The probable error is thus approximately 1 per cent of the range. The addition of four range PEs may increase the safety zone by as much as 80 per cent: in the case of 105 mm shells fired at 10 000 m, from 500 to 900 m; or for 155 mm shells fired at 15 000 m, from 800 to 1 400 m.

5. VT = a proximity fuze which causes the projectile to explode before hitting the ground, thereby increasing effectiveness against personnel and light matériel but avoiding craters.

6. FAC = 'forward air controller'.

7. 'Barrel Roll' denoted armed reconnaissance operations against infiltration routes in Laos.

8. LORAN = 'Long Range Navigation', an electronic navigation system employing radio beacons on the ground.

9. SAR = 'search and rescue'.

10. A later document confirmed this practice of paying a bonus per sortie and identifies the CIA as the source of money; following the cease-fire agreements, the pilots were faced with a serious loss of income, but after some negotiation the CIA agreed to pay them for *not* flying the sorties (US Senate Foreign Relations Committee, 1973).

11. VC = 'Viet Cong', US jargon for the Peoples Liberation Armed Forces; NVA = 'North Vietnamese Army', US term for regular forces of the PLAF originating in the Democratic Republic of Viet Nam (North Viet Nam).

12. Commission III of the Diplomatic Conference on International Humanitarian Law made significant progress at its Second Session in 1975 in restricting attacks against certain kinds of target, including cities, dams, crops and nuclear power stations. At the second session of the Conference of Government Experts on Certain Conventional Weapons, held in Lugano in 1976, some progress was achieved on the question of mines and booby traps.

Bibliography and references

Aebi, F., Brönnimann, E. & Mayor, J., 1977, Some observations on the behaviour of small caliber projectiles in soap targets. *Acta Chirurgica Scandinavica,* Supplement 477, pp. 49–57.

Ahearn, A. M., 1966, Viet Cong medicine. *Military Medicine* **131** (3), pp. 219–221.

Allen, H. R., 1972, *The Legacy of Lord Trenchard.* Cassell, London.

Allen, W. G. B., 1951, Automatic rifles. *Army Quarterly* (UK) **63** (1), pp. 50–54.

Amato, J. J , Billy, L. J., Gruber, R. P. *et al.,* 1970, Vascular injuries. An experimental study of high and low velocity missile wounds. *Archives of Surgery* **101**, pp. 167 ff.

Amato, J. J., Rich, N. M., Billy, L. J. *et al.,* 1971, High velocity arterial injury. A study of the mechanism of injury. *Journal of Trauma* **11,** pp. 412 ff.

Amnesty International, 1971, *Report of an Inquiry into Allegations of Ill-treatment in Northern Ireland.* London.

Applegate, R., 1969, Riot control 1969. *Ordnance* (September–October), pp. 180–184.

Applegate, R., 1971, Nonlethal police weapons. *Ordnance* (July–August), pp. 62–66.

Archer, D. H. R. (ed.), 1976, *Jane's Infantry Weapons 1976.* Macdonald & Jane's, London.

Artz, C. P., Bronwell, A. W. & Sako, Y., 1955, Experiences in the management of abdominal and thoraco-abdominal injuries in Korea. *American Journal of Surgery* **89,** pp. 773 ff.

Austria, Sweden & Switzerland, experts of, 1977, *Terminal Ballistics and Wounding Effects of Small Calibre Projectiles.* Joint paper presented at the fourth session of the Diplomatic Conference on International Humanitarian Law Applicable in Armed Conflicts, Geneva.

Baldwin, H. W., 1967, Laser and a silent plane tested for Army of future. *New York Times* (17 October).

Baldwin, H. W., 1973, The strategy of the old bombers. *New York Times* (19 January).

Barnes, F. C., 1965, *Cartridges of the World.* Follett, Chicago.

Bartleson, C. J., 1968, Retinal burns from intense light sources. *American Industrial Hygiene Association Journal* **29** (1), pp. 415–424.

Batchelor, J. & Hogg, I., 1972, *Artillery.* Scribner, New York.

Baxter, R. R., 1973, Criteria of prohibition of weapons in international law. *Festschrift für Ulrich Scheunes,* Berlin, p. 50.

Beebe, G. W. & DeBakey, M. E., 1952, *Battle Casualties, Incidence, Mortality and Logistic Considerations.* Thomas, Springfield, Illinois.

Beer, A., 1975, Überlegungen zu einer Einheits-Handfeuerwaffe. *Truppendienst* (2), pp. 115–119.

Beller, W. S., 1968, *The American Arsenal.* Putnam, New York.

Beller, W. S., 1969, *Arsenal for the Brave: A History of the US Army Munitions Command, 1962–1968.* Washington, DC.

Ben-Hur, N. & Soroff, H., 1975, Combat burns in the 1973 October war and the anti-tank missile burn syndrome. *Burns* **1,** pp. 217–221.

Benner, R. L., 1968, *Recent Advances in High Fragmenting Steels.* Technical report 3833. US Army Picatinny Arsenal, Dover, New Jersey.

Benzinger, T., 1950, Physiological effects of blast in air and water. In *German Aviation Medicine in World War II,* vol. 2, chapter 14-B. Surgeon General, US Air Force, US Government Printing Office, Washington, DC.

Berlin, R. H., 1977, Energy transfers and regional blood flow changes following missile trauma. (To be published.)

Berlin, R., Gelin, L. E., Janzon, B., Lewis, D. H., Rybeck, B., Sandegård, J. & Seeman, T., 1976, Local effects of assault rifle bullets in live tissues. *Acta Chirurgica Scandinavica,* Supplement 459.

Berlin, R., Janzon, B., Rybeck, B., Sandegård, J. & Seeman, T., 1977, Local Effects of assault rifle bullets in live tissues. Part 2: Further studies in live tissues and relations to some simulant media. *Acta Chirurgica Scandinavica,* Supplement 477, pp. 1–48.

Berndt, 1897, *Die Zahl im Kriege. Statistische Zahlen aus der neueren Kriegsgeschichte im Kriege.* Vienna.

Beyer, H. G., 1898–1899, Observations on the effects produced by the 6-mm. rifle and projectile. An experimental study. *Journal of the Boston Society of Medical Sciences* **3** (January), pp. 117–136.

Beyer, J. C. (ed.), 1962, *Wound Ballistics.* Office of the Surgeon General, Department of the Army, Washington, DC.

Biles, R. E., 1972, *Bombing as a Policy Tool in Vietnam: Effectiveness.* A staff study based on the Pentagon Papers, prepared for the use of the Committee on Foreign Relations, United States Senate. US Government Printing Office, Washington, DC.

Billroth, T., 1859, *Historische Studien über die Beurteilung und Behandlung der Schusswunden.* Reimer, Berlin.

Bircher, H., 1899, *Die Wirkung der Artilleriegeschosse.* Sauerlander, Aarau (Switzerland).

Black, A. N., Burns, B. D. & Zuckerman, S., 1941, An experimental study of the wounding mechanism of high velocity missiles. *British Medical Journal* **2,** pp. 872–874.

Blix, H., 1974, Current efforts to prohibit the use of certain conventional weapons. *Instant Research on Peace and Violence* (Tampere Peace Research Institute, Finland) **4** (1), pp. 21–30.

Bloch, I. S., 1899, *The Future of War in its Technical, Economic and Political Relations,* translated and abridged edition. London, 1899; Boston, 1902; republished by Garland Publishing, Inc., 1971.

Blomqvist, G., 1976, Fuel air explosives. *Arménytt* (Sweden) (4), pp. 20–23.

Bluntschli, J. C., 1874, *Das Moderne Kriegsrecht der zivilisierten Staaten,* 2nd edition. Beckschen, Nördlingen (Germany).

Bordwell, P., 1908, *The Law of War between Belligerents.* Chicago.

Born, G., 1976, Laserwaffen – sind sie realisierbar? *Wehrtechnik* (7), pp. 22–25.

Born, M., 1964, What is left to hope for? *Bulletin of the Atomic Scientists* (April), pp. 2–5.

Boys, C. V., 1893, On electric spark photographs; or photography of flying bullets, etc., by the lights of the electric spark. *Nature* **47,** pp. 415–421, 440–446.

Braxton Hicks, H., 1900, The use of explosive bullets by the Boers. *British Medical Journal* **1,** p. 1313.

Breitenecker, R., 1969. Shotgun wound patterns. *American Journal of Clinical Pathology* **52** (September), pp. 258–269.

Brendt, W., 1967, Danger: Booby traps. *Infantry* (May–June), pp. 42–43.

De Breucker, J., 1974, La déclaration de Bruxelles de 1874 concernant les lois et coutumes de la guerre. *Chronique de Politique étrangère* **27** (1), pp. 3–87.

Brüel, P. V. & Olesen, H. P., 1973, Infrasonic measurements. *B. K. Technical Review* **3,** pp. 14–25.

Bruns, P. von, 1889, *Die Geschosseinwirkung der neuen Kleinkaliber-Gewehre. Ein Beitrag zur Beurteilung der Schusswunden in künftigen Kriegen.* Lauppschen, Tübingen.

Bruns, P. von, 1898, Inhumane Kriegsgeschosse. *Archiv für klinische Chirurgie* **57,** pp. 602–607.

Bruns, P. von, 1899, *Über die Wirkung der neuesten englischen Armeegeschosse.* Tübingen.

Bruns, P. von, 1915, Die Dumdumgeschosse und ihre Wirkung. *Bruns Beiträge zur klinischen Chirurgie* **96,** p. 7.

Brussels Conference on the Rules of Military Warfare (1874). Command No. 1. (1875) C.1128. HMSO, London.

Busk, H., 1860, *The Rifle and How to Use it.*

Byrnes, D. P., Crockard, H. A., Gordon, D. S. & Gleadhill, C. A., 1974, Penetrating craniocerebral missile injuries in the civil disturbances in Northern Ireland. *British Journal of Surgery* **61** (3), pp. 169–176.

Callender, G. R. & French, R. W., 1935, Wound ballistics. Studies in the mechanism of wound production by rifle bullets. *The Military Surgeon* **77** (4), pp. 177–201.

Cassese, A., 1975, Weapons causing unnecessary suffering: Are they prohibited? *Rivisto di Diritto Internazionale* **58,** pp. 12–42.

Chapelier, G. & Van Malderghem, J., 1971, Plain of Jars. Social changes under five years of Pathet Lao administration. *Asia Quarterly* (1).

Charters, A. C. & Charters, A. C., 1976, Wounding mechanism of very high velocity projectiles. *Journal of Trauma* **16** (6), pp. 464–470.

Chase, M., 1973, Long range planning for 40 mm ammunition. Mortar Ammunition Manufacturers Conference, 28–29 March, vol. 2. US Army Munitions Command, Dover, New Jersey.

CINCPAC (US Commander in Chief Pacific), 1971, *Proceedings of CINCPAC Fifth Conference on War Surgery,* 29 March–2 April. Tokyo.

Clague, T. E., 1972, Dust explosion mechanisms. *Birmingham University Chemical Engineer* **23** (2), pp. 45–50.

Clemedson, C.-J., 1949, An experimental study of air blast injuries. *Acta Physiologica Scandinavica* **18,** Supplement 61.

Clemedson, C.-J., 1966, Detonationsskador. *Försvars- och Katastrofmedicin,* chapter 24. Stockholm.

Clemedson, C.-J., Frankenberg, L., Jönsson, A., Petterson, J. & Sundqvist, A.-B., 1969, Dynamic response of thorax and abdomen of rabbits in partial and whole body blast exposure. *American Journal of Physiology* **216** (3), pp. 615–620.

Clemedson, C.-J., Falconer, B., Frankenberg, K., Jansson. A. & Wennerstrand, J., 1973, Head injuries caused by small calibre, high velocity bullets. An experimental study. *Zeitschrift für Rechtmedizin* **73,** pp. 103–114.

Clowes, W., 1588, *A prooved practice for all young Chirurgeons.* Cadman, London.

Coates, J. F., 1972, Non-lethal police weapons. *Technology Review* **74** (7), pp. 49–56.

Coates, K., Limqueco, P. & Weiss, P. (eds.), 1971, *Prevent the Crime of Silence.* Reports from the sessions of the International War Crimes Tribunal founded by Bertrand Russell. Allen Lane, The Penguin Press, London.

Cohen, —., 1967, *A "flash bulb" approach to some Vietnam defense problems.* RM-5293-PR, RAND Corporation, Santa Monica, California.

Collins, J. A., Gordon, W. C., Hudson, T. L., Irvin, R. W., Kelly, T. & Hardaway, R. M.,

1968, Inapparent hypoxemia in casualties with wounded limbs: Pulmonary fat embolism? *Annals of Surgery* **167** (4), pp. 511–520.

Compton, E. (ed.), 1971, *Report of the enquiry into allegations against the security forces of physical brutality in Northern Ireland arising out of events on the 9th August, 1971*. UK Home Office, HMSO, London.

Copes, W., 1976, *A comparison of the "effectiveness" of air delivered napalm and high explosives when used in the close air support role*. Statement on behalf of US Delegation at the Conference of Government Experts on the Use of Certain Conventional Weapons, Lugano, 28 January–26 February 1976.

Council on Economic Priorities, 1970, *Efficiency in Death: The Manufacturers of Anti-Personnel Weapons*. Harper & Row, Perennial, New York.

Cranz, C. & Becker, K., 1921, *Handbook of Ballistics* (translated from German), 2nd ed. HMSO, London.

Crevecoeur, P., 1973, Anti-personnel hand grenades: Some recent European developments. *International Defense Review* **6** (3), pp. 372–374.

Crossman, E. C., 1915, Dum-dum bullets. *Scientific American* (17 April).

Crossman, J., 1966, Grenades, now and then. *Ordnance* (July–August).

Curreri, P. W., Asch, M. J. & Pruitt, B. A., Jr., 1970, The treatment of chemical burns: Specialized diagnostic, therapeutic and prognostic considerations. *Journal of Trauma* **10** (8), pp. 634–642.

Davis, D. M., 1973, Airborne guns and rockets. *Ordnance* (March–April), pp. 388–391.

Deane-Drummond, A., 1975, *Riot Control*. Royal United Services Institute for Defence Studies, London.

DeBakey, M. E. (ed.), 1955, *General Surgery, Surgery in World War II*, vol. 2. Medical Department, United States Army, Office of the Surgeon General, Department of the Army, Washington, DC.

Dedijer, V. (ed.), 1967, *Tribunal Russell: Le Jugement de Stockholm*. Gallimard, Paris.

Dellinger, D., 1966, North Vietnam: Eyewitness report. *Liberation* (December), pp. 7–8.

Delorme, E. & Chavasse, P., 1892, Etude comparative des effets produits par les balles de fusil gros de 11 mm. et du fusil Lebel de 8 mm. *Archives de médicine et pharmacologie militaires* **17,** pp. 81–112.

De Muth, W. E., 1966, Bullet velocity and design as determinants of wounding capability. *Journal of Trauma* **6** (2), pp. 222–232.

De Muth, W. E., 1969, Bullet velocity as applied to military rifle wounding capacity. *Journal of Trauma* **9** (1) pp. 27–38.

De Muth, W. E. & Smith, J. M., 1966, High velocity bullet wounds of muscle and bone. The basis of rational early treatment. *Journal of Trauma* **6** (6), pp. 744–755.

Dennis, J. A., 1975, MEROC demonstrates fuel/air explosive use neutralization capabilities. *Army Research and Development News Magazine* (US) **16** (1), pp. 12–13.

Dennis, J. A., 1976, SLUFAE: Long-range minefield breaching system tested. *Army Research and Development News Magazine* (US) (May–June), pp. 14–15.

Dent, C. T., 1900, Small-bore rifle bullet wounds and the "humanity" of the present war. *British Medical Journal* (19 May), pp. 1209–1213.

Derry, T. K. & Williams, T. I., 1960, *A Short History of Technology: From the Earliest Times to A.D. 1900*. The Clarendon Press, Oxford.

Desaga, H., 1950a, Blast injuries. In *German Aviation Medicine in World War II*, vol. 2, chapter 14-D. Surgeon General, US Air Force, US Government Printing Office, Washington, DC.

Desaga, H., 1950b, Experimental investigations of the action of dust. In *German Aviation*

Medicine in World War II, vol. 2, chapter 13-B. Surgeon General, US Air Force, US Government Printing Office, Washington, DC.

Diffenbaugh, W. G., 1965, Military surgery in the Civil War. *Military Medicine* (May), pp. 490–496.

Dimond, F. C. & Rich, N. M., 1967, M-16 rifle wounds in Vietnam. *Journal of Trauma* **7** (5), pp. 619–625.

Divine, D., 1966, *The Broken Wing: A Study in the British Exercise of Air Power.* Hutchinson, London.

Dobbyn, R. C., Bruchey, W. J. & Shubin, L. D., 1975, *An evaluation of police handgun ammunition: Summary report.* LESP-RPT-0101.01. (mimeographed). Law Enforcement Standards Program, National Institute of Law Enforcement and Criminal Justice, US Department of Justice.

Dodd, N. L., 1973, New British weapons. *National Defense* (September–October), pp. 92, 94, 98.

Dudley, H. A., Knight, R. J., McNeur, J. C. & Rosengarten, D. S., 1968, Civilian battle casualties in South Vietnam. *British Journal of Surgery* **55** (5), pp. 332–334.

Duffet, J. (ed.), 1968, *Against the Crime of Silence.* Proceedings of the Russell International War Crimes Tribunal. Bertrand Russell Peace Foundation and O'Hare Books, New York & London.

Dunant, H., 1862, *A Memory of Solferino.* Translated and published by the American National Red Cross, Washington, DC., 1959.

Dunn, D. J. & Sterne, T. E., 1952, *Hand Grenades for Rapid Incapacitation.* BRL R-806. Ballistic Research Laboratories, Aberdeen Proving Ground, Maryland.

Dupuy, R. E. & Dupuy, T. W., 1970, *The Encyclopedia of Military History.* Macdonald & Jane's, London.

Dziemian, A. J., Mendelson, J. A. & Lindsey, D., 1961, Comparison of the wounding characteristics of some commonly encountered bullets. *Journal of Trauma* **1**, pp. 341–353.

Eibl-Eibesfeldt, I., 1975, *Krieg und Frieden aus der Sicht der Verhaltensforschung.* Piper, Munich.

Egner, D. O., Shank, E. B., Wargovich, M. J. & Tiedemann, A. F., 1973, *A Multidisciplinary Technique for the Evaluation of Less Lethal Weapons,* vol. 1. US Army Land Warfare Laboratory, Aberdeen Proving Ground, Maryland.

Egner, D. O. & Williams, L. W., 1975, *Standard Scenarios for the Less Lethal Weapons Evaluation Model.* US Army Human Engineering Laboratory, Aberdeen, Maryland.

Ellis, J., 1976, *The Social History of the Machine Gun.* Pantheon, New York.

Ezell, E. C., 1969, *The Search for a Lightweight Rifle: The M14 and M16 Rifles.* Unpublished doctoral dissertation, Case Western Reserve University, Cleveland, Ohio.

Falk, R. A. (ed.), 1968, *The Vietnam War and International Law,* vol. 1. Princeton University Press, Princeton, New Jersey.

Falk, R., Kolko, G. & Lifton, R. (eds.), 1971, *Crimes of War.* Random House, New York.

Falla, S. T., 1940, Effect of explosion-blast on lungs. *British Medical Journal* **2**, pp. 255–256.

Fauchille, P., 1921, *Traité de Droit international public,* vol. 2. Rousseau, Paris.

Ferretti, F., 1976, Zap! *New York Times Magazine* (4 January), pp. 13–16.

Finck, P. A., 1965, Ballistic and forensic pathologic aspects of missile wounds. Conversion between Anglo-American and Metric-System units. *Military Medicine* **130** (5), pp. 545–569.

Fisher, J. B., 1946, *Incendiary Warfare.* McGraw-Hill, New York.

Fleck, D., 1973, Beiträge zur Weiterentwicklung des humanitären Völkerrecht für bewaffnete Konflikte. *Veröffentlichungen des Instituts für Internationales Recht an der Universität Kiel* **71.**

Foley, C., 1972, Pentagon reveals secrets of US "death-ray" arms. *Observer* (London) (3 September).

Fosbery, G. V., 1869, Explosive bullets and their application to military purposes. *Journal of the Royal United Services Institution* **12,** pp. 15–27.

French, R. W. & Callender, G. R., 1962, Ballistic characteristics of wounding agents. In *Wound Ballistics* (J. C. Beyer, ed.) US Army, Office of the Surgeon General, Washington, DC.

Fried, J. H. E., 1972, The electronic battlefield and the dictates of public conscience. *Revue belge de Droit international,* pp. 431–454.

Fuller, J. F. C., 1932, *War and Western Civilization: 1832–1932. A Study of War as a Political Instrument and Expression of Mass Democracy.* Duckworth, London.

Futrell, R. F., 1961, *The United States Air Force in Korea, 1950–1953.* Duell, Sloan and Pearce, New York.

Ganzoni, N., 1975, *Die Schussververletzung im Krieg.* Huber, Bern.

Garner, J. W., 1920, *International Law and the World War,* vol. 1. Longmans, Green, London.

Gestewitz, H.-R., 1968, Über die Geschädigtenstrukturen, die Organisation der medizinischen Hilfe und den Transport Geschädigter infolge des See–Luftkrieges der Vereinigten Staaten von Nordamerika gegen die Demokratische Republik Vietnam von 1965 bis 1967. *Zeitschrift für Militärmedizin* **9** (5), pp. 259–262.

Gestewitz, H.-R. & Schwarzer, R. (eds.), 1975, *Feldchirurgie.* Militärverlag der DDR, E. Berlin.

Glasstone, S. (ed.), 1962, *The Effects of Nuclear Weapons.* US Government Printing Office, Washington, DC.

Goddard, C., 1935, Stopping power. *The Military Surgeon* **76** (2), pp. 57–71.

Gorman, J. F., 1969, Combat arterial trauma. Analysis of 106 limb-threatening injuries. *Archives of Surgery* **98** (February), pp. 160–164.

Grant, U.S., 1885, *Personal Memoirs.* New York.

Gravel, M., 1971, *The Pentagon Papers. Senator Gravel Edition.* Beacon Press, Boston.

Graves, W., 1975, New life for the troubled Suez Canal. *National Geographic Magazine* **147** (6), pp. 792–817.

Green, C. McL., Thomson, H. C. & Roots, P. C., 1955, *Planning Munitions for War. United States Army in World War II.* Technical Services, Department of the Army, Washington, DC.

Greenway, H. D. S., 1977, Israel links U.S. arms to its survival. *International Herald Tribune* (15 February).

Guide to Viet Cong Ammunition, 1971. Normount Technical Publications, Forest Grove, Oregon.

Gurney, R. W., 1944, *A New Casualty Criterion.* Report No. 498. Ballistic Research Laboratories, Aberdeen Proving Ground, Maryland.

Guthrie, G. J., 1815, *On Gunshot Wounds of the Extremities.* Longman, London.

Hadfield, G., 1941, Problems of blast injuries. *Lancet* **1,** pp. 110–111.

Hadfield, G., Ross, J. M., Swain, R. H. A. & Djury-White, J. M., 1940, Blast from high explosive. *Lancet* **2,** pp. 478–481.

Hammon, W. M., 1971, Analysis of 2187 consecutive wounds of the brain from Vietnam. *Journal of Neurosurgery* **34** (February), pp. 127–131.

Händel, S. & Jansson, P., 1974, Infraljudet – förekomst och verkningar. *Läkartidning* (Sweden) **71** (16), pp. 1635–1639.

Hardaway, R. M., 1969, Clinical management of shock. *Military Medicine* **134** (9), pp. 643–654.

Harrison, E. A., 1973, *Biological Effects of Microwaves. A Bibliography with Abstracts.* Com-73-11720. National Technical Information Service, Springfield, Virginia.

Hartmann, F. von, 1876, *Kritische Versuche.* Baetel, Berlin.

Harvey, E. N., Knorr, I. M., Oster, G. & McMillen, J. H., 1947, Secondary damage in wounding due to pressure changes accompanying the passage of high velocity missiles. *Surgery* **21**, pp. 218–239.

Harvey, E. N., McMillen, J. H., Butler, E. G. & Puckett, W. O., 1962, Mechanism of wounding. In *Wound Ballistics* (J. C. Beyer, ed.). Office of the Surgeon General, Department of the Army, Washington, DC.

Harvey, F., 1967, *Air War, Vietnam.* Bantam, New York.

Harvey, W. J., 1972, Picatinny Arsenal claims amazing destructive power for grenade designed for individual soldier to serve numerous combat needs. *Army Research and Development News Magazine* (US) (August), pp. 16–17.

Havelock, H. M., 1867, *Three Main Military Questions of the Day.* London.

Hayward, J. F., 1955, *European Firearms.* HMSO, London.

Heiney, O. K., 1973, Advanced gun propellants. *National Defense* (September–October), pp. 152–157.

Henderson, H., 1974, RAF bombs in Ethiopia. Letter to the *Sunday Times* (London) (10 February).

Henderson, N. P., 1943, German explosive bullets. *British Medical Journal* **1,** pp. 170–171.

Hinde, R. A., 1966, *Animal Behavior.* McGraw-Hill, New York.

Hirshman, S., 1973, Long range planning for 60 mm, 81 mm & 4.2 inch mortar shell parts. Mortar Ammunition Manufacturers Conference, 28–29 March, vol. 1. US Army Munitions Command, Dover, New Jersey.

Hitchman, N. A., 1952, *Operational Requirements for an Infantry Hand Weapon.* Technical Memorandum ORO-T-160. Project Balance, Operations Research Office, Johns Hopkins University, Maryland.

Hobart, F. W. A., 1971*a,* The next NATO rifle. *International Defense Review* **4** (1), pp. 67–70.

Hobart, F. W. A., 1971*b,* The Armalite AR-18 rifle, A trials report. *International Defense Review* **4** (3), pp. 274–275.

Hobart, F. W. A., 1972, The infantry light machine gun – 7.62 or 5.56? *International Defense Review* **5** (2), pp. 261–264.

Hobart, F. W. A., 1973*a,* Fin stabilization or spin? *Ordnance* **5** (7), pp. 313–315.

Hobart, F. W. A., 1973*b,* Postwar Czech small arms. *Ordnance* **5** (8), pp. 350–353.

Hobart, F. W. A., 1973*c,* The Imp – A weapon for the 80s? *International Defense Review* **6** (4), pp. 505–506.

Hobart, F. W. A. (ed.), 1974, *Jane's Infantry Weapons 1975.* Macdonald & Jane's London.

Hobart, F. W. A., 1975*a,* Letter to the editor. *International Defense Review* **8** (1).

Hobart, F. W. A., 1975*b,* Russian small arms and machine guns. *International Defense Review* **8** (1), pp. 48–53.

Hobart, F. W. A., 1975*c,* The HK 36 assault rifle. *National Defense* (January–February), pp. 276–277.

Hobart, F. W. A., 1975*d,* Sterling submachine guns. *National Defense* (March–April), pp. 356–357.

Hoff, A. von, 1969, *Feuerwaffen,* 2 vols. Klinkhardt & Biermann, Brunswick (FR Germany).

Hogg, I. V. & Batchelor, J., 1976, *The Machine Gun*. Purnell's History of the World Wars (Special). BPC, London.

Hogg, O. F. G., 1970, *Artillery: Its Origin, Heyday and Decline*. Hurst, London.

Holland, T. E., 1908, *The Laws of War on Land*. Clarendon Press, Oxford.

Hood, R. A. & Kyriakides, K., 1971, Some subjective effects of infrasound. British Acoustical Society Meeting, *Infrasound and Low Frequency Vibrations*, Salford University, 26 November 1971, pp. 71–107.

Hoopes, T., 1969, *The Limits of Intervention*. McKay, New York.

Hopkinson, D. A. W. & Watts, J. C., 1963, Studies in experimental missile injuries of skeletal muscle. *Proceedings of the Royal Society of Medicine* (UK) **56,** pp. 461–468.

Horsley, V., 1894, The destructive effects of small projectiles. *Nature* **50** (1283), pp. 104–108.

Hughes, B. P., 1974, *Firepower: Weapons Effectiveness on the Battlefield, 1630–1850*. Arms & Armour Press, London.

Hughes, C. W., 1971, Acute vascular injuries: civilian and military. *Journal of Trauma* **11** (2), pp. 189–190.

Huntington, S. P., 1968. In *No More Vietnams. The War and the Future of American Foreign Policy* (R. M. Pfeffer, ed.). Adlai Stevenson Institute of International Affairs and Harper & Row, New York.

Indonesia, 1976, *Study of comparison between the effects caused by 7.62 mm and 5.56 mm calibre bullets shot in a block of soap*. COLU/204. Working paper submitted by the Indonesian experts to the Conference of Government Experts on the Use of Certain Conventional Weapons, Lugano, 28 January–26 February 1976.

International Committee of the Red Cross, 1955, *Draft Rules for the Protection of the Civilian Population from the Dangers of Indiscriminate Warfare*. Geneva.

International Committee of the Red Cross, 1958a, *Draft Rules for the Limitation of the Dangers Incurred by the Civilian Population in Time of War*, 2nd edition. Geneva.

International Committee of the Red Cross, 1958b, *Final Record Concerning the Draft Rules for the Limitation of the Dangers Incurred by the Civilian Population in Time of War*. XIXth International Conference of the Red Cross, New Delhi, October–November 1957. Geneva.

International Committee of the Red Cross, 1969, *Reaffirmation and Development of the Laws and Customs Applicable in Armed Conflicts*. Report submitted to the XXIst International Conference of the Red Cross. Geneva.

International Committee of the Red Cross, 1972a, vol. 1, *Basic Texts*. Conference of Government Experts on the Reaffirmation and Development of International Humanitarian Law Applicable in Armed Conflicts, Second Session, 3 May–3 June 1972. Geneva.

International Committee of the Red Cross, 1972b, vol. 2, *Commentary*. Conference of Government Experts on the Reaffirmation and Development of International Humanitarian Law Applicable in Armed Conflicts, Second Session, 3 May–3 June 1972. Geneva.

International Committee of the Red Cross, 1972c, *Report of the Work of the Conference*, 2 vols. Conference of Government Experts on the Reaffirmation and Development of International Humanitarian Law Applicable in Armed Conflicts, Second Session, 3 May–3 June 1972. Geneva.

International Committee of the Red Cross, 1973a, *Draft Additional Protocols to the Geneva Conventions of August 12, 1949*. Geneva.

International Committee of the Red Cross, 1973b, *Draft Additional Protocols to the Geneva Conventions of August 12, 1949: Commentary*. Geneva.

International Committee of the Red Cross, 1973c, *Weapons that may Cause Unnecessary Suffering or Have Indiscriminate Effects*. Report on the Work of Experts. Geneva.

International Committee of the Red Cross, 1974, *Report on the Work of the Conference of Government Experts on the Use of Certain Conventional Weapons, Lucerne, 24.9–18.10 1974*. Geneva.

International Committee of the Red Cross, 1976, *Conference of Experts on the Use of Certain Conventional Weapons, Second Session, Lugano, 28.1–26.2 1976*. Geneva.

James, T., 1971, Gunshot wounds of the South African War. *South African Medical Journal* (9 October), pp. 1089–94.

Jane's Infantry Weapons 1975 (F. W. A. Hobart, ed.), 1974. Macdonald & Jane's, London.

Jane's Infantry Weapons 1976 (D. H. Archer, ed.), 1976. Macdonald & Jane's, London.

Jane's Weapon Systems 1972/73 (R. T. Pretty & D. H. Archer, eds.), 1972. Jane's Yearbooks, London.

Jane's Weapon Systems 1974/75 (R. T. Pretty & D. H. Archer, eds.), 1974. Macdonald & Jane's, London.

Jane's Weapon Systems 1976 (R. T. Pretty, ed.), 1976. Macdonald & Jane's, London.

Janzon, B., 1973, *A Concept Formulation of a Rule for the Limitation of the Development of Some Fragmentation Weapons which may Cause Superfluous Injury According to International Law*. FOA 2 report A 257-M2, D4(D7). National Defence Research Institute, Stockholm.

Janzon, B., 1974, *Calculations of the Behaviour of Small Calibre, Spin Stabilized Projectiles Penetrating a Dense Medium*. FOA task No. M270 (mimeographed). National Defence Research Institute, Tumba, Sweden.

Janzon, B., 1975, *Stridsdelsfysik* [Warhead physics]. National Defence Research Institute, Stockholm.

Janzon, B. & Norrvi, Y., 1975, Skotthål i tvål visar verken av vapen. *FOA Tidning* (Stockholm) (December), pp. 9–11.

Jernberg, E., 1971, *Report from Certain Investigations as regards Physiological Effects of Small Arms Ammunition* (mimeographed). Swedish Army Matériel Administration, Stockholm.

Joenniemi, P. & Rosas, A., 1975, *International Law and the Use of Conventional Weapons*. Research Report No. 9. Tampere Peace Research Institute, Finland.

Johannsohn, G., 1977, Fuel air explosives revolutionize conventional warfare. *International Defense Review* **9** (6), pp. 992–996.

Johnson, D. L., 1973, Effects of infrasound on respiration. Aerospace Medical Association, Annual Scientific Meeting, 7–10 May 1973.

Johnson, G. B. & Lockhoven, H. B., 1965, *International Armament*. International Small Arms Publishers, Cologne.

Johnson, H. E., 1974, Assessing Soviet progress in small arms research and development. *Army Research and Development News Magazine* (US) **15** (6), pp. 31–32.

Johnson, T. M., 1970, The AK 47. *Army* (US) **20** (6), pp. 41–45.

Jones, E. L., Peters, A. F. & Gasior, R. M., 1968, Early management of battle casualties in Vietnam. *Archives of Surgery* **97** (1), pp. 1–26.

Kalshoven, F., 1973, *The Laws of Warfare*. Henry Dunant Institute, Geneva, and Sijthoff, Leiden.

Kalshoven, F., 1975, The Conference of Government Experts on the Use of Certain Conventional Weapons, Lucerne, September 14 to October 18, 1976. In *Netherlands Yearbook of International Law* **6**, pp. 77–102.

Kanegis, A., Klare, M., Knopp, F. *et al.*, 1970, *Weapons for Counterinsurgency*. Local

Research Action Guide No. 1. National Action/Research on the Military Industrial Complex, American Friends Service Committee, Philadelphia, Pennsylvania.

Keith, A. & Rigby, H. M., 1899, Modern military bullets: A study of their destructive effects. *Lancet* **2**, pp. 1499–1507.

Kitching, J., 1975, Land mine warfare. *International Defense Review* **7** (5), pp. 591–694.

Kocher, Th., 1875, *Über die Sprengwirkung der modernen Kleingewehr-Geschosse,* vol. 1. Schwabe, Basel.

Kocher, Th., 1880, *Über Schusswunden. Experimentelle Untersuchungen über die Wirkungsweise der modernen Kleingewehr-Geschosse.* Vogel, Leipzig.

Köhler, R., 1897, *Die Modernen Kriegswaffen.* Enslin, Berlin.

Korfmann, M., 1973, The sling as a weapon. *Scientific American* **229** (October), pp. 35–42.

Kosar, F., 1974, Die Bewaffnung der israelischen Armee im Yom-Kippur Krieg. *Truppendienst* (3), pp. 239–243.

Kovaric, J. J., Aaby, G., Hamit, H. F. & Hardway, R. M., 1969, Vietnam casualty statistics: February–November 1967. *Archives of Surgery* **98** (February), pp. 150–152.

Krause, F., 1905, Sling contrivances for projectile missiles. *Annual Report 1004,* pp. 619–639. The Smithsonian Institution, Washington, DC.

Krauss, M., 1957, Studies in wound ballistics: Temporary cavity effects in soft tissues. *Military Medicine* **120**, pp. 221 ff.

Krauss, M., 1971, *Explosives Detecting Dogs.* AD-736 829 (mimeographed). US Army Land Warfare Laboratory, Aberdeen Proving Ground, Maryland.

Krepon, M., 1974, Weapons potentially inhumane: The case of cluster bombs. *Foreign Affairs* **52** (3), pp. 595–611.

Ksander, Y., 1971a, *Soviet Chemical Laser Research.* R-921/1-ARPA. RAND Corporation, Santa Monica, California.

Ksander, Y., 1971b, *Soviet Chemical Laser Research: Pulse Lasers.* R-921-ARPA. RAND Corporation, Santa Monica, California.

Kussbach, E., 1976, Die Brüsseler Deklarationen 1874 über die Gesätze und Gebräuche des Krieges. *Österreichische Militärische Zeitschrift* (6), pp. 469–472.

Kussbach, E., 1977, Internationale Bemühungen um die Beschränkung des Einsatzes bestimmter konventionellen Waffen. *Österreichische Zeitschrift für Öffentliches Recht und Völkerrecht* **28**, pp. 1–50.

Küttner, H., 1900, *Unter dem Deutschen Rothen Kreuz im Südafrikanischen Kriege.* Hirzel, Leipzig.

LaGarde, L. A., 1900, Gunshot injuries by the weapons of reduced calibre. *Bulletin of the Johns Hopkins Hospital* (January).

LaGarde, L. A., 1914, *Gunshot Injuries.* Bale, Sons & Dickinson, London.

Lancet, 1899, The new British Service bullet (editorial). (4 February), p. 319.

Lancet, 1899, Dum-dum bullets (editorial). (10 June), p. 1573.

Lancet, 1900, The alleged poisonous copper-coated Mauser bullets (editorial). **1**, pp. 1741–1742.

Latina, J. A., 1975, The incidence of post-operative wound infections during the Vietnam conflict. *Military Medicine* **140** (5), pp. 354–355.

Latour, C., 1974, Small arms. *NATO's Fifteen Nations* (June–July), pp. 63–71.

Lebowitz, R. M., 1972, *The Sensitivity of Portions of the Human Central Nervous System to "Safe" Levels of Microwave Radiation.* R-983-RC (March). RAND Corporation, Santa Monica, California.

Le Gall, P., 1974, The MDF.1 Multi-mode Anti-personnel Grenade. *International Defense Review* **7** (2), pp. 230–232.

Lescaze, L., 1976, U.S. offers concussion bomb and secret scanners to Israel. *International Herald Tribune* (14 October).

Leventhall, H. G., 1973, Man-made infrasound: Its occurrence and some subjective effects. Colloquium on Infrasound, Paris, 24–27 September.

Levitsky, S., James, P. M., Anderson, R. W. & Hardaway, R. M., 1968, Vascular trauma in Vietnam battle casualties: An analysis of 55 consecutive cases. *Annals of Surgery* **168** (5), pp. 831–836.

Lewis, B. R., 1956, *Small Arms and Ammunition in the United States Service.* The Smithsonian Institution, Washington, DC.

Liddell Hart, B. H., 1946, *The Revolution in Warfare.* Faber & Faber, London.

Littauer, R. & Uphoff, M. (eds.), 1972, *The Air War in Indochina,* revised ed. Beacon Press, Boston.

Litwin, M. S., Fine, S., Klein, E. & Fine, B. S., 1969, Burn injury after carbon monoxide laser irradiation. *Archives of Surgery* **98** (February), pp. 219–222.

Liszka, L., 1973, Kraftwerk sänder ut oerhört starkt ohörbart buller. *Forskning och framsteg* (Sweden) (3), pp. 3–4.

Longmore, T., 1877, *Gunshot Injuries: Their History, Characteristic Features, Complications and General Treatment, with Statistics concerning Them as They have been met with in Warfare.* Longmans Green, London.

Lorenz, K., 1966, *On Aggression.* Methuen, London.

Lowe, J. R., 1968, EOD in Vietnam. *Ordnance* (July–August), pp. 71–76.

Ludvigsen, E. C., 1975, 'Short war' view cause for concern. *Army* (US) (October), pp. 117–123.

Lumsden, M., 1975, 'Conventional' war and human ecology. *Ambio* **4** (5–6), pp. 223–228.

Lavaas, J., 1959, *The Military Legacy of the Civil War.* Chicago.

MacCormac, W., 1895, Some points of interest in connexion with the surgery of war. *Lancet* **2,** pp. 290–292.

MacCormac, W., 1900, The wounded in the present war. *Lancet* **1,** pp. 1485–1488.

MacCormac, W., 1900, Notes from Sir William MacCormac. *Lancet* **1,** *passim.*

Mach, E. von & Salcher, P., 1887, *Photographische Fixierung der durch Projectile in der Luft eingeleiten Vorgänge.* Der Kaiserliche Academie der Wissenschaft zu Wien.

MacLeod, N. A., 1967, Genesis of the Claymore. Letter to *New Scientist* (5 January), p. 44.

Magis, S. F., 1967, *Material Selection for Naturally Fragmenting Munitions, Summary Report.* US Naval Weapons Laboratory, Technical memorandum No. T-13/67. Dahlgren, Virginia.

Maiman, T. H., 1960, Stimulated optical radiation in ruby masers. *Nature* **187,** p. 493.

Makins, G. H., 1900, Some impressions of military surgery in South Africa. *British Medical Journal* **1,** p. 344.

Malinverni, G., 1974, Armes conventionelles modernes et droit international. *Schweizerisches Jahrbuch für internationales Recht* **30,** pp. 28–30.

Manucy, A., 1949, *Artillery through the Ages.* National Park Service Interpretative Series History No. 3. US Government Printing Office, Washington, DC.

Mardell, T. & Söderberg, B., 1975, *In Service of Peace: Middle East 1975.* Keterpress, Jerusalem.

Margolis, R. J., 1974, Stun guns, bean bags and dumdums. *Washington Post* (8 December).

Marsden, J. N., 1975, Defeat of tactical minefields. *National Defense* (September–October), pp. 127–129.

278

Martens, C. de., 1858–61, *Causes célèbres de droit des gens,* 5 vols.

Martin, J., 1974, *Armes à feu de l'armée française 1860 à 1940.* Crepin-Leblond, Paris.

Martin, J. & Campbell, E. H., 1946, Early complication following penetrating wounds of the skull. *Journal of Neurosurgery* **3,** p. 58.

Massu, J., 1972, *La vraie bataille d'Alger.* Plon, Paris.

Matthew, T. P., 1858, History of wounds and injuries. In *Medical and Surgical History of the British Army which served in Turkey and the Crimea during the War against Russia in the Years 1854–55–56,* vol. 2, pp. 253–396. Harrison, London.

Maughon, J. S., 1970, An inquiry into the nature of wounds resulting in killed in action in Vietnam. *Military Medicine* **135,** pp. 8–13.

McBride, A., 1976, *The Zulu War.* Osprey, London.

McMillen, J. H. & Gregg, J. R., 1945, *The Energy, Mass and Velocity which is required of Small Missiles in order to produce a Casualty.* Missile Casualties Report No. 12. Office of Scientific Research and Development, Division of Medical Sciences, National Research Council (US).

Medinger, P., 1935, The effects of projectiles upon vital tissues: Stopping power. *Military Surgeon* **76** (2), pp. 57–71.

Mendelson, J. A. & Glover, J. L., 1967, Sphere and shell fragment wounds of soft tissues: Experimental study. *Journal of Trauma* **7** (6), pp. 889–914.

Meyer-Arendt, J. R., 1968, Efficiency and limitations of lasers as weapons. *American Journal of Optometry and Archives of the American Academy of Optometry* (March), pp. 188–191.

Meyrowitz, H., 1968, Réflexions à propos du centenaire de la Déclaration de Saint-Petersbourg. *Revue internationale de la Croix-Rouge* (600), pp. 541–555.

Miles, J. R., 1974, *Incendiary Weapons and International Law.* Unpublished dissertation.

Millar, R., Rutherford, R. H., Johnston, S. & Malhotra, V. K., 1975, Injuries caused by rubber bullets: A report on 90 patients. *British Journal of Surgery* **62,** pp. 480–486.

Milsom, J., 1970, *Russian Tanks, 1900–1970.* Arms & Armour Press, London.

Mironov, A., 1976, Liken hittades med ansikten förvridna av fasa på fartyget (translated from Russian). *Östersundsposten* (Sweden) (11 October).

Mohr, G. C., Cole, J. N., Guild, E. & Von Gierke, H. E., 1965, Effects of low frequency and infrasonic noise on men. *Aerospace Medicine* **36,** pp. 817–824.

Morin, A., 1872, *Les Lois relatives à la Guerre selon le Droit des Gens Modernes,* 2 vols. Cosse, Marchal & Billard, Paris.

Moritz, A., 1943, Mechanisms of head injury. *Annals of Surgery* **117** (4), pp. 562–575.

Mounter, L. A., 1973, Soviet design philosophy: Research and its impact on weapons systems development. *Army Research and Development News Magazine* (US) (September–October), pp. 14–15.

Mullins, L. E., 1965, The mines at Messines. *Military Review* **45** (4), pp. 18–24.

Myatt, F., 1974, *The Soldier's Trade: British Military Developments,* 1660–1914. Macdonald & Jane's, London.

Nancrede, C. B., 1899, The effects of modern small arms projectiles, as shown by the wounded of the Fifth Army Corps during the campaign resulting in the capture of Santiago de Cuba. *Transactions of the American Surgical Society* **17.**

Neel, S., 1973, *Medical Support of the U.S. Army in Vietnam.* Vietnam Studies Series. US Department of the Army, Washington, DC.

Nimier, H. & Laval, E., 1899, *Les Projectiles des Armes de Guerre, leur Action vulnérante.* Paris.

Norrvi, Y., 1975a, Billig bränsle & luft = dödande tryckvåg. *FOA Tidning* (Stockholm) **13** (2), pp. 8–11.

Norrvi, Y., 1975*b*, FOA-prov med FAE-laddningar. *FOA Tidning* (Stockholm) (December), pp. 16–17.

Nunes-Vais, A., 1974, A new dimension in mine warfare. *Army Research and Development News Magazine* (US) (July–August), pp. 22–23.

Oakeshott, R. E., 1960, *The Archaeology of Weapons: Arms and Armour from Prehistory to the Age of Chivalry*. Butterworth, London.

Oberdorfer, D., 1975, Seoul marks 25th anniversary of War. *International Herald Tribune* (27 June).

O'Brien, D. D., 1973, Missile wounds, Belfast 1971. *Proceedings of the Royal Society of Medicine* **66** (March), pp. 292–296.

Ochsner, W. W. A., Jacob, S. W. & Mansberger, A. R., 1958, A new preparation for the study of experimental shock from massive wounds: I. Standardization. *Surgery* **43**, pp. 703–707.

Odenberg, F. W., 1975, Hülsenlose munition. *Wehrtechnik* (8), pp. 896–898.

Ogilvie, W. H., 1944, *Forward Surgery in Modern War*. Butterworth, London.

Ogston, A., 1899, Continental criticism of English rifle bullets. *British Medical Journal* (25 March), pp. 752–757.

Ogston, A., 1899, The Peace Conference and the dum-dum bullet. *British Medical Journal* (29 July), pp. 278–281.

Oppenheim, L., 1955, *International Law*, 7th. ed. (H. Lauterpacht, ed.). Longmans, London.

Otis, G. A., 1876, *The Medical and Surgical History of the War of the Rebellion*, vol. 2, part 2. US Government Printing Office, Washington, DC.

Owen, J. I. H. (ed.), 1975, *Brassey's Infantry Weapons of the World 1975*. Brassey's London.

Painter, H. W., 1974, Picatinny Arsenal in research and development. *Army Research and Development News Magazine* (US) (January–February).

Partington, J. R., 1960, *A History of Greek Fire and Gunpowder*. Heffer, Cambridge (UK).

Paust, J. J., 1974, Weapons regulation, military necessity and legal standards: Are contemporary Department of Defense "practices" inconsistent with legal norms? *Denver Journal of International Law and Policy* **4** (2), pp. 229–235.

Payne, R., 1966, *Lawrence of Arabia*. Robert Hale, London.

Pengelley, R. B., 1973, Internal security – Some recent British developments. *International Defense Review* **6** (5), pp. 620–623.

Petty, C. S., 1969, Firearms injury research. *American Journal of Clinical Pathology* **52** (3), pp. 277–288.

The Physiologic Effects of Wounds, 1952. Board for the Study of the Severely Wounded, North African–Mediterranean Theatre of Operations. Office of the Surgeon General, Department of the Army, Washington, DC.

Pleasants, H., 1938, *The Tragedy of the Crater*. Reprinted by Eastern National Park & Monument Association, Philadelphia, Pennsylvania, 1975.

Porritt, A., 1953, The treatment of war wounds. In *Surgery* (Z. Cope, ed.), pp. 9–30. History of the Second World War, United Kingdom Medical Series. HMSO, London.

Pretty, R. T. (ed.), 1976, *Jane's Weapon Systems 1976*. Macdonald & Jane's, London.

Pretty, R. T. & Archer, D. H. R. (eds.), 1972, *Jane's Weapon Systems 1972/73*. Jane's Yearbooks, London.

Pretty, R. T. & Archer, D. H. R. (eds.), 1974, *Jane's Weapon Systems 1974/75*. Macdonald & Jane's, London.

Prokosch, E., 1972, *The Simple Art of Murder: Antipersonnel Weapons and their*

Developers. National Action/Research on the Military Industrial Complex, American Friends Service Committee, Philadelphia, Pennsylvania.

Prokosch, E., 1976, Antipersonnel weapons. *International Social Science Journal* **28** (2), pp. 341–358.

Prouty, L. F., 1972, *The Secret Team: The CIA and its Allies in Control of the United States and the World*. Prentice-Hall, Englewood Cliffs, New Jersey.

Rathbun, F. F., 1963, The rifle in transition. *Army* (US) **14** (1), pp. 1925.

Reed, L., 1973, The ethics of using anti-personnel weapons in war. In *Unterwegs zum Frieden* (R. Weiter & V. Zsifkovits, eds.), pp. 481–492. Herder, Vienna.

Rich, N. M., 1968, Wounding power of various ammunition. *Resident Physician* (US) (February), pp. 72–74.

Rich, N. M., Johnson, E. V. & Dimond, F. C., 1967, Wounding power of missiles used in the Republic of Vietnam. *Journal of the American Medical Association* **199** (1), pp. 157–168.

Riffin, P. V., 1972, *High Fragmentation Steels for Artillery and Tank Munitions*. Report SP 72–17. US Army Materials and Mechanics Research Center, Watertown, Massachusetts.

Rinehart, J. S. & Pearson, J., 1954, *Behavior of Metals Under Impulsive Loads*. American Society for Metals, Cleveland, Ohio.

Rinehart, J. S. & Pearson, J., 1963, *Explosive Working of Metals*. Macmillan, New York.

Robinson, C. A., 1973*a*, Fuel air explosives. Services ready joint development plan. *Aviation Week & Space Technology* **98** (8), pp. 42–46.

Robinson, C. A., 1973*b*, Soviets begin fuel–air explosive tests. *Aviation Week & Space Technology* **99** (17), p. 24.

Robinson, R. S., 1973, Salvo Squeezebore: A novel ammunition concept. *Ordnance* (March–April), pp. 384–387.

Roane, L. W., 1973, Dual cycle rifle: U.S. Army small arms systems agency developing new concept. *Army Research and Development News Magazine* (US) (May–June), pp. 22–24.

Rogers, B. W., 1974, *Cedar Falls–Junction City: A Turning Point*. Vietnam Studies. US Department of the Army, Washington, DC.

Rogers, H. C. B., 1975, *A History of Artillery*. Citadel, Secaucus, New Jersey.

Rohne, H., 1894, Studie über den Schrapnellschuss der Feldartillerie. *Archiv der Artillerie- und Ingenieur-Offiziere* **101**, p. 385.

Rolin-Jaequemyns, G., 1870, La Guerre actuelle dans ses Rapports avec le Droit international. *Revue de Droit international et de législation comparée* **4**. Van Dooselaere, Ghent.

Rosenblad, E., 1974, *Prohibited Weapons – Treaties and Bibliography*. Documentation and Data, 6. Bibliographical Institute, Royal Swedish Library, Stockholm.

Rosenhead, J., 1976, A new look at less "less lethal" weapons. *New Scientist* **72** (1031), pp. 672–674.

Rössle, R., 1950, Pathology of blast effects. In *German Aviation Medicine in World War II*, vol. 2, chapter 14-C. Surgeon General, US Air Force, US Government Printing Office, Washington, DC.

Rusca, F., 1915. *Deutsche Zeitschrift für Chirurgie* **132**, p. 315.

Russell, B., 1967, *War Crimes in Vietnam*. Allen & Unwin, London.

Ryabchikov, V., 1977, Civil defence of the USSR. *Soviet Military Weekly* (February), pp. 46–67.

Rybeck, B., 1974, Missile wounding and hemodynamic effects of energy absorption. *Acta Chirurgica Scandinavica,* Supplement 450.

281

Sandoz, Y., 1975, *Des armes interdites en droit de la guerre*. Doctoral thesis, University of Neuchâtel. Grounauer, Geneva.

Sayle, M., 1973, The end of a demolition job in Indo-China. *Sunday Times* (London) (19 August).

Schell, J., 1968, *The Military Half*. Knopf, New York.

Schildt, R., 1972, Mortality rate in quantified combined injuries. *Strahlentherapie* **144** (1), pp. 40–49.

Schwarzenberger, G., 1968, *International Law*, vol. 2. Stevens, London.

Schwarzenberger, G., 1974, The law of armed conflict: A civilized interlude? In *The Yearbook of World Affairs*, pp. 293–309. London Institute of World Affairs & Stevens, London.

Scientific American, 1914, The Dumdum bullet. (3 October.)

Scott, F., 1971, To strike unseen. *Royal United Servicemen's Journal* (June), pp. 30–35.

Scott, J. B. (ed.), 1915, *The Hague Conventions and Declarations of 1899 and 1907*. Carnegie Endowment for International Peace and Oxford University Press, New York.

Scott, J. B. (ed.), 1916, *Instructions to the American Delegates to the Hague Peace Conferences and their Official Reports*. Carnegie Endowment for International Peace and Oxford University Press, New York.

Scott, J. B. (ed.), 1920, *The Proceedings of the Hague Peace Conferences: Translation of the Official Texts*, vol. 1, *The Conference of 1899*. Carnegie Endowment for International Peace and Oxford University Press, New York.

Scott, R., 1974, *Projectile Trauma: An Enquiry into Bullet Wounds* (mimeographed). Trauma Unit, Chemical Defence Establishment, Porton Down, England.

Security Planning Corporation, 1972, *Nonlethal Weapons for Law Enforcement*. A report to the National Science Foundation, Washington, DC.

Sellier, K., 1969, *Schusswaffen und Schusswirkungen: Ballistik, Medizin und Kriminalistik*. Lübeck.

Senkus, N. J., 1967, A new radar for the infantry. *Infantry* (US) (September–October), pp. 58–59.

Shallice, T., 1973, The Ulster depth interrogation techniques and sensory deprivation research. *Cognition* **1**, pp. 385–405.

Shank, E. B., Thein, B. K., Campbell, D. & Wargovich, M. J., 1974, *A Comparison of Various Less Lethal Projectiles*. Technical Report 71–79. US Army Land Warfare Laboratory, Aberdeen, Maryland.

Sheehan, N. (ed.), 1971, *The Pentagon Papers*. Bantam, New York.

Shellnut, R. J. & Jenkins, E. R., 1971, *Long-range Shotshell*. US Patent No. 3, 599,568 (17 August).

Shoup, D. M., 1969, The new American militarism. *Atlantic Monthly* (April), pp. 51–56.

Sidorenko, A. A., 1970, *The Offensive*. Military Publishing House of the Ministry of Defence, Moscow, translated and published under the auspices of the US Air Force.

Sie, I. S. L., 1972, The military rifle of today and tomorrow. *NATO's Fifteen Nations* (June–July), pp. 88–97.

Simeone, F. A., 1963, Shock, trauma and the surgeon. *Annals of Surgery* **158** (5), pp. 759–774.

Skodny, D., 1970, Progress in ammunition. *Ordnance* (January–February), pp. 428–481.

Slessor, J., 1956, *The Central Blue*. Cassell, London.

Sliney, D. H. & Palmisano, W. A., 1968, The evaluation of laser hazards. *American Industrial Hygiene Association Journal* **29** (1), pp. 425–431.

Smith, W., 1969, *Small Arms of the World*, 9th revised ed. Stackpole, Harrisburg, Pennsylvania.

282

Snellman, B., 1966, Projektilverkan. *Försvars- och Katastrofmedicin* (Stockholm).

Spaight, J. M., 1924, *Air Power and War Rights*. Longmans Green, London.

Spencer, C. C., 1908, *Gunshot Wounds*. Hodder & Stoughton, London.

Stanley, A. T., 1967, Caltrops: tactical antipersonnel obstacles. Interim report covering the period May 6 to August 4, 1966. US Army Engineer Research and Development Laboratories, Fort Belvoir, Virginia. (Author's abstract in *Technical Abstracts Bulletin* (1), 1967.)

Stark, P. R., 1968, Interchangeable arms? *Ordnance* (September–October), pp. 183–184.

Stein, E., 1971, Impact of new weapons technology on international law: Selected aspects. *Recueil des Cours* **133** (2), Sijthof, Leiden.

Stettbacher, A., 1968, *Spreng- und Schiesstoffe*. Rascher, Zurich.

Stevenson, W. F., 1897, *Wounds in War: The Mechanism of their Production and Treatment*. Longmans, Green, London.

Stockholm International Peace Research Institute, 1971, *The Problem of Chemical and Biological Warfare*, vol. 1. Almqvist & Wiksell, Stockholm.

Stockholm International Peace Research Institute, 1973, *The Problem of Chemical and Biological Warfare*, vol. 2. Almqvist & Wiksell, Stockholm.

Stockholm International Peace Research Institute, 1974, *World Armaments and Disarmament, SIPRI Yearbook 1974*. Almqvist & Wiksell, Stockholm.

Stockholm International Peace Research Institute, 1975a, *Incendiary Weapons*. Almqvist & Wiksell, Stockholm, and MIT Press, Cambridge, Massachusetts.

Stockholm International Peace Research Institute, 1975b, *World Armaments and Disarmament, SIPRI Yearbook 1975*. Almqvist & Wiksell, Stockholm.

Stockholm International Peace Research Institute, 1976a, *The Law of War and Dubious Weapons*. Almqvist & Wiksell, Stockholm.

Stockholm International Peace Research Institute, 1976b, *The Ecological Consequences of the Second Indochina War*. Almqvist & Wiksell, Stockholm.

Stockholm International Peace Research Institute, 1976c, *World Armaments and Disarmament, SIPRI Yearbook 1976*. Almqvist & Wiksell, Stockholm.

Stone, I. F., 1952, *The Hidden History of the Korean War*. Monthly Review Press, New York.

Styles, S. G., 1976, Bombs and bomb beaters. *International Defense Review* **8** (5), pp. 817–819.

Suckow, S., 1976, Humanitarian Law Conference: A progress report. *ICJ Review* (16), pp. 51–60.

Suter, K. D., 1975, Modernizing the laws of war. *Australian Outlook* **29** (2), pp. 211–219.

Svensson, C., 1974, *Luftstötvågsinducerad lungskada – Matematisk modell*. Fort F/F rapport 103:42 (May). National Defence Research Institute, Stockholm.

Swearington (Chief Warrant Officer), 1969, *Staff study on pernicious characteristics of U.S. explosive ordnance* (mimeographed). US Marine Corps (October).

Switzerland, Groupe de recherches ballistiques, Armée Suisse, 1976, *Essais de tir, Armes de petit calibre, 5.56 mm et 7.62 mm*. Report presented by the Swiss delegation at the second session of the Conference of Government Experts on the Use of Certain Conventional Weapons, Lugano, 28 January–26 February 1976.

Thein, B. K., Shank, E. B. & Wargovich, M. I., 1974, *Analysis of a bean-bag-type projectile as a less lethal weapon* (draft report). US Army Land Warfare Laboratory, Aberdeen Proving Ground, Maryland.

Thiess, A. M., 1963, Beobachtungen über Gesundheitsschädigungen durch Einwirkung von Äthylenoxid. *Archiv für Toxikologie* **20**, pp. 127–140.

Thiess, A. M. & Goldmann, P., 1968, Kasuistische Mitteilung über eine ausgedehnte bullös-toxische Dermititis durch Spuren von Äthylenoxid. *Arbeitsmedizin, Sozialmedizin, Arbeitshygiene* **3** (2), pp. 29–31.

Thoresby, F. P., 1966, Cavitation: The wounding process of the high velocity missile, a review. *Journal of the Royal Army Medical Corps* (UK) **112**, pp. 89–99.

Thoresby, F. P. & Darlow, H. M., 1967, The mechanisms of primary infection of bullet wounds. *British Journal of Surgery* **54**, pp. 359–361.

Thoresby, F. P. & Matheson, J. M., 1967, Gas gangrene of the high velocity missile wound. *Journal of the Royal Army Medical Corps* (UK) **113**, pp. 31–39.

Thoresby, F. P. & Watts, J. C., Gas gangrene of the high-velocity missile wound. *British Journal of Surgery* **54**, pp. 25–29.

Tresckow, A. von, 1975, Landminen. *Soldat und Technik* **18** (8), pp. 388–400.

Tompkins, J. S., 1966, *The Weapons of World War III: The Long Road Back from the Bomb.* Doubleday, New York.

Treves, 1900, The wounded in the present war: Report to the Royal Medical and Chirurgical Society, 8 May 1900. *British Medical Journal* (12 May), pp. 1156–1162.

Trooboff, P. D. (ed.), 1975, *Law and Responsibility in Warfare: The Vietnam Experience.* University of North Carolina Press, Chapel Hill, North Carolina.

Truckenmiller, W. C., 1964, Developing cast shell. *Ordnance* (March–April).

Turney-High, H. H., 1971, *Primitive War: Its Practice and Concepts.* University of South Carolina Press, Columbia, South Carolina.

UK War Office, Departmental Committee on Small Arms, 1898, *Further trial of Dum Dum bullets and of bullets to R. L. Designs Nos. 9063B and 9063*.* Report No. 17. The War Office, London.

UK Ministry of Defence, 1974, *British Defence Equipment Catalogue,* 6th ed. Defence Sales Organisation, Combined Services Publications, London.

United Nations, 1973*a*, *Napalm and Other Incendiary Weapons and all Aspects of their Possible Use.* Report of the Secretary-General, A/8803/Rev. 1. New York.

United Nations, 1973*b*, *Existing Rules of International Law concerning the Prohibition or Restriction of Use of specific Weapons.* Survey prepared by the Secretariat, A/9215, 2 vols. New York.

Urlanis, B., 1971, *Wars and Population.* Progress Publishers, Moscow.

US Air Force Armament Laboratory, 1970, *Guide* [to non-nuclear munitions and associated munitions under cognizance of AFATL], part 1. Eglin Air Force Base, Florida.

US Army Concept Team in Vietnam, 1968, *Grenade Launcher, 40 mm Automatic, XM174.* APO, San Francisco.

US Army Materiel Command, 1969, *Arsenal for the Brave: A History of the United States Army Materiel Command 1962–1968.* US Army Materiel Command, Washington, DC.

US Army Munitions Command, 1970, *Cartridges, 40 mm: Multiple Projectile, XM576E1 & XM576E2.* Draft technical manual 1310-209-12. Dover, New Jersey.

US Army Munitions Command, 1972, *Laboratory Posture Report.* Research, Development and Engineering Directorate, Dover, New Jersey.

US Army Munitions Command, 1973, *Laboratory Posture Report.* Research, Development and Engineering Directorate. Dover, New Jersey.

US Army Project Manager for Selected Ammunition, 1972, *Program Achievements 1962–1972.* PMSA submission for US Army Materiel Command tenth anniversary. Dover, New Jersey.

US Bureau of Naval Personnel, 1970, *Aviation Ordnanceman 3 & 2.* Rate Training Manual, NAVPERS 10345-C.

US Commander in Chief Pacific, 1968, *Report on the War in Vietnam.* US Government Printing Office, Washington, DC.

US Defense Supply Agency, 1971, *Supply Bulletin SB 708–30,* (June), p. 21. Department of Defense Ammunition Code. US Department of the Army, Washington, DC.

US Department of the Army, 1956, *The Law of Land Warfare.* Field Manual 27-10. Washington, DC.

US Department of the Army, 1962, *Barriers and Denial Operations.* FM 31-10 (14 August). Headquarters, Department of the Army, Washington, DC.

US Department of the Army, 1964, *Land Mines.* Technical Manual TM 9-1345-200 (8 June). Headquarters, Department of the Army, Washington, DC.

US Department of the Army, 1965, *Jungle Training and Operations.* Field Manual No. 31-30 (23 September). Headquarters, Department of the Army, Washington, DC.

US Department of the Army, 1966, *Bombs and Bomb Components.* Technical Manual TM 9-1325-200. Washington, DC.

US Department of the Army, 1966, *Individual Weapons and Marksmanship.* ROTCM 145–30. Washington, DC.

US Department of the Army, 1967, *Artillery Ammunition: Guns, Howitzers, Mortars and Recoilless Rifles.* Technical Manual TM 9-1300-203. Washington, DC.

US Department of the Army, 1969, *Jungle Operations.* Field Manual FM 31-35. Washington, DC.

US Department of the Army, 1971, *Identification List.* Supply Catalog SC 1305/30-IL. Washington, DC.

US Department of the Army, 1972, *40 mm Grenade Launchers M203 and M79.* Field Manual FM 23-31. Washington, DC.

US Departments of the Army and the Navy, 1971, *Grenades, Hand and Rifle.* TM 9-1330-200/oP 3833, rev. 1, vol. 1/TM-1330-15/1. Washington, DC.

US Departments of the Army, the Navy & the Air Force, 1967, *Handling, Maintenance, Storage and Inspection (Including Repair Parts and Special Tool Lists). Dispenser and Bomb, Aircraft: CBU-1A/A, CBU-2/A, CBU-2B/A, CBU-2C/A, CBU-3/A, CBU-3A/A, CBU-8A/A, CBU-9/A, CBU-9B/A, CBU-12/A, CBU-12A/A, and CBU-26/A.* TM 9-1325-202-50/1/NAVAIR 11-5A-2, vol. 1/TO 11A1-5-1-7, with revisions. Washington, DC.

US Departments of the Army, the Navy, and the Air Force, 1970, *Adapter, Cluster Bomb: ADU-253/B, ADU-253A/B, ADU-253B/B, ADU-256/B, ADU-256A/B, ADU-256B/B, ADU-272A/B, ADU-272B/B, ADU-285A/B, ADU-285B/B and Bomb Cluster, Fragmentation: CBU-22/B.* TM 9-1325-207-5/TO 11A1-5-15-2. Washington, DC.

US Department of the Navy, 1970, *Aviation Ordnanceman 3 & 2.* Rate Training Manual NAVPERS 10345-C. Washington, DC.

US Department of the Navy, 1972*a*, *Description, Safety, Service, and Handling Instructions (Intermediate), Airborne Rockets.* Technical Manual NAVAIR 11-85-5, rev. 1. Washington, DC.

US Department of the Navy, 1972*b*, *Unpacking, Assembly, and Maintenance Instructions, Intermediate, Aircraft Dispenser and Bombs CBUs -24/B, -29/B, -49/B, -24A/B, -29A/B, -49A/B, -24/B (Mod), -29/B (Mod), -49/B (Mod), -24C/B, -49C/B, -62/B, and -63/B.* Technical Manual NAVAIR 11-5A-1. Naval Air Systems Command, Washington, DC.

US Department of State, 1976, *Licenses for Export of Arms to Foreign Police Forces,* 2 vols. Office of Munitions. Washington, DC.

US House of Representatives Committee on Appropriations, 1971, *Department of*

Defense Appropriations for Fiscal Year 1972. Hearings, part 4. US Government Printing Office, Washington, DC.

US House of Representatives Committee on Appropriations, 1972, *Department of Defense Appropriations for Fiscal Year 1973*. Hearings, part 4, p. 193. US Government Printing Office, Washington, DC.

US House of Representatives Committee on Appropriations, 1973, *Department of Defense Appropriations for 1974*. Hearings, part 7. US Government Printing Office, Washington, DC.

US Military Academy, 1968–9, *Ordnance Engineering: Vol. 2, Ballistics: Book 2, Exterior Ballistics and Terminal Ballistics*.

US Senate Committee on Appropriations, 1971, *Department of Defense Appropriations for Fiscal Year 1972*. Hearings, part 1. US Government Printing Office, Washington, DC.

US Senate Committee on Appropriations, 1971, *Department of Defense Appropriations, Fiscal Year 1972*. Hearings, part 4. US Government Printing Office, Washington, DC.

US Senate Committee on Appropriations, 1974, *Department of Defense Appropriations, Fiscal Year 1975*. Hearings, part 3, p. 860. US Government Printing Office, Washington, DC.

US Senate Committee on Armed Services, 1974, *Fiscal Year 1975 Authorization for Military Procurement, Research and Development, and Active Duty, Selected Reserve and Civilian Personnel Strengths*. Hearings, Ninety-third Congress, Second Session. US Government Printing Office, Washington DC.

US Senate Committee on Foreign Relations, 1969, *Briefing on Vietnam*. Hearings. US Government Printing Office, Washington, DC.

US Senate Committee on Foreign Relations, 1970, *Moral and Military Aspects of the War in Southeast Asia*. Hearings. Ninety-first Congress, Second Session. US Government Printing Office, Washington, DC.

US Senate Committee on Foreign Relations, 1970, *Cambodia: December 1970*. A Staff Report. US Government Printing Office, Washington, DC.

US Senate Committee on Foreign Relations, 1971, *Impact of the Vietnam War*. Prepared by the Foreign Affairs Division, Congressional Research Service, Library of Congress. US Government Printing Office, Washington, DC.

US Senate Committee on Foreign Relations, 1971, *Laos: April 1971*. Staff report for the Subcommittee on US Security Agreements and Commitments Abroad. US Government Printing Office, Washington, DC.

US Senate Committee on Foreign Relations, 1972, *Vietnam Commitments, 1961*. Staff study based on the Pentagon Papers, No 1. US Government Printing Office, Washington, DC.

US Senate Committee on Foreign Relations, 1973, *Thailand, Laos, Cambodia, and Vietnam: April 1973*. Staff report prepared for the use of the Subcommittee on US Security Agreements and Commitments Abroad (11 June). US Government Printing Office, Washington, DC.

US Senate Committee on the Judiciary, 1968, *Civilian Casualty and Refugee Problems in South Vietnam*. Findings and Recommendations of the Subcommittee to Investigate Problems Connected with Refugees and Escapees. US Government Printing Office, Washington, DC.

US Senate Committee on the Judiciary, 1970, *Refugee and Civilian War Casualty Problems in Indochina*. Staff Report prepared for the use of the Subcommittee to Investigate Problems Connected with Refugees and Escapees. US Government Printing Office, Washington, DC.

US Senate Committee on the Judiciary, 1974, *Relief and Rehabilitation of War Victims in Indochina: One Year after the Ceasefire*. Study Mission report prepared for the use of the Subcommittee to Investigate Problems Connected with Refugees and Escapees, Ninety-third Congress, Second Session. US Government Printing Office, Washington, DC.

US War Department, 1943, *Unexploded Bombs, Organization and Operation for Disposal*. Field Manual 9-40. US Government Printing Office, Washington, DC.

[Viet Nam] Juridical Sciences Institute, 1968, *US War Crimes in Vietnam*. Vietnam State Commission of Social Sciences, Hanoi.

Virgilo, R. W., 1970, Intrathoracic wounds in battle casualties. *Surgery, Gynecology and Obstetrics* **130**, p. 609.

Wade, N., 1972, Technology in Ulster: Rubber bullets hit home, brainwashing backfires. *Science* **176** (9 June), pp. 1102–1106.

Wargovich, M. J., Egner, D. O., Busey, W. M., Thein, B. K. & Shark, E. B., 1975, *Evaluation of the Physiological Effects of a Rubber Bullet, a Baseball, and a Flying Baton*. Technical Memorandum 24-75. US Army Human Engineering Laboratory, Aberdeen, Maryland.

Webster, C. & Frankland, N., 1961, *The Strategic Air Offensive against Germany, 1939–1945*, 4 vols. HMSO, London.

Weeks, J., 1972, *Infantry Weapons*. Illustrated History of World War II Series. Pan/Ballantine, London.

Weller, J., 1966, *Weapons and Tactics: Hastings to Berlin*. Vane, London.

Weller, J., 1967, *Fire and Movement*. Crowell, New York.

Weller, J., 1968, Enemy weapons in Vietnam. *Ordnance* (September–October).

Weller, J., 1968, Good and bad weapons for Vietnam. *Military Review* **48** (10), pp. 56–64.

Weller, J., 1972, Mechanized infantry. *Infantry* (September), pp. 32–33.

Weller, J. 1973, The Galil rifle – an Israeli weapon system. *National Defense (September–October), pp. 142–145*.

Westing, A. H., 1972, The super bomb. *American Report* **2** (45), p. 3.

Westing, A. H., 1975, The unexploded munitions problem: An American legacy to Indochina that still wounds and kills. *Sunday Rutland* (Vermont) *Herald & Times Argus* (14 December).

Whelan, T. J., Burkhalter, W. E. & Gomez, A., 1968, Management of war wounds. In *Advances in Surgery* (E. E. Welch, ed.), vol. 3, pp. 227–350. Yearbook Medical Publishers, Chicago.

White, C. S. & Richmond, D. R., 1959, *Blast Biology*. US Atomic Energy Commission.

White, W. D., 1974, *U.S. Tactical Air Power: Missions, Forces, and Costs*. The Brookings Institution, Washington, DC.

Widhofner, H., 1974a, Leichte Infanteriewaffen von Morgen. *Truppendienst* (1), pp. 13–14.

Widhofner, H., 1974b, Leichte Infanteriewaffen von Morgen (II). *Truppendienst* (2), pp. 109–112.

Wilson, L. B., 1921, Dispersion of bullet energy in relation to wound effects. *Military Surgeon* **49** (3), pp. 241–251.

Winchester, J. H., 1966, New weapons in the Vietnam War. *NATO's Fifteen Nations* **11** (October–November), pp. 91–94.

Wiseman, R., 1705, *Eight Chirurgical Treatises*, 4th ed. London.

Woodruff, C. E., 1898, The causes of the explosive effects of modern small-calibre projectiles. *New York Medical Journal* **68**, pp. 593–601.

Wolff, L. H. *et al.*, 1955, Timelag and the multiplicity factor in abdominal injuries. In

General Surgery, vol. 2, pp. 103–112. US Army Surgery in World War II Series. Office of the Surgeon General, Department of the Army, Washington, DC.

Worley, M. L., 1959, *New Developments in Army Weapons, Tactics, Organization, and Equipment*, 2nd ed. Stackpole, Harrisburg, Pennsylvania.

Wulff, T., 1975, *Krig och humanitet* [War and humanity]. Folk och Försvar, Stockholm.

Wulff, T., Janzon, B., Ohlson, L.-O., Petré, T. & Rybeck, B., 1973, *Conventional Weapons: Their Deployment and Effects from a Humanitarian Aspect. Recommendations for the Modernization of International Law*. A Swedish Working Group study. Royal Swedish Ministry of Foreign Affairs, Stockholm.

Yelshin, N., 1977, Soviet small arms. *Soviet Military Review* (2), pp. 15–17.

Yen Thanh, 1974*a*, Greenness [*sic*] and the patients. *South Viet Nam in Struggle* (4 March).

Yen Thanh, 1974*b*, Paddies on old no-man's land. *South Viet Nam in Struggle* (1 April).

Zuckerman, S., 1940, Experimental study of blast injury to the lungs. *Lancet* **2** (24 August), pp. 219–238.

Zuckerman, S., 1941, Problems of blast injuries. *British Medical Journal* **1**, pp. 94–96.

Zuckerman, S. *et al.*, 1941, Discussion of the problem of blast injuries. *Proceedings of the Royal Society of Medicine* **34**, pp. 171–188.

Index

A

'Air Method' 20
Air power, increasing use of, by USA 46
Aircraft (US) developed for anti-personnel use in Indo–China War
—, armament of 32–33
—, armament systems of 34
American Society for International Law 226
Ammunition
—, artillery 5–6, 11–12, 138–141
—, —, Beehive 139, 140
—, —, canister 6, 139, 140
—, —, examples of, listed by country 137, 139
—, development of 5–8, 77–81
—, Gyrojet 107
—, manufacturers of, for small arms, listed by country 115–119
—, mortar 132–136
—, —, examples of, listed by country 135–136
—, musket 53, 54
—, pistol 81–83
—, —, ballistic characteristics of, listed by type 81
—, rifle
—, —, ballistic characteristics of, listed by type 79
—, —, intermediate-power 22–23, 87–90
—, —, —, ballistic characteristics of, listed by type 88
—, —, reduced calibre 90–96, 104–105
—, —, safety zone for 113
—, Salvo 106
—, Salvo Squeezebore (SSB) 106–107
—, sub-machine-gun 81–83
—, technology, trends in 110–111
Amnesty International 205
Amron Corporation 105
Applied Electro-Mechanics Company 203

B

Ardagh, *Sir* John 216, 217
Area denial 35
Area of effect 140
Armée-Universal-Gewehr (AUG) 101, 102, 103
Arms race, impact of Viet Nam War on 42–44
Artillerie Inrichtigen 96
Artillery 11–12, 17–18, 22, 24, 27, 138–141, 249, 260–261
—, safety zone for 140, 141
Australia 102
Austria 7, 8, 94, 99
Austro–Hungarian Government 219
Automated battlefield 39, 43, 51

Balearic Islands, mercenary slingers from 4
Ballista 4, 5
Ballistics, wound. *See* Wound ballistics
Ballistite 8
Batons 108. *See also* Shok Baton
Battle
— of the Aisne (1914) 18
— of Arogee (1867–68) 15
— of Pleven (1877) 8
— of Solferino (1859) 11
— of Waterloo (1815) 5
Berdan, Hiram (*Colonel*) 79
Beretta Company 100
Berlin, post-World War II disposal of unexploded munitions in 198
Blast 12, 164–177, 181
—, biological effects of 166–169, 176
Bloch, Ivan S. 13, 16, 17, 213
Bluntschli, J. C. 212
Bomb(s) 18, 27, 46, 137, 145–162, 223
—, block-buster 171
—, cluster 29–31, 46, 146–161, 162, 180, 223, 226
—, —, Giboulée 43, 160
—, —, Lazy Dog 124